The Paraphilias

The Paraphilias

Changing Suits in the Evolution of Sexual Interest Paradigms

J. PAUL FEDOROFF, MD, FRCPC
Professor of Psychiatry; Criminology; and Law
Director, Sexual Behaviours Clinic
Integrated Forensic Program, The Royal
Head, Division of Forensic Psychiatry
University of Ottawa
Past-President International Academy of Sex Research

OXFORD
UNIVERSITY PRESS

OXFORD
UNIVERSITY PRESS

Oxford University Press is a department of the University of Oxford. It furthers the University's objective of excellence in research, scholarship, and education by publishing worldwide. Oxford is a registered trade mark of Oxford University Press in the UK and certain other countries.

Published in the United States of America by Oxford University Press
198 Madison Avenue, New York, NY 10016, United States of America.

CIP data is on file at the Library of Congress
ISBN 978-0-19-046632-9

Dedication

This book was written with the encouragement of my late wife, Beverley Fedoroff, RN (1964–2015). She regularly accompanied me to annual conferences of the American Academy of Psychiatry and the Law and the International Academy of Sex Research. Conversation and debates we had in the evenings following those and other scientific meetings greatly influenced my thinking. It was her idea that I accept the invitation to be the sole author of this book as she correctly pointed out my views are often unique. At times I have regretted following her advice to be the sole author, as most of my work has been collaborative. However, in the end, she was as usual, completely correct in insisting I sit down and say exactly what I think and why. I will always be grateful to her for being, as she put it, my greatest fan. She has always been to me a constant source of inspiration. In dilemmas, she consistently took the optimistic view and taught me to live by her three-part motto: "Do not expect everyone to agree with you; if you are right, no one important will care; and live every day to the fullest."

This book is my attempt to fulfill her wish.

Contents

About the Book Cover

The cover is an unfinished painting that Beverley worked on from time to time. It is based on a photograph I took through an open window in a restaurant in Puerto Rico. We had been at the 35th annual meeting of the International Academy of Sex Research and we had snuck out of the hotel to have lunch together. Our table was at the back of the restaurant, and the window overlooked a narrow beach and then, the sea. As the waves rhythmically broke as they reached the beach, Beverley commented that while the shore looked like a straight line from a distance, it was actually a constantly changing mixture of sand, rock, and sea. We talked about how change in nature is constant, especially for complex systems. She loved the photograph, and her project to copy it in a painting took on a life of its own. She would finish one part and then decide to alter it. Eventually I realized that her project, like the shore in the photograph, was meant to constantly change and never end.

I would like to acknowledge the assistance of Patricia Foster, Graphic Designer, for advise on the book cover.

Preface

This book is based on approximately 30 years of experience concerning the assessment and treatment of paraphilias and unconventional sexual interests. In that time, thousands of papers on these topics have been published. There are also many books about problematic sexual behaviors, most focusing on sex crimes or so-called hypersexuality and/or sexual addiction. Together, these publications present a grim and pessimistic prognosis for anyone who has unusual sexual interests of any type. This book is intended to respectfully challenge that view.

Specifically, this book is intended to review what is known about paraphilias and to challenge current popular opinions about the nature of paraphilias and their prognosis. In the process, analyses of current and past paradigms are presented together with new ways to understand, investigate, and provide meaningful assistance to people with paraphilias.

This book has a unique design. There are many similarities concerning how each of the paraphilias is assessed and treated. Also, one of the criticisms of treatment programs that have not been as productive as hoped was reliance on a "treatment manual" that interfered with therapists' abilities to tailor treatment to the specific needs of the individual seeking treatment (Fedoroff & Marshall, 2010). Therefore, in order to minimize repetition, and in order to avoid a "manualized" approach, Chapters 1 and 2 deal with general issues of perspective, assessment, and treatment. This is followed by chapters on each of the paraphilic disorders as listed in the Fifth edition of the *Diagnostic and Statistical Manual of Mental Disorders* (American Psychiatric Association, 2013). Each of those chapters can be read independently with reference to Chapters 1 and 2 as needed. The final chapter attempts to integrate the main themes of this book and to suggest ways the field may move forward. In addition, each of the paraphilia chapters includes a table consisting of references from the past 10 years. These are not intended to be exhaustive and not all are endorsed; rather, they are intended to provide starting points for readers who would like more in-depth information or alternative views to the ones expressed in this book.

It is said that according to "Rule 34 of the Internet," for every topic on the Internet there is a pornographic example (and usually a website) of it somewhere on the World Wide Web. For most of the paraphilias listed in Chapter 10, this is true. However, readers are cautioned that just because there is a website that claims to explain the sexual interests of an obscure paraphilia, it does not mean that the owner of the website has experience with the paraphilia or knows anything about it. Learning about sex by watching pornography is not recommended. Readers are also cautioned that some apparently authoritative web and social media sites are authored by people with their own agendas. Caution is needed especially for sites that include *ad hominem* comments or apparently definitive statements with no supporting data.

The opinions expressed in this book are those of Dr. Fedoroff and not necessarily shared by the institutions where he has worked or by the colleagues with whom he has collaborated.

References

American Psychiatric Association. (2013). *Diagnostic and statistical manual of mental disorders* (5th ed.). Arlington, VA: American Psychiatric Publishing.

Fedoroff, J. P., & Marshall, W. L. (2010). Paraphilias. In D. McKay, J. S. Abramowitz, & S. Taylor (Eds.), *Cognitive behavioral therapy for refractory cases* (pp. 369–384). Washington, DC: American Psychological Association.

Acknowledgments

In the past 18 years that I have worked in the Sexual Behaviours Clinic (SBC) at the Royal and at the University of Ottawa, I have had the benefit of working with students, some of whom have chosen to take time from their busy lives to work on SBC projects and/or become employees in the Clinic. I acknowledge several in particular:

Susan Curry, BA Hons: Susan had already set up the SBC database before I arrived at the Royal and has been instrumental in protecting its integrity. She is a statistician in the best sense of the word, skeptical of anything without verified empirical evidence.

Natasha Knack, BA Hons summa cum laude: Natasha joined the SBC as a volunteer following a criminology elective. She is literally the voice and author of many of the SBC's newest audiotaped SBC stimuli. She became a research assistant, then coordinator in the SBC and Institute of Mental Health Research (IMHR). She has spearheaded the SBC's "prevention project," which aims to recruit people with paraphilias who want treatment but do not know where to find it. This is a website she created for a funded research project to encourage people to get treatment and which provides information about the SBC. She is now in a master's program in Clinical Forensic Psychology at Carleton University but still very much involved in the SBC. The link she would want all to know about, which explains more about the SBC is: https://sexualbehavioursclinic.ca.

Thanh Ly, BSc cum laude: Thanh joined the SBC as a volunteer and is now a research assistant in the SBC's research program. She has been invaluable in her role of telling patients about new research studies, conducting literature reviews, and presenting new research at international conferences. She has quietly established herself as one of the most important members of the SBC responsible for many of its successes, including this book.

Lisa Murphy, BSc, MA (Crim) Magna cum laude: Lisa joined the SBC via a criminology elective. She is now program coordinator of the SBC and runs the SBC's phallometry lab. She is a prolific traveler as well as writer and presenter of the latest SBC discoveries. This brief tribute in no way summarizes how important she has been to the success and future of the SBC. The SBC owes much of its success to her.

Rebekah Ranger, BA, BSc cum laude: Rebekah joined the SBC as a student in psychology and criminology and has become a research assistant in the SBC and IMHR. She has specialized in research involving people with intellectual disabilities who also have problematic sexual interests. She has also made a name for herself as an expert in the area of "Other specified paraphilias."

Sam Rice, BA cum laude, MA (Crim): Sam joined the SBC as a criminology student. Her hard work in organizing information about the SBC provided the groundwork that eventually led to the SBC being named the top academic clinical research program and awarded the American Psychiatric Association Gold award in 2015. She now works in innovative programs to assist addicts and disadvantaged people.

Deborah Richards, BA, CMHM, MA (Psych): Deborah established and leads a program for people with intellectual disabilities and problematic sexual behaviors at the Association of Community Living Wieland. That clinic predates the current SBC and permits the SBC to provide service to most of Ontario. She is a champion and advocate for the disadvantaged, a successful researcher and teacher, and an inspiration.

Heather Tarnai-Feeley, MSW: Heather has been a co-therapist in the SBC during the development of its current treatment model. In addition to providing exquisite support to SBC patients in terms of financial and housing needs she has been invaluable in providing a model in group demonstrating how men and women, while acknowledging gender differences, can interact professionally, respectfully and non-sexually.

Each of these people has contributed to the SBC far beyond any requirements of their universities or the Royal. We have learned from each other. From my frequent discussions with them, I am confident they will be the first to challenge my views the minute new data suggest the need. I am not only happy about that, I expect it and will always respect them for their courage to pursue careers that have taken them to the edge of current knowledge about problems that most people prefer to avoid or ignore. Thank you.

I also thank my many teachers and mentors who are too numerous to list. Of particular note are Drs. John Bancroft, John Bradford, Fred Berlin, Ray Rosen, Paul McHugh, Philip Slavney, and John Money. Finally, I acknowledge all my thousands of patients and their spouses, partners and relatives who have volunteered for numerous research projects, tolerated rescheduled appointments, patiently explained the intimate aspects of their lives, explained perceived gaps in the SBCs resources, told me when I was wrong, and most importantly, provided evidence to support the hypothesis that people with paraphilic interests can change not only by not reoffending but also by establishing new healthy sexual interests and lifestyles and new identities as people with *former* sexual problems replaced by fully consensual sexual interests.

About the Author

J. Paul Fedoroff is a Full Professor of Forensic Psychiatry, Criminology, and Law. He is a Past President of the International Academy of Sex Research and the Canadian Academy of Psychiatry and the Law. He is also Director of the Sexual Behaviours Clinic at the Royal and Head of the Division of Forensic Psychiatry in the Department of Psychiatry at the University of Ottawa in Canada.

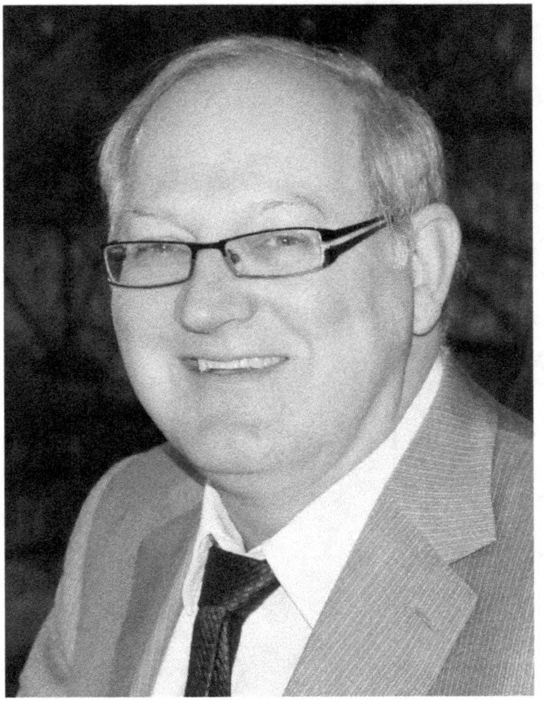

1

Perspectives and Paradigms

An Introduction to the Paraphilias

Every generation thinks it invented sex.

—Muriel Elaine Fedoroff

Introduction

Paraphilias are sexual interests that differ from "normal." This book challenges the widespread belief that paraphilias cannot be changed and therefore cannot be successfully treated. To many, suggesting that a person with a primary sexual interest in children can change their sexual interest to adults is heretical. So be it. However, clinicians and scientists are obliged to question and challenge beliefs that fail to adequately explain what they see in their clinics and labs.

Specifically, scientists need to change their paradigms when new ones provide better explanations of the data and better predictions of the new data (Kuhn, 1962). Clinicians need to provide the best possible care for their patients, even if it contradicts what their teachers told them. Readers are invited to reconsider the oft-repeated dogma which states that all paraphilias are immutable. Is there a scientific basis for this claim? Are the observed data better explained if paraphilias can change? Does this new paradigm permit better predictions about new observations?

From a scientific perspective, readers should scrutinize each statement in this book and consider not only what observations support them but also what observations or experiments could disprove them. Similarly, readers should consider how much evidence is required to accept that the null hypothesis has been disproven or at least brought into question. From a clinical perspective, readers should consider whether the possibility that paraphilias can change is better for patients and whether there is any danger in telling them there is no evidence they cannot get better. Conversely, what is the effect of telling patients there is no hope they will ever get better?

Terminology

This book is about people with problematic sexual interests and behaviors. People with these problems are typically referred to in frankly stigmatizing and denigrating terms. In this book, "person first" terminology is used to emphasize that a person's sexual interests are only one of many characteristics that may define that person.

Although important, a person's sexual interests are an inadequate and misleading way to describe the totality of who a person is. Therefore, terms such as "pedophile" or "deviant" are not used in this book. For brevity, the phrase "person with a paraphilia" is meant to include anyone with a problematic sexual interest (acknowledging that many unconventional sexual interests do not cause actual harm to anyone). Also, unless otherwise noted, any gender-specific terms should be read as literary devices rather than claims about men or women. In addition, phrases, terms, and definitions that are acceptable today can become stigmatizing or worse in the future. It is hoped that future readers will understand that terms used in this book are ones that are currently accepted in most circles and are not intended to offend or imply anything specific about any specific person. This book also uses "gender" and "sex" as adjectives. Various sources use these terms in different ways. In this book, *gender* refers to a person's subjective experience of being male or female in terms of their perception of what their society defines as being a man or woman, boy or girl. In this book, male and female *sex* refers to the state of having an XY or XX genotype, respectively. It is recognized that like almost all variables used to describe humans, there are variations. For example, some people have XXY or XYY or XO karyotypes. Similarly, in some cases, the genetic karyotype may not result in the typical phenotype (e.g., men with androgen insensitivity syndrome, who have an XY karyotype, may have a female phenotype due to receptors that are unresponsive to androgens).

In this book, people seeking or in treatment in the Sexual Behaviours Clinic (SBC) are referred to as "patients." Again, this is a convenience term for many that could be applicable. For example, many referrals to the SBC are from lawyers whose clients are before the courts. Because the assessor in those cases is acting as an agent of the lawyer, the person being assessed could properly be termed a "client." However, unlike many programs that defer treatment until all legal issues have been resolved, the SBC offers treatment to everyone who wants it, regardless of their legal status. This means that many "clients" also become "patients."

Case Reports

Several clinical case reports are presented in this book. All are based on actual accounts of patients treated by the author but not all were treated in the SBC or even in Canada. In fact, most case reports are composites of several patients and have been written so that even if a patient reads a case report based on them, they will not be sure they are the person being described. More importantly, the cases are written in a manner to ensure that no one reading this book will be able to positively identify a person they know. All unpublished case reports in this book have been reviewed by the Royal's ethics committee and approved for publication in this book. If you are a patient reading this book and you read a case report that sounds like you, you can rest assured, it is not you—just another person like you.

Paradigms and Perspectives

In this book, the word "paradigm" is used to describe a way of organizing the way data are understood. Although scientists tend to speak of "dominant paradigms" and "paradigm shifts" when a new paradigm becomes dominant, this book argues that it is possible and acceptable to consider more than one paradigm at once. In fact, because each paradigm permits a different perspective, being able to entertain more than one paradigm is better.

There are few areas in mental health more influenced by the paradigm of the observer than sexuality. "Every generation thinks it invented sex," meaning each generation creates its own paradigm to understand and explain sexuality. Unfortunately, it also seems that each generation thinks the next generation needs to be protected from its own understanding of the true nature and complexity of sex and sexuality. In North America, children are still taught about "birds and bees." Adolescents are mainly taught about sexually transmitted infections and the dangerousness of heterosexual vaginal intercourse without "protection." Typically, education about sexual variations is avoided or presented as "deviant." This pattern has influenced and continues to influence the way people think about sex and the way they think about "problematic" sex.

Classifications of sexual variation have consistently come up short due to the tendency of authors to view the problem(s) from a single perspective (Fedoroff, 2009). Near the end of the last century, McHugh and Slavney (1998) proposed four "perspectives" that have influenced the way clinicians think about mental phenomena. At the *beginning* of the last century, those four perspectives represented four paradigms held by four very influential sexologists: Richard von Krafft-Ebing, Alfred Binet, Magnus Hirschfeld, and Sigmund Freud. The following is a brief review of the four paradigms.

Disease Perspective

The disease perspective is the one most familiar to physicians. It is based on the concept of "disease," which is defined as a broken part either in anatomy (e.g., a broken bone) or in physiology (e.g., diabetes due to inadequate insulin production). The concept of "cure" is based on the disease perspective. Even from within the single perspective of "disease," the way problems are conceptualized influences how "curable" the problems are perceived to be. There is a tendency to think of anatomical diseases as ones that go away when the broken part is fixed. Therefore, people tend not to think of a fractured tibia due to a ski accident as a disease and do not refer to a person as "cured" when their cast is removed and they return to the slopes. Some diseases due to broken anatomic structures are permanent. One example is dementia pugilistica, which is a disease of boxers caused by repeated blows to the head that result in closed-head brain trauma. However, even in traumatic brain injury, the extent to which the syndrome is thought of as a disease is due more to presumed changes in brain physiology than to broken anatomical parts. This means that dementia pugilistica is more often thought of as a disease due to physiologic changes in dopamine production by the boxer's substantia nigra, which causes parkinsonian symptoms, rather than due to the head trauma itself.

Diseases that result in abnormal physiology are more often thought of as chronic and therefore "incurable." Even if the symptoms are alleviated, as long as the physiologic problems are not fixed, the person is still labeled as having the disease. So, a person with diabetes is still diagnosed with diabetes even if they are treated with insulin and have normal blood glucose levels. This is because they still have the physiologic abnormality of inadequate endogenous insulin.

Patients with cancer often have both a physiologic abnormality (cancer cells) and an anatomic abnormality (e.g., breast lump). The field of oncology has evolved from describing "cancer" as an incurable disease that can at best be "managed" to describing cancer as a disease with multiple causes that if detected early and treated properly can be changed. Patients in sustained remission are described as having "no evidence of disease" (NED). If a woman with stage 1 breast cancer goes 5 years without recurrence, she is described as having "no evidence of disease," which is equivalent to cure. After 5 years, if she shows signs of another breast tumor, most experts consider it to be a new cancer and not a "recurrence."

In the case of paraphilias, if a patient no longer has any signs or symptoms of paraphilic interest, from a modern disease perspective, the person should be labeled as having NED. If they eventually relapse and show signs again, doesn't it make more sense to say they have acquired a new paraphilia rather than saying the paraphilia is "incurable"?

In the early 1900s, Richard von Krafft-Ebing (1840–1902) disguised his case histories of men and women with variations in sexual interest by writing them in Latin (Krafft-Ebing, 1886/1999). He identified masturbation as an activity that caused mental illness, especially "sexual deviations." He defined sexual deviations as any sexual activity that did not contribute to procreation of the species. Remarkably, more than 100 years later, the Fifth edition of the *Diagnostic and Statistical Manual of Mental Disorders* (DSM-5; American Psychiatric Association [APA], 2013) adopted an almost identical definition: "The term *paraphilia* denotes any intense and persistent sexual interest other than sexual interest in genital stimulation or preparatory fondling with phenotypically normal, physically mature, consenting human partners" (p. 685). The DSM-5 distinguishes between people who meet the criteria for a paraphilia and those who meet the criteria *and*, due to the paraphilia, either suffer from "clinically significant distress or impairment in social, occupational, or other important areas of functioning" or, in the case of paraphilias that involve potentially criminal acts, "has acted on these sexual urges with a non-consenting person." People who meet these secondary criteria are defined as people with a paraphilic *disorder*.

The DSM-5 definition has been, and continues to be, criticized (Fedoroff, 2011; Moser, 2011, 2016; First, 2014). One of the most significant criticisms is that the DSM-5, like Krafft-Ebing's more than 100-year-old definition, is a definition of exclusion. DSM-5 paraphilic disorders are any "intense or persistent sexual interest" in anything besides activities leading to genital stimulation with consenting partners who look normal and that causes someone distress.

Krafft-Ebing was a physician and psychiatrist, so it is not surprising that he primarily used the disease perspective to describe and explain variants in sexual interests and behaviors. Most of his observations involved patients who had been convicted of sex crimes and subsequently incarcerated or who were patients of medical colleagues who also used a disease perspective to assess and treat their very troubled patients.

So, what was the "broken part"? Krafft-Ebing noted that all the patients he interviewed or observed or received medical information about had one common characteristic: They all masturbated. He speculated that masturbation causes an imbalance in "bodily humors" resulting in the disease of "sexual deviance," analogous to the way diabetes is a disease caused by an imbalance between endogenous insulin and blood glucose.

Krafft-Ebing's explanation of paraphilias and criminal sexual acts is an example of mistaking correlation for causation. The observation that men in custody for sex crimes engage in masturbation does not prove that masturbation is the cause of sexual deviations (as Krafft-Ebing referred to them). We now know there is absolutely no direct causal relationship between masturbation and problematic sexual behaviors of any type. It is notable that Krafft-Ebing undoubtedly was aware of situations in which masturbation did not cause unusual sexual interests. However, the disconfirming data were explained away. The fact that incidents in which exceptions to the proposed explanation did not cause Krafft-Ebing to refute or dismiss the theory that masturbation causes paraphilias underscores how paradigms can influence what is seen as important and permit false paradigms to persist.

This pattern of explaining away or ignoring data that do not fit the paradigm (e.g., men who masturbate but who do not become sexually deviant) has been named the Semmelweis reflex after Dr. Semmelweis, a physician who was fired because he told doctors to wash their hands before the discovery of germs and the invention of "germ theory" (Fedoroff, Curry, Ranger, & Bradford, 2016).

Behavioral Perspective

Krafft-Ebing's explanation of problematic sexual interests and behaviors as being the result of a physiologic imbalance due to masturbation did not satisfy the dermatologist Ivan Bloch (1872–1922), the psychologist Alfred Binet (1857–1911), or the neurologist Albert Moll (1862–1939). Binet was an early behaviorist, then known as an "associationist." Unlike Krafft-Ebing, associationists noticed there were people who masturbated who did not end up in prison. They also noticed that masturbation can be pleasurable and "rewarding." He and others therefore argued that it was not masturbation per se that was the problem. Instead, they suggested that people with unconventional sexual interests had learned or acquired their interests due to a maladaptive (learned) association between orgasm and an unconventional stimulus or scenario.

In other words, associationists argued that masturbation can facilitate an association between non-procreative situations and the powerful reward of orgasm. A paradigm that explains paraphilias as the product of faulty or maladaptive learning is a powerful one. All people experience a change in the salience of sexual issues as they age from childhood to adolescence to adulthood. Other acquired human characteristics, such as language, hobbies, and habits, are learned, so it makes intuitive sense that sexual interests can also be learned and therefore be behaviorally modifiable.

Furthermore, as Moll (1897, as cited in Sulloway, 1983, p. 304, as cited in Fedoroff, 2008, p. 568) noted,

> Were a single sexual experience, and indeed, the first sexual experience to induce a lasting association between sex drive and the object of their first sexual experience, then we would have to find sexual perversion everywhere. Where are there to be found people who initially satisfied their sexual impulse in a normal manner?

Moll's comment helps illustrate how the behavioral perspective can be misunderstood. The fact that problematic sexual interests are not acquired after a single pairing does not negate the behavioral perspective. Similarly, the fact that problematic sexual interests do not "extinguish" in a classical or operant or second-order conditioning schedule does mean that learning is not an important factor.

A second misunderstanding is the assumption that the only significant "reward" for sexual activity is orgasm. In fact, sex can be rewarding on multiple levels that are independent of orgasm. In many cases, the pursuit of sexual arousal and the experience of becoming sexually aroused provide greater reward than the pleasure derived from orgasm. This fact may also explain why the significant negative reinforcements and punishments resulting from problematic sexual behaviors do not appear to decrease or extinguish paraphilic interests like other "learned" behaviors.

Case Report 1.1

Nurses frequently commented with approval about a couple attending the bariatric surgery clinic. The patient was a woman with "morbid obesity" who had become so heavy that she required a specially constructed, reinforced wheelchair. She was brought to appointments by her devoted husband, who was a small man. He could barely be seen when he pushed her wheelchair from behind. They were described as a devoted couple, and he had stuck with her through numerous failed attempts to lose weight. The woman was accepted for gastric bypass surgery. After the procedure, her weight loss was dramatic, and everyone cheered the day she stood up on her own. The nurses were therefore surprised when the patient arrived for her next appointment crying. "What is wrong?" they asked. "He left me," she replied.

In North American culture, being thin and fit is sexy. However, some "devotees" (see Chapter 10, this book) are sexually aroused by disability. Nurses in this clinic assumed the patient's husband would become more "devoted" when his wife became more classically sexually attractive. Unfortunately for the patient, they were wrong.

Here is a situation in which the care providers failed to consider what would be rewarding to the patient's husband. The clinical team was understandably working within a disease perspective in which being overweight is a problem that merits surgical treatment. However, the patient's husband was more interested in his wife when she was disabled than when she was independent. What may have been rewarding to the nurses was not rewarding to him.

The lesson here is to be careful about assuming what is rewarding (positively or negatively) when assessing behavioral explanations or interventions. It is also important to note that the woman's husband may not have realized how important his wife's disability was to him. If asked, he may not have said it was important, especially if part of his interest was sexually motivated.

Dimensional Perspective

At the same time that Krafft-Ebing was championing a disease perspective and Binet was arguing for a behavioral explanation, Magnus Hirschfeld (1868–1935) offered a third explanation for problematic sexual interests (Hirschfeld, 1933/

1935). He astutely noted that people can be ranked on a continuous scale on virtually any nondichotomous scale. For example, people can be ranked in terms of height, weight, intelligence, and so on, as well as virtually any sexual variable aside from fairly dichotomous variables such as chromosomal sex (e.g., XX or XY).

Hirschfeld was primarily interested in orientation and anticipated the Kinsey scale, an excellent example of a dimensional description of a sexual variable. In the Kinsey scale (Kinsey, Pomeroy, & Martin, 1948/1998), the concept of sexual orientation was transformed from dichotomous (homosexual vs. heterosexual) to a scale ranging from 0 to 6 (0 = interest only in heterosexual partners and 6 = interest only in homosexual partners). Often overlooked is the fact that the Kinsey scale also includes a default ranking of "no socio-sexual contacts or reactions."

The dimensional perspective explains people with paraphilias as examples of normal population extremes. For example, for an unrelated diagnosis, people with intellectual disability were defined in the DSM-IV as people with intelligence more than 2 standard deviations below the population norm (APA, 1994, p. 46). A dimensional perspective explains people with pedophilia as people who are aroused by youth to a greater and more extreme extent than the interest in youth shown by the average person who does not have pedophilia.

The dimensional perspective has the appearance of being less stigmatizing because it avoids dealing with causes directly. People are simply categorized as "variants of normal." However, categorization based on a variable without attention to other factors has limitations. Although they both may be the same height, there is a difference between a person who is short because his parents were short and a person who is short due to growth hormone deficiency. This is an example of how dimensional and disease perspectives can intersect. A second limitation of the dimensional perspective is the danger of conflating variables. For example, orientation is often referred to as sexual orientation even though there is a difference between degree of sexual interest in sexual acts with the same sex and romantic interest in the same sex.

Life Story Perspective

A fourth person commenting on the development of sexual interests was the neurologist Sigmund Freud (1856–1939). As the creator of psychoanalysis, his influence on clinicians' views about mental illness was, and continues to be, difficult to overestimate. Despite creating a paradigm based on an uncontrolled and small number of cases, Freud continues to have the highest H factor of any scientist tracked by the Web of Science. Although many of the details of psychoanalysis, such as the Oedipus complex, have become less salient in modern times, his observation that people cannot resist ascribing meaning to events is fundamental to all modern psychotherapies. Freud himself was influenced by his contemporaries, including Moll, Hirschfeld, and especially Krafft-Ebing. Krafft-Ebing sent Freud each new edition of his magnum opus, *Psychopathia Sexualis*, and in turn commented on Freud's conceptualizations of sexuality (Freud, 1962).

The life story perspective is powerful because people have an innate need to explain their feelings and actions. A good example is the concept of "sexual addiction." Some people find the idea of addiction to be helpful in explaining their interests even though sex has none of the characteristics of an addictive substance. The problem with the life story perspective is that the search for meaning can take on a life of its own. Patients often present with the hope that by analyzing their childhood and life story, they will discover the cause of their paraphilic interests. A problem with this approach is that it can delay recovery. How does anyone know when they have uncovered the correct or true meaning?

In the SBC, when patients request therapy to review their childhood in search of the "cause" of their paraphilia, they are invited to adopt a different approach. They are asked to start with the SBC recommendations but assured that once they are better, a review of their childhood can be arranged. Unfailingly, once patients recover, they say they are too busy enjoying their new lives to want to spend time reviewing their childhood. The point here is that it is important for clinicians not to lose sight of the goals of treatment, which should be (in order) (1) immediate cessation of illegal or problematic behaviors, (2) stabilization of lifestyle, (3) enhancement of nonproblematic sexual interests and behaviors, and (4) stabilization of the new healthy lifestyle to the point that the problematic sexual behaviors are no longer of interest. The patient should not feel they have "given up" anything of value but instead feel they have gained a new sexual identity in which their sexual interests are both lawful (consensual) and pleasurable to the point that returning to their previous problematic behaviors would be an aversive experience.

A New Paradigm

Advocates of each of the four perspectives reviewed previously jostled for legitimacy during the 20th century. Unfortunately, most chose a single perspective and ignored the others. In 1986, psychologist John Money (1921–2006) presented a fifth paradigm that combined perspectives and ideas that were popular at the time. He presented his ideas in a book with a singularly lengthy title: *Lovemaps: Clinical Concepts of Sexual Erotic Health and Pathology, Paraphilia and Gender Transposition in Childhood, Adolescence and Maturity* (Money, 1986). In his book, he argued that every person has a "lovemap," which is defined as the characteristics of a person or situation that are maximally sexual arousing to the individual. As can be seen from the subtitle of *Lovemaps*, Money included gender identity within the concept of lovemap. In fact, he combined more than just gender identity. Specifically, he included gender role, orientation, and sexual interest, although these ideas were not always explicitly set out and, in fact, were often comingled.

Money's concept of lovemap comingled two powerful scientific concepts, popular in the 1970s and 1980s. The first was based on the phenomenon of "imprinting," for which Konrad Lorenz (1903–1989) received a Nobel Prize in 1973 (Lorenz, 1935). Lorenz was able to show that newborn geese would "pair-bond" with objects other than their mother if exposed to the moving objects during a "critical period" after hatching. The second was the establishment of "critical periods" in the development of optic neural pathways and neural specificity, for which Roger Sperry, David Hubel, and Torsten Wiesel shared a Nobel Prize in 1981.

Money suggested that in humans, sexual interest is imprinted during a critical period to form a "lovemap." He explained paraphilic interests as faulty imprinting, or "vandalized lovemaps." This idea has had surprising longevity given the fact that imprinting, especially sexual imprinting, has never been demonstrated in humans and the fact that the idea of immutable neural pathways has now been replaced by the idea of neural plasticity.

Characteristics of Sexuality

It has been argued (Fedoroff, 2016) that human sexuality is more accurately described by five independent and orthogonal characteristics:

1. Genetic: One way to describe human sexuality is *genetic*. It is known that males have an XY genetic karyotype and females have an XX karyotype. However, many variations are possible. People with androgen insensitivity syndrome have an XY genotype but a female phenotype because they do not respond to the masculinizing effects of testosterone. People with an XXY genotype (Klinefelter syndrome) have an essentially masculine appearance but have underdeveloped testes. People with an XO genotype (Turner syndrome) have a female phenotype but, like most people with Klinefelter syndrome, are infertile.
2. Gender identity and gender role: *Gender identity* refers to the subjective sense of being male or female, which is established in children by age 6 years (although some experts claim gender identity can be evidenced when people are as young as age 2 years). Once established, children self-identify as being a "boy" or a "girl." They also learn how to present themselves and act socially in a way that reinforces their sense of being a boy or girl, and this is termed *gender role*.
3. Orientation: Orientation is often presented as a characteristic defined by the gender or sex of the person whom the person finds sexually arousing. However, it is now known that men who have sex with men are not necessarily gay, and having sex with a woman does not make a gay man straight. Similarly, gay men who lose their sex drive do not renounce their "gayness." Most people can recall their orientation as children before they were

Table 1.1 Aspects of Sexuality and Their Mutability

Aspect	Characteristic	Mutability	Comment
Genetic	Determined by genes at conception	Nil	XX = female XY = male
Gender	Identity: Self-concept Role: Public presentation	Little Voluntary	Controversial
Orientation	Gender(s) of affection	Little to moderate	Often confused with sexual interest
Drive	Strength of wish to engage in sex act(s)	Highly changeable	Highly modifiable by a variety of methods
Interest	What the person finds sexually arousing	Moderate to high	Paraphilias defined solely by persistent interest

aware of their sexual interest. In this book, *orientation* is defined by the sex and gender(s) of the people for whom a person has romantic (as opposed to sexual) feelings. Of course, it is possible to love the same person in whom one has a sexual interest, but love interests and sexual interests are two different things. This is an important concept because disputes about the mutability of sexual interests are often confused with the unethical idea of "therapy" designed to change love interests.

4. Sex drive: *Sex drive* refers to how much a person wants to have sex. The drive to have sex is experienced as a feeling. Whether a person, in fact, wants to have sex is influenced by many factors besides lust, such as moral and cultural beliefs, experience, health, and medications.
5. Sexual interest: *Sexual interest* refers to what a person wants to do when they have sex and with whom they want to do it. The DSM-5 defines paraphilias as persistent unconventional sexual interests, and paraphilic disorders are defined as harmful sexual interests.

The five aspects of sexuality are summarized in Table 1.1.

The Mutability of Sexual Interests

The five characteristics of sexuality described previously differ concerning how easily they can be changed. For example, a person's karyotype is defined at conception and is not changeable, so a person's chromosomal sex is unchangeable and people with abnormal karyotypes, while treatable, are not curable. Gender identity can change, especially in childhood, and gender role is certainly modifiable. However, in most cases, both gender identity and role, once established, tend to be permanent characteristics. Orientation, like gender identity, once established, tends to be permanent, although the concept of orientation fluidity has gained in popularity.

In contrast, sex drive is highly changeable. People are accustomed to experiencing changes in sex drive due to circumstances. Sex drive is modifiable, and people often take steps to consciously change their sex drive (e.g., taking a cold shower, thinking about income taxes, or watching pornography and masturbating).

Although sexual interests are less easy to change than sex drive, they are certainly more changeable than genes, gender, or orientation. When someone comments that paraphilias cannot be changed, it is important to consider whether they are confusing sexual interests with genes or gender or orientation, which cannot (or should not) be changed.

This book is an attempt to summarize thoughts and observations about paraphilias and other unconventional sexual interests and behaviors accumulated during the past 30 years. The book focuses on the paraphilias listed in the APA's DSM-5 but clearly relates to the many sexual interests not mentioned in any of the five editions of the DSM or 10 versions of the *International Classification of Diseases* (ICD). The main treatments used in the SBC are summarized in Chapter 2.

Several years ago, a list of paraphilias was published (Fedoroff, 2003). An updated version of that list is presented in Table 1.2 to provide a handy reference. A column titled "J. Money Classification" has been added to record a classification system that Money suggested but which has not been widely adopted. It is a complex classification system that is described in detail in his numerous writings, including *Lovemaps* (Money, 1986). Money's classification system is based on a life story perspective (discussed previously). It is important to note that some of the classifications in Table 1.2 may not be official Money classifications and are presented to show how I would classify them based on what I know of Money's teachings. At the end of this book, three modified versions of Table 1.2 are presented for consideration.

Table 1.2 Paraphilias in the Literature with Money's (1986) Likely Classification

Paraphilia	Core Interest/Act	J. Money Classification
Abasiophilia	Disability	Eligibility
Acoustophilia	Sounds	Solicitation/courtship
Acrophilia	Heights	Eligibility
Acrotomophilia	Amputees	Eligibility/sacrificial
Agalmatophilia	Statues	Fetish
Agnophilia	Fighting (observing)	Predatory
Agrexophilia	Being heard having sex	Solicitation/courtship
Algolagnia	Pain	Sacrificial
Amaurophilia	Blindness	Solicitation/courtship
Anasteemaphilia	Height difference	Eligibility
Andriomimetophilia	Women with male features or dressed as men	Fetish

Table 1.2 Continued

Paraphilia	Core Interest/Act	J. Money Classification
Anlilagnia	Older women by younger men	Eligibility
Anthropophagy	Eating human flesh	Predatory
Apodysophilia	Undressing	Solicitation/courtship
Apotemnophilia	Becoming an amputee	Sacrificial
Aquaphilia	Water	Fetish
Arachnophilia	Spiders	Fetish
Aretifism	Bare feet	Fetish
Asphyxiophilia	Asphyxiation	Sacrificial
Autagonistophilia	Being on display	Solicitation/courtship
Autoandrophilia	Females being males	Eligibility
Autoassassinophilia	Being hunted	Predatory
Autoerotic self-asphyxia	Self-strangulation	Sacrificial
Autogynephilia	Being female or having female features	Fetish
Autohemofetishism	Self-bleeding	Sacrificial
Autonepiophilia	Diapers	Fetish
Autophagiophilia	Self-ingestion	Sacrificial
Biastophilia	Rape	Courtship/predatory
Candaulism	Spouse with another partner	Multiple
Capnolagnia	Smoking	Fetish
Catherophilia	Catheterization	Fetish
Celebriphilia	Celebrities	Eligibility
Chremastistophilia	Sex for money	Mercantile
Chronophilia	Age discrepancy	Multiple
Coprophilia	Feces	Fetish
Crush fetish	Crushing creatures	Sacrificial
Dacnolagnomania	Murder	Sacrificial
Dacryphilia	Emotional distress, crying	Sacrificial
Dendrophillia	Trees or foliage	Fetish
Dermatophilia	Skin/leather or fur	Fetish
Devotee	Disability	Eligibility/sacrificial
Dippoldism	Spanking children of partner	Sacrificial
Doraphilia	Smell of fur	Fetish
Dysmorphilia	Discrepant size	Fetish
Ecouteurism	Overhearing sex	Solicitation/courtship
Emetophilia	Vomiting	Sacrificial
Entomophilia	Insects	Fetish
Ephebophilia	Early adolescent	Eligibility
Eproctophilia	Flatulence	Fetish
Erotophonophilia	Murder	Sacrificial
Exhibitionism	Exposing to strangers	Solicitation/courtship
Faunoiphilia	Watching animal mating	Fetish

(continued)

Table 1.2 Continued

Paraphilia	Core Interest/Act	J. Money Classification
Feederism	Feeding	Fetish/eligibility
Formicophilia	Ants	Fetish
Frotteurism	Rubbing strangers	Solicitation/courtship
Gerontophilia	Elderly	Eligibility
Gonophilia	Knees	Fetish
Gynemimetophilia	Male with breasts	Eligibility
Harpazophilia	Being robbed	Mercantile
Hebephilia	Late adolescent	Eligibility
Heirophilia	Religious objects	Fetish
Hematophilia	Blood	Fetish
Heterophilia	Heterosexuals by a non-heterosexual person	Eligibility
Hodophilia	Foreign venues/vacations	Solicitation/courtship
Homeovestism	Same-sex clothing	Fetish
Homilophilia	Religious speeches/sermons	Sacrificial
Hoplophilia	Guns	Fetish
Hybristophilia	Criminals	Eligibility/sacrificial
Hygrophilia	Body fluids	Fetish
Hyphephilia	Fabrics	Fetish
Iatronudia	Medical doctors	Eligibility
Incest	Relative(s)	Eligibility
Infantophilia	Infants	Eligibility
Katoptronophia	Mirrors	Fetish
Kleptophilia	Stealing	Mercantile
Klismaphilia	Enemas	Fetish
Lactophilia	Lactation	Fetish
Lust murder	Murder	Sacrificial
Macrophilia	Giants	Eligibility
Maiesiophilia	Pregnancy	Eligibility
Maschalagnia	Armpits	Fetish
Mask fetishism	Masks or removal of masks	Eligibility
Masochism	Being controlled	Sacrificial
Masochism	Loss of control	Sacrificial
Mechanophilia	Cars	Fetish
Melissophilia	Bee stings	Sacrificial
Melolagnia	Music	Mixed
Menophilia	Menstruation/tampons	Fetish
Microphilia	Smallness	Fetish/eligibility
Morphophilia	Discrepant size	Fetish/eligibility
Mucophilia	Mucous	Fetish
Mysophilia	Filth	Fetish
Nanophilia	Short partner	Eligibility
Narratophilia	Erotic talk	Solicitation/courtship
Nasophylia	Noses	Fetish

Table 1.2 Continued

Paraphilia	Core Interest/Act	J. Money Classification
Necrobestialism	Dead animals	Sacrificial
Necrophilia	Death	Sacrificial
Necrophilia	Corpses	Sacrificial
Nosophilia	Terminal illness	Sacrificial
Odaxelagnia	Biting	Predatory
Olfactophilia	Odors	Fetish
Omorashi	Full bladder	Fetish
Partialism	Body part	Fetish
Pecattiaphilia	Sin	Sacrificial
Pedophilia	Children	Eligibility
Pedovestism	Wearing children's clothes	Mixed
Phobophilia	Fear	Sacrificial
Picquerism	Stabbing	Sacrificial
Pictophilia	Photographs	Fetish
Podophilia	Feet	Fetish
Pseudozoophilia	Partner posing as an animal	Fetish
Public masturbation	Public but no wish to be seen	Solicitation/courtship
Pygmalionism	Statues	Fetish
Pyrophilia	Fire	Fetish
Retifism	Shoes	Mixed
Rhabdophilia	Flagellation	Fetish
Sadism	Control	Sacrificial
Saliromania	Degradation of appearance	Sacrificial
Salirophilia	Perspiration	Mixed
Scotopic syndrome	Being castrated (male)	Mixed
Scoptophilia	Consensual viewing	Sacrificial
Somnophilia	Sleeping sexual partner	Solicitation/courtship
Stethnolagiophilia	Female bodybuilders	Solicitation/courtship
Stigmatophilia	Piercings/tattoos/uniforms	Fetish
Stitophilia	Food	Fetish/eligibility
Symphorophilia	Disasters	Fetish
Taphophilia	Buried alive	Sacrificial
Telephone scatologia	Obscene phone calls	Sacrificial
Teratophilia	Deformity	Solicitation/courtship
Thesauromania	Collecting belongings of partner	Eligibility/sacrificial
Timophilia	Wealth or status	Fetish
Toucherism	Touching	Eligibility
Transvestism	Clothes of the opposite gender	Solicitation/courtship
Transvestophilia	Transvestite partner	Fetish
Trichophilia	Hair	Fetish
Undinsim	Water or urine	Fetish

(*continued*)

Table 1.2 Continued

Paraphilia	Core Interest/Act	J. Money Classification
Urophilia	Urine	Fetish
Vampirism	Blood	Fetish
Vomerophilia	Vomiting	Fetish
Vorarephilia	To consume or be consumed	Sacrificial
Voyeurism	Spying	Sacrificial
Wannabee	To be disabled	Solicitation/courtship
Xenophilia	Strangers/other races	Acrotemnophilia
Zelophilia	Feeling jealous	Eligibility
Zoophilia	Animals	Eligibility
Zoosadism	Control of animals/harm	Eligibility

Conclusion

There is more than one way to look at sex. Observers should be aware of the perspective they use to assess data and of the paradigm(s) they use to make sense of them. This is important because it influences not only what is seen but also how what is seen is weighted. Sexology has a history of being poor at communication between its experts, with a tendency to dismiss anyone with a different perspective or paradigm. It is hoped this book will encourage a new look at the data and the prospects for the successful treatment of those paraphilias that require treatment.

References

American Psychiatric Association. (1994). *Diagnostic and statistical manual of mental disorders* (4th ed.). Washington, DC: Author.

American Psychiatric Association. (2013). *Diagnostic and statistical manual of mental disorders* (5th ed.). Arlington, VA: American Psychiatric Publishing.

Fedoroff, J. P. (2003). Paraphilic worlds. In S. B. Levine (Ed.), *Handbook of clinical sexuality for mental health professionals* (pp. 401–424). New York, NY: Routledge.

Fedoroff, J. P. (2008). Treatment of paraphilic sexual disorders. In D. L. Rowland & L. Lacocci (Eds.), *Handbook of sexual and gender identity disorders* (pp. 563–585). Hoboken, NJ: Wiley.

Fedoroff, J. P. (2009). The paraphilias. In M. G. Gelder, N. C. Andereasen, J. J. Lopez-Iber, Jr., & J. R. Beddes (Eds.), *The new Oxford textbook of psychiatry* (2nd ed., pp. 832–842). Oxford, UK: Oxford University Press.

Fedoroff, J. P. (2011). Forensic and diagnostic concerns arising from the proposed DSM-5 criteria for sexual paraphilic disorder. *Journal of the American Academy of Psychiatry and the Law, 39*(2), 238–241.

Fedoroff, J. P. (2016). Managing versus successfully treating paraphilic disorders: The paradigm is changing. In S. B. Levine, C. B. Risen, & S. E. Althof (Eds.), *Handbook of clinical sexuality for mental health professionals* (pp. 345–361). New York, NY: Taylor & Francis.

Fedoroff, J. P., Curry, S., Ranger, R. C., & Bradford, J. M. W. (2016). Regression to the mean or the Semmelweis reflex? Invited commentary. *Archives of Sexual Behavior, 45*(7), 1869–1870. doi:10.1007/s10508-016-0786-3

First, M. (2014). DSM-5 and paraphilic disorders. *Journal of the American Academy of Psychiatry and the Law, 42*, 191–201.

Freud, S. (1962). *Three essays on the theory of sexuality* (J. Strachey, Trans.). New York, NY: Basic Books.

Hirschfeld, M. (1935). *Men and women: The world journey of a sexologist* (O. P. Green, Trans.). New York, NY: Putnam. (Original work published 1933)

Kinsey, A. C., Pomeroy, W. B., & Martin, C. E. (1998). *Sexual behavior in the human male*. Bloomington, IN: Indiana University Press. (Original work published 1948)

Krafft-Ebing, R. von. (1999). *Psychopathia sexualis*. Bloat Books. ISBN:0-9650324-1-8 (Original work published 1886)

Kuhn, T. S. (1962). *The structure of scientific revolutions*. Chicago, IL: University of Chicago Press. ISBN:0-226-45808-3

Lorenz, K. (1935). Der Kumpan in der Umwelt des Vogels: Der Artgenosse als auslösendes Moment sozialer Verhaltensweisen. *Journal für Ornithologie, 83*, 137–215, 289–413.

McHugh, P. R., & Slavney, P. R. (1998). *The perspectives of psychiatry* (2nd ed.). Baltimore, MD: Johns Hopkins University Press.

Money, J. (1986). *Lovemaps: Clinical concepts of sexual/erotic health and pathology, paraphilia, and gender transposition in childhood, adolescence, and maturity*. New York, NY: Prometheus. ISBN:0-8290-1589-2

Moser, C. (2011). Hypersexual disorder: Just more muddled thinking. *Archives of Sexual Behavior*, 40, 227–229. doi:10.1007/s10508-010-9690-4

Moser, C. (2016). DSM-5 and the paraphilic disorders: Conceptual issues. *Archives of Sexual Behavior, 45*(8), 2181–2186. doi:10.1007/s10508-016-0861-9

2
Assessment, Treatment, and Management of Paraphilic Disorders

> I know some people say I can't be cured but fortunately I do not understand them. I am not much of a reader.
>
> —A Sexual Behaviours Clinic patient with pedophilia and dyslexia discussing the loss of his pedophilic interests

Introduction

Many books, chapters, and articles concerning the assessment and treatment of the paraphilias have been published. Most are limited due to a lack of clarity about what is being treated and a failure to fully recognize the heterogeneity of the treatment population(s). For example, *Psychopathia Sexualis* by Krafft-Ebing (1886/1999) is a *tour de force* in case studies but provides little, if any, information about treatment approaches and even less about successful treatment outcomes. The second edition of *Sexual Deviance* by Laws and O'Donohue (2008) provides chapters on the main *Diagnostic and Statistical Manual of Mental Disorders*, fourth edition, text revision (American Psychiatric Association, 2000) paraphilias, with each chapter providing a review of theories concerning a specific paraphilia followed by a discussion of treatments for that paraphilia. Unfortunately, the recommended treatments do not always flow logically from what would be expected from the literature reviewed. Expectations of treatment success are also typically modest in Laws and O'Donohue's anthology of treatments. This is not intended as a criticism of the second edition but, rather, a suggestion that the current book has the benefit of a knowledge base established by Laws and O'Donohue that permits and supports the establishment of a fresh look at the nature and treatability of the paraphilias. Current and past treatments for paraphilic disorders were more recently summarized in Murphy, Bradford, and Fedoroff (2014) and Fedoroff (2016).

In this book, assessment issues are incorporated in each chapter. This is because the Sexual Behaviours Clinic's (SBC) approach to assessment is that it should be ongoing and subject to revision based on response to treatment. The SBC assessment process has been previously described in detail (Fedoroff, 2010, 2016). A brief overview of the SBC's approach to assessment is presented here.

Initial Assessment

Before the assessment begins, new patients are provided with a document that summarizes the reporting laws in Ontario so they are aware of these laws and can make an informed decision about proceeding with the assessment (for more information about reporting laws, see Chapter 6, this book). Next, patients are asked to complete a 40-page computerized intake questionnaire either via emailed or in the SBC lab. Some patients do not have computers (now fairly rare) or have legal conditions against using computers that can access the Internet, so they are invited to complete the questionnaire in the lab. Importantly, everyone is asked if they have any difficulties with reading, writing, or computers. Patients who are illiterate or who have dyslexia or intellectual disabilities are respectfully assisted in completing the questionnaire. It is not uncommon for people who have been labeled as "oppositional" or "in denial" by other agencies to in fact be illiterate. Rather than tell other assessors about their illiteracy, they simply refuse to complete forms or scribble "yes" and "no" answers. A rule in the SBC is to always investigate why patients are reluctant to do something before labeling them as "difficult." Often, the reluctance has to do with embarrassment or shame that once appropriately addressed changes the patient's attitude toward the assessment.

Completion of the intake questionnaire typically takes approximately 1½ hours. Before patients begin to complete the questionnaire, they are asked four questions:

1. Whose idea was it to come to the SBC?
2. Do *you* agree it is a good idea?
3. What is the reason you have come to the SBC today?
4. Do *you* want treatment?

It is SBC policy to offer treatment after the first visit with a caution to the patient that the treatment plan will be modified once the full assessment is completed. Patients are then referred to one of the five SBC groups that meet every week (discussed later). In this way, all SBC patients can begin to receive treatment within 7 days from the day they walk through the door of the SBC.

The next visit involves reviewing all the information in the intake questionnaire. Some patients prefer to answer questions on a computer, whereas others prefer to speak to the interviewer. By combining the process of answering questions on a computer with an in-person interview to review the questionnaire, the benefits of questionnaire answers (e.g., can be done in private, the patient has time to think about their answers, and the patient does not put their name on the questionnaire so they can feel more free to answer questions honestly) are combined with the benefits of in-person interview answers (e.g., the patient's understanding of the question can be verified, the meaning of the patient's answer can be verified, the patient can change their answers or add to them, and all the information is recorded in a standardized format suitable for research studies). The questionnaire itself is comprehensive and includes questions about family history, personal history, substance use, legal history, medical and psychiatric history, as well as extensive questions about the person's sexual history and current sexual interests and behaviors and problems. A complete mental status exam is also performed by the examining psychiatrist. As much collateral information as possible is collected and reviewed, including police synopses of any charges or convictions, judge's reasons for judgment, reports from children's aid and probation and parole, and past medical and psychiatric charts. In addition, people who know the patient are interviewed, with the patient's permission.

Phallometric Testing

The SBC offers penile plethysmographic (PPG) testing to men. The premise of the test is that blood flow to a man's penis will increase when he is sexually aroused. Several methods of detecting an increase in penile blood flow have been explored since the 1950s when the technique was first developed by Kurt Freund to test the veracity of army conscripts who were hoping to avoid the draft in (then) Czechoslovakia by claiming they were homosexual. Measurement of changes in penile blood flow in response to standardized stimuli are often referred to as "phallometric testing." Details of this procedure have been published elsewhere and are discussed in Chapter 6 of this book (Fedoroff, Kuban, Bradford, 2009; Murphy, Ranger, Fedoroff, et al., 2015; Murphy, Ranger, Stewart, et al., 2015).

Note that there are inherent problems in phallometry. The most important is that the premise that penile blood flow is directly correlated to sexual arousal is not always true. Men can get penile erections when they are not aroused (e.g., when they are asleep), and they can fail to get erections even when they are sexually aroused (e.g., due to erectile dysfunction). To at least partially deal with this problem, men are shown a variety of stimuli so their responses to a theme (e.g., adult men) can be compared to their responses to a different theme (e.g., girls). Tables on the sensitivity and specificity of phallometric testing have been published with sensitivity for pedophilia ranging from 42% to 100% and specificity ranging from 80% to 100% (Fedoroff et al., 2009). It is generally agreed that the sensitivity and specificity for distinguishing PPG response to men versus women is better than for children, likely because the phenotypic appearance of children varies considerably depending on the age of the child. Phallometric testing should never be used to determine guilt or innocence. In the SBC, it is used as another source of information to assist in tailoring treatment to the specific needs of the individual patient. One interesting observation is that patients sometimes use PPG results to explain why they want treatment: "Well doc, I would never do the things with children that they say I did, but I can't argue with the [PPG] numbers. Sign me up [for treatment]."

Vaginal Photoplethysmography

The SBC will be offering vaginal photoplethysmography (VPP) to assist in assessing the sexual arousal patterns of women (Knack, Murphy, Ranger, Meston, & Fedoroff, 2015). VPP is based on the observation that blood flow in the walls of the vagina increases during sexual arousal in a manner analogous to the increase in penile blood flow in men during sexual arousal. Changes in vaginal wall blood flow can be measured using a small photoelectric instrument that the woman being tested inserts into her vagina before being presented with sexual stimuli. It is generally agreed that the correlation between vaginal wall blood flow and subjective sexual arousal is even less perfect than it is in men. However, as with PPG, it can provide another set of data to assist in designing a treatment plan for women. As with PPG in men, VPP in women should never be used to determine guilt or innocence. Other methods that have been investigated to measure sexual arousal in women include measuring vaginal lubrication and/or change in temperature, laser Doppler imaging, and labial and clitoral photoplethysmography (reviewed by Kukkonen, 2014). However, to date, none of these techniques has been used to measure sexual arousal patterns in forensic cases.

Visual Reaction Time

Assessments using visual reaction time (VRT) are based on the well-established phenomenon that people tend to look at pictures of people they find sexually arousing longer than they look at pictures of people who they find less sexually arousing. By measuring how long a patient looks at slides of men, women, boys, and girls, an estimate can be made of how sexually appealing each category of slides is to the person being tested. Some have claimed that the test is as good as PPG at determining sexual arousal patterns (Abel, Huffman, Warberg, & Holland, 1998).

In the SBC, VRT is offered when patients want an independent test of the accuracy of their PPG test. In general, with the exception of cases in which the man has severe erectile dysfunction, PPG and VRT results tend to be in agreement.

Polygraphs

Many assessment and treatment programs include polygraph interviews in the assessment process (Grubin, Kamenskov, Dwyer, & Stephenson, 2019). There is little question that people who know they are going to be polygraphed are more disclosing of information (Grubin, 2010). However, the SBC does not use polygraphy. Instead, the SBC works to create an environment in which patients feel free to discuss their progress or lack of progress in therapy. Patients are told they will never be criticized or "breached" for discussing problematic sexual interests; in fact, they are encouraged to do so. Patients quickly learn this is true from attending group therapy sessions in which group members regularly discuss issues relating to persistent problematic sexual interests. Again, acting on criminal interests is never condoned. In this environment, polygraphy seems unnecessary. It also helps the SBC avoid stepping into the real or perceived role of detective.

Other Physiologic Methods of Assessing Sexual Interest

Several physiologic measures associated with sexual arousal are under investigation, including thermography, pupillary dilatation, visual eye tracking, electroencephalography (EEG), and functional magnetic resonance imaging. Preliminary studies suggest that preconscious EEG changes may occur before conscious sexual arousal occurs (Knott, Impey, Fisher, Delpero, & Fedoroff, 2016; Kirenskaya, A & Kamenskov, 2019), and changes in brain blood flow associated with sexual arousal may be detectable (Cheng, Secondary, Burke, Fedoroff, & Dwyer, 2015). Another avenue of investigation is whether the gaseous neurotransmitter nitric oxide, associated with penile tumescence, can be detected in association with sexual arousal.

Although all these, and other, methods to assess sexual arousal have some use, none compares to the information attainable from open conversation with patients who understand that the program is there to help them.

Planning the Treatment

Once the information has been collected, the patient is provided with a verbal formulation of what has been found, a differential diagnosis, a working diagnosis, and proposed treatment options. Remarkably, most treatment protocols for people with paraphilia-related problems do not explicitly state the aim of treatment. Instead, proxy estimates of success are offered, the most frequent being rates of recidivism, often approximated by rearrest rates. This is because most treatments programs ignore the possibility that modifying the sexual interests that define the problem is a valid and achievable treatment goal.

The problem is exacerbated by the fact that people with paraphilic disorders rarely seek help through a direct route. Consider a person with depression. That person typically has consulted with their friends and romantic partner(s), who advised the person to see a physician or other mental health professional, usually with an assurance that with treatment, they will get better soon (M. Komrad, 2012). In most cases, they will go for help and get it. According to the most recent CANMAT guidelines for bipolar disorders (Yatham et al., 2018, P. 121), "With treatment, 19%–25% of patients will experience a recurrence every year, compared to 23%–40% of those on placebo" (Vazquez, Holtzman, Lolich, Ketter, & Baldessarini, 2015, cited in abstract).

In contrast, people with paraphilic disorders typically tell no one about their concerns. When they are "caught," they attempt to avoid letting anyone know, especially their friends or romantic partner(s). People who do know about the problem assure the person there are no effective treatments. Not surprisingly, the person typically does not seek help until they become hopeless and therefore depressed, leading to the depression scenario described previously. Alternatively, if the paraphilic disorder involves a sexual interest in criminal activity, they often are arrested and again are assured treatment prospects are hopeless—even though the recidivism rate (defined as subsequent charge or rearrest regardless of conviction) for sex offenders (regardless of treatment received) is 13.7% after 5 years of opportunity (Hanson & Morton-Bourgon, 2005).

Approximately 15 years ago, the SBC of the Integrated Forensic Program of the Royal took the unprecedented approach of changing its paradigm from one of hopeful management to an active treatment program with the goal of curing people with problematic paraphiliac interests. In fairness, the paradigm shift was gradual and not fully articulated at the time. In 2001, the idea that paraphilias could not be cured was shared by many SBC clinicians and staff members who had been educated under the paradigm of the time, which was that paraphilias were incurable. However, the SBC was also a clinical research program, and the data, even then, did not support the idea that all paraphilic interests and the people who had them were immutable.

The following is a summary of the SBC approach to treatment. It is not intended to be a treatment manual or substitute for formal training in individual, couple's, group, or pharmacotherapy. As indicated in Chapter 1, the SBC has avoided use of treatment manuals due to the absence of evidence that treatment manuals increase treatment efficacy. Instead, this chapter is intended to provide information about how the SBC works, based on 15 years of experience. Other descriptions of the philosophy of the SBC are available (Fedoroff, 2003, 2008, 2009, 2010; Fedoroff, Murphy, & Ly, 2018). Details of the approach to assessment in the SBC have also been published (Murphy & Fedoroff, 2017). The following is a more specific summary of the SBC approach to therapy, but it is important to remember that a critical element in successful treatment is individualization of the treatment to the needs of the patients and their families. For this reason, every patient who attends SBC group therapy is also seen individually approximately every 3 months in order to check on progress and modify treatment based on how well it is working.

Step 1: A Systematic and Expedited Intake

Given the differences between the ways people with nonparaphilic psychiatric disorders and people with paraphilic psychiatric disorders arrive at the therapist's office, the approaches to therapy are understandably different. An essential first step is to convince the person seeking treatment for a paraphilic disorder that treatment is both available and extremely effective. This is done by reassuring the person they have come to the right place. It is important to remember the person has almost certainly already been told the situation is hopeless, often by people with little or no clinical experience in treating paraphilias or by people who have adopted a paradigm that does not include the possibility of successful treatment—for example, adherence to the now debunked belief that neural pathways, once established during a critical period, are immutable.

The SBC is fortunate because most new patients have already heard positive comments about the program. Increasingly, many new patients arrive with the report that they chose the SBC precisely because it was criticized by others whose programs seem less effective.

It also helps if the program's initial assessment approach is nonjudgmental, comprehensive, and calm. Being nonjudgmental and comprehensive are qualities that any therapy program should have. *Calmness* refers to the fact that most new SBC patients arrive in a state of crisis. They have just been "caught" by their spouse, cautioned by a police office, arrested, or recently released from custody. It is vital for the program to deal with immediate problems expeditiously but without adding to the acute stress experienced by the patient.

This is one reason the SBC avoids having a waiting list by typically seeing new patients within 24 hours of first contact and offers treatment the same week. Patients are invited to voluntarily participate in the SBC via a program of interventions that are not crisis based. This process is assisted by use of the comprehensive anonymized computerized intake assessment described previously.

Although treatment is offered immediately, final diagnosis is deferred until after the information is collected and reviewed. This process has the effect of immediately calming the patient and providing them with a sense of hope.

It is important to note that the SBC is intentionally an out-patient program. This is because it is difficult or impossible to avoid coercion in a jail or prison. This is important because sex crimes are sex crimes not because they involve sex but, rather, because they involve nonconsent and/or unlawful coercion. For this reason, SBC clinicians make a point of always providing the opportunity for SBC patients to provide signed, witnessed informed, voluntary, revocable consent. Assessment and treatment in the SBC is always voluntary and has the goal of successful reintegration into society, including a normalization of any criminal paraphilic interests and behaviors.

Step 2: A Scientific Approach

After preliminary information has been collected, the differential diagnosis is reviewed with a focus on the reason the possible diagnoses are being entertained.

The scientific method of the SBC is explained. Specifically, the first step is to define the problem based on the data available. Next, hypotheses are developed to explain the data, and then a series of interventions are proposed to test the hypothesized solutions to the problem. Patients are reassured they do not need to believe the hypotheses for the interventions to be effective and worthwhile. All that is required is for them to voluntarily enact or comply with the intervention and to honestly report how successful it was. It is important to emphasize that if the intervention does not work, it will still provide information about the problem that will make selection of the next intervention easier and more likely to be effective.

Step 3: Realistic Optimism

Provide evidence that the person will get better. It is helpful to tell the person their problem is not unique. If the therapist has seen a similar case or if it has been described in the literature, the therapist should say so. No matter how common the paraphilia is, (e.g., pedophilia or shoe fetishism), people tend to think they are the first of their kind. This is because people often have difficulty admitting they have a paraphilia, especially after they recover. As a result, self-reports of recovery from paraphilic disorders are rare. Group therapy is highly effective in helping patients admit they have a problem and accepting it is not hopeless. This is especially true if the group is an open one in which new group members are mixed with group members who have been receiving treatment for some time.In these "mixed" groups, other group members can provide first-person testimony about the efficacy of treatment; confirm that things do get better; and confirm that cure, or at least "no evidence of the disorder," is a reasonable and expected treatment objective.

In the case of paraphilic disorders involving sexual interest in criminal acts, it is crucial to establish the fact that successful treatment of the person is of benefit to both the person and the community. This obvious fact is often a novel revelation to people with paraphilias, treatment providers, and law enforcement authorities, all of whom are prone to think in terms of "us" versus "them" or "good guys" versus "bad guys." In truth, no one wants to have an abnormal or dysfunctional sexual interest. The efficacy of treatment increases when the person seeking treatment understands that the therapist has a fiduciary duty to work in their best interests which fortunately is what society wants, or at least what society should want.

The Problem with the Risk–Need–Responsivity Model

Currently, treatment protocols based on the risk–need–responsivity (RNR) model are widely advocated (Bonta & Wormith, 2013). However, the SBC avoids strict adherence to the RNR model. In Canada, the phrase "risk, need, responsivity" has become the mantra of officials in charge of designing treatment programs in Canadian correctional institutes. The RNR model is based on work by respected researchers but is not recommended because it states that intensity of intervention should be based on the estimated risk posed by the person seeking treatment. This is an example of a misapplication of the disease perspective, which suggests that more severe disease should receive more intensive treatment (and vice versa).

Although the RNR model may appeal to bureaucrats who mistakenly think it is wise to scrimp on treatment for low-risk offenders to save resources and therefore money, it makes no sense if cure and prevention are the aims of treatment. In fact, it has been argued that devoting resources to prevention and early intervention is far more effective than attempting to treat people who typically are considered high risk (e.g., repeated recidivists) (Knack, Winder, Murphy, & Fedoroff, 2019). It also confuses risk of reoffense with the "severity" of the paraphilic disorder. In an aggregated study involving 7,740 sex offenders (Hanson, Harris, Helmus, & Thornton, 2014), the risk that "high-risk" offenders would reoffend was shown to decrease every year that they did not reoffend.

The "N" in RNR refers to the notion that treatment should target criminogenic factors or "needs" (e.g., problems with drug use). Although this approach is partially effective, the SBC places at least as much attention on establishing healthy, noncriminogenic factors akin to what is advocated by the "good lives" method of treatment (Ward & Brown, 2004). For example, most RNR treatment programs take the view that people with pedophilia must give up on the idea of having sex with another person, based on the false view that people with pedophilia can never change their pedophilic interests. In contrast, the SBC encourages people with pedophilia to associate their sexual feelings and fantasies with adults.

The "R" in RNR refers to "responsivity"—that is, the need to alter treatment based on how well the treatment is working. The SBC strongly advocates this approach. Unfortunately, many RNR programs impose the program's needs on the patient rather than modifying treatment to meet the specific needs of the patient. For example, a treatment program that emphasizes respect for punctuality will not work for patients who cannot tell time and who do not own wristwatches. A treatment program that requires written homework will not work for patients with dyslexia. Many patients labeled as "unmotivated" or "oppositional" in correctional RNR programs become highly motivated and cooperative when their dyslexia is identified and accounted for in the treatment plan.

Step 4: Consider All the Options

The fourth step in the SBC program is to review possible treatment interventions. At this stage, it is important to assure the person that treatment is entirely voluntary. In addition to being ethical, modeling respect for consent is crucial. A variety of recommended treatment options together with the risks and benefits of the treatment and the decision to exert the right to decline treatment(s) should be offered. Usually, more than one treatment intervention is potentially useful, and the possibility of combining treatments should also be offered. Some treatment options for consideration are presented next.

Individual Psychotherapies

More than 500 types of individual psychotherapies have been described (Norcross, VandenBos, & Freedheim, 2011). In 1991, Frank and Frank reviewed the psychotherapies then in existence and concluded that the factor most associated with treatment efficacy is how much the *therapist* believes in the treatment.

Psychotherapies That Do Not Appear to Work

Psychoanalysis Some psychotherapies have little evidentiary support. For example, there is little or no evidence that psychoanalytic therapies are effective or practical in the treatment of paraphilic disorders. This fact is often a disappointment to people with paraphilic disorders who present for help with the expectation that this will involve an in-depth and lengthy review of their childhood to uncover the traumatic event(s) that led to the development of their paraphilic interests.

It is important to respect the person's life-story perspective and explanation for how they got the way they are now. However, to follow this route to solve the presenting problem is a mistake because it can delay change, and there is no way to know when the correct explanatory "event" has been discovered. For example, a person with transvestic fetishism may recall a Halloween when his older sister dressed him as a girl. However, there is no evidence that mischievous older sisters cause transvestic fetishism.

Also, spending time uncovering childhood events may convey the false impression that the process of recovery will take a long time and, more importantly, permit the person with the paraphilic disorder to rationalize continuing to engage in problematic sexual acts. In the SBC, patients are reminded that all sexual behaviors are voluntary and that all members of society are expected to limit their sexual behaviors to the requirements of the law and social expectations.

Relapse Prevention In the 1970s, relapse prevention therapies (RPTs) were developed to treat people with addictions to substances (especially alcohol; Marlatt & Donovan, 2005). They, in turn, were adapted to treat sex offenders (Laws, 1989). A major premise of RPT is that it is easier to resist temptations when they are further away. In RPT, "triggers" and patterns of behavior leading to the problematic behaviors are identified. People are then taught to identify triggers and patterns of behavior and escape routes they can take to avoid going down the problematic path.

This method makes sense and can be effective, especially if the fact that the person is responsible for their behaviors is emphasized. It is less effective if the person seeking treatment is not disabused of the notion that the paraphilic interest itself can be changed. The strengths and limitations of RPT in the treatment of sex offenders are reviewed elsewhere (Fedoroff & Marshall, 2010).

Many people with paraphilic disorders present with the belief that they are "addicted" to paraphilic acts. This is largely due to the prevalence of addiction paradigms in society, especially in North America, where institutions such as the Betty Ford Clinic and self-help programs such as Alcoholics Anonymous (AA) are widely hailed (despite a lack of scientific support) and the concept of "sexual addiction" is routinely offered by celebrities as an explanation and/or excuse for their sexual indiscretions.

The Problem with "Sex Addiction" It is important to respect the perspective of the person seeking help provided that the perspective does not interfere with getting better. People who self-identify as "sex addicts" often have other dependencies that are true addictions (e.g., alcohol dependency), and there is a tendency for a person with a true drug addiction to explain their sexual problems as addictions.

In the SBC, the definition of nonbehavioral addictions is explained as an acquired dependence on a nonphysiologic (or external) substance to which the addict gains tolerance in the sense of needing more to achieve the same effect and for which there are characteristic withdrawal symptoms when the substance is stopped. The difference is explained between a drug addiction, in which tolerance and withdrawal effects can be documented, and "sex addiction," in which "tolerance" does not occur and there are no physiologic withdrawal symptoms.

In the case of so-called sex addicts, it is particularly important to establish the motivation for seeking treatment. A useful question is, "If you were single, would you be here?" If the answer is "no," it raises the likelihood that the actual problem is a relationship problem, involving the patient and whomever insisted the patient seek therapy. Often, so-called sex addicts are better characterized as people with sexual frustration(s), often caused by feelings of guilt about sex.

Interventions That Do Appear to Work

Taking Responsibility Immediately In the SBC, the idea of avoiding acting on a theoretically irresistible (paraphilic) addiction is replaced with the idea that sexual behaviors are always under voluntary control and that paraphilic behaviors are less pleasurable than nonparaphilic goals. A common analogy is a comparison of "unhealthy fast food," which may be attractive, with healthy and/or gourmet food, which may require more effort to prepare but ultimately is much more enjoyable. A second analogy is to compare playing tennis with an unwilling child to playing tennis with a willing, age-matched, opponent. It is easy for patients to understand that sexual relations with a consenting partner will be better than with a nonconsenting partner in the same way that playing tennis with someone who is unwilling or unable to hit the ball back is less enjoyable. They also easily agree that forcing anyone to engage in any activity is wrong.

Also, people with paraphilic interests are invited and expected to stop all problematic paraphilic acts immediately. They are helped to understand that having paraphilic interests is different from having an addition to a drug. Importantly, they are reassured there is no need to "taper" paraphilic behaviors because there are no adverse physiologic effects from stopping paraphilic acts "cold turkey." Stopping the problematic sexual behaviors is not only eminently possible but also healthy and the *first* step to getting better. This intervention is important not only to stop harm to innocent victims but also to establish that SBC therapists are there to help, which means insisting on no more victims, ever.

Circles of Support and Accountability The slogan "no more victims" was coined by Circles of Support and Accountability (CoSA) (Azoulay, Murphy, Winder, & Fedoroff, 2019). CoSA programs recognize that although it is stressful to go into custody, it can also be very stressful to be released from custody, especially if the person has been in custody for a lengthy period. The SBC has seen patients who went into custody before there was the Internet, cell phones, and bank machines. CoSA provides a group of trained volunteers who help the person find accommodation, get furniture and food, get medications, and get to appointments. These vital issues are often completely neglected by the criminal justice system but are highly significant in terms of reducing rates of recidivism (Wilson, Cortini, & McWhinnie, 2009). Affiliation with a CoSA group has been shown to reduce rates of sexual recidivism in high-risk offenders by 83% over an average follow-up period of 35 months. Given that, if they do happen, most offenses occur within the first 12 months, this is a significant intervention.

Motivated Behaviors Patients who claim they cannot resist their sexual urges are educated about motivated behaviors (Toates, 2009). These are acts that are motivated by physiologic mechanisms. Some, such as breathing, are indeed impossible to resist. The urge to sleep can be resisted for a day or two but then becomes irresistible. Others, such as eating, are possible to resist acting on for days or even weeks. Sex is comparatively weakly motivated. Unlike breathing or eating, it is possible to live without sex, and in fact, the urge to have sex decreases the longer it is not acted upon.

Group Therapies

The SBC relies heavily on group psychotherapy to treat people with paraphilic disorders. However, patients also receive individual therapy for concurrent problems, such as substance abuse, depression, and anxiety, and to double-check on the progress being made.

Good Lives Model

An example of a more optimistic model of treatment, compatible with the SBC approach is the good lives model (GLM; Ward & Brown, 2004). This model conceptualizes healthy sexuality as the natural outcome of success in achieving life goals. It is compatible with other treatment models and has been presented as an enhancement to ongoing treatments (Andrews, Bonta, & Wormith, 2011; Ward, 2002). Some patients have difficulty changing their self-identity from that of "sex offender" to that of "former sex offender" or "recovered." GLM principles are helpful in achieving this aim. Some patients elect to be treated with medications to reduce their sex drives while they focus on improving their lives, and more do so when they are reminded that the treatment is voluntary and they can stop the medication whenever they wish.

Couple's Therapy

Sex is inherently an interactive activity. Therefore, therapy designed to change a person's sexual interests and activities needs to take the person's romantic and sexual partner(s) into account. To engage the patient's partner, it is important to avoid appearing to blame the partner. Blame is never a useful therapeutic device. In the SBC, partners are invited to join the person seeking treatment in the role of being an authority about the person: "Thanks for joining us today Ms. X, you probably know more about your husband than anyone else." Spouses rarely disagree with this assessment and are comfortable in this role. They generally welcome being consulted, especially when there has been a breakdown in trust between the spouse and the person seeking treatment.

At the first meeting with the spouse and person seeking treatment, the spouse is assured they are not the patient and that no clinical chart is being opened on them. To enhance the impression that the patient is the focus of treatment, they are always seen together with the patient. Next, rules of confidentiality are reviewed. It is explained that what the person seeking treatment says in private meetings with the therapist is confidential between the therapist and the person seeking treatment. However, there are no rules against the therapist receiving information from anyone else, including the spouse. The spouse is told they should feel free to call if they are concerned that treatment is not working or going in the wrong direction.

The way significant others are integrated into the therapeutic program has evolved during the past 15 years. Although celibacy and choosing to live as a single person are legitimate lifestyles, they usually are not the ideal goals of people with paraphilias. Instead, people with problematic paraphilias are encouraged to establish trusting, respectful, and honest intimate relationships that enhance healthy sexual lifestyles. This option requires the willing participation of at least one "significant other."

Case Report 2.1

One day, the wife of a man who had sought treatment in the SBC gave Dr. Fedoroff a lecture:

> Doc, I can see what you have done for my husband. He is now in individual and group therapy. He is getting medication that has helped his depression. He has completed an addictions program and is now sober. He has completed an occupational therapy assessment and now is in school to train for a career that makes him excited to get up every morning. You have found him a medical doctor, and he has had a sleep study that diagnosed sleep apnea for which he is now on CPAP [continuous positive airway pressure] that has cured his insomnia, decreased his irritability and given him more energy. But doc, what are you doing for me?

The fact was, besides improving the nature and quality of her husband, the SBC was not doing anything to help her. So, the SBC established "spouses" groups for the adult sexual and romantic partners of the men and women in treatment in the SBC. As per hospital policy, each spouse received a full psychiatric assessment, a chart was opened, and weekly groups were scheduled.

The groups were a disaster. People did not show up or dropped out after the first one or two sessions. Unlike the SBC groups for people with paraphilias and paraphilic disorders, people in the spouse's group seemed unmotivated and even embarrassed to be in a group "with other people who know why I am here." Something was wrong. The answer is now apparent: Spouses of people seeking treatment in the SBC are not patients. They are married to patients.

As a result of that realization, the SBC program for spouses changed dramatically. Instead of treating spouses like patients, they were treated the way they should be: as healthy and vital members of society who happen to be in love with people receiving treatment in the SBC. To do this, the groups were changed so that people in treatment in the SBC attended and invited their spouses to attend as guests. Because they were not patients, the guests did not need to have an intake interview or to have a clinical chart opened. The sessions were intended to be primarily educational and not strictly therapy sessions, so they intentionally were scheduled to occur just once every 3 months.

While couple's therapy sessions in which the person with problematic sexual interests and/or behaviors (the patient) and their spouse (who is not a patient) remain a crucial component of SBC treatment, the spouse's group underwent a significant change.

Friends and Family Group

Not long after the SBC had changed the spouse's groups as described previously, Dr. Fedoroff received another lecture from another SBC patient:

> Doc, I have heard about the spouse's group, and it sounds fantastic. The guys in the group say it has given them a chance to show their partners what they do every Tuesday night and it has given their partners a place where they can talk about what is bugging them. For someone whose wife was thinking about leaving because all her friends said she should, it is amazing to see what happens when they meet women who have not only stayed, but who say staying was the best decision they ever made. Or, at least that is what I have heard. The problem is, I can't go to the groups because I don't have a spouse or even a girlfriend.

He paused for a minute and then said, "But I do have a sister." Of course, he was right.

So, the SBC changed the group from being a "spouses" group to a "friends and family" group. The change has been dramatic because it makes the group accessible to more people (only approximately 30% of the people treated in the SBC have spouses or long-term partners). The Friends and Family group is very popular and has assisted in providing new perspectives on the impact of both treated and untreated paraphilic disorders.

Secondary Victims

The Friends and Family group led to the creation of the term used frequently in SBC sessions, "secondary victims." It is understood that people who commit sex crimes have victims. However, people often forget that sex offenders victimize not only the people with whom they have nonconsensual sex but also all the people around them. Consider the innocent brother of a sex offender. One day he is going about his regular business. The next day his boss is questioning her judgment in having hired him. The spouse of one offender said she had moments when she envied her husband because he got to disappear into a jail cell while she was left to endure the looks of her neighbors and the accusations of her friends, especially after she said she planned to stay with her husband.

The Friends and Family group has proven to be extremely popular, and the sessions are dramatic in ways regular group sessions rarely are. One reason is that the patients who invite their friends and family are very much taking a risk because they are inviting the people whom they care about and on whom they depend the most into the only place where they have been able to talk about their secret problems without recrimination. Patients who do take the risk are almost universally happy they did so. A primary benefit is that the group provides a way for patients to demonstrate to their friends and family that they have taken their problems seriously. Similarly, a theme among people accused of committing sex crimes is a wish they could be trusted again. Bringing friends and family members to a group such as the Friends and Family group is a way to start earning back that trust. As one example of the efficacy of the group, in a recent session, one of the women announced that she and her partner (who was an SBC patient) had become engaged to be married. There was applause, then another woman announced that she and her boyfriend (who was an SBC patient) had also decided to get married. More applause. Then a third couple in the room announced their engagement. In each case, the relationship had begun with the woman knowing about her boyfriend's criminal past and was fully aware of what his paraphilic interests had been before treatment.

Case Report 2.2

One evening during a Friends and Family group meeting, a new guest who had been sitting quietly spoke up. She disclosed that she had recently gone to the police to report that she had been sexually assaulted by a family member when she was a little girl. With tears in her eyes, and while looking at each of the patients in the room, she said, "You should be proud of yourselves for doing what I wish the person who abused me should have done!" The room went quiet. The patients were speechless. They had been sitting with a woman not realizing she was the victim of abuse. She had spoken, and her anger at the man who abused her was evident. However, what came through was her acceptance that the men in this room were in the process of change that deserved praise.

Patient-Specific Groups

In addition to the Friends and Family group, the SBC offers several groups explicitly designed for SBC patients and clients. She had not only (at least partially) forgiven them, she was praising them.

Adult Interest Group

A mainstay of treatment for men and women who have been accused of sexual interest in children is the SBC's Adult Interest group (AIG). The group has evolved during the past 15 years due to practical considerations and in response to constant feedback from the people it serves. In the process, the SBC has shown that most of the traditional rules about group therapy are not valid. For example, textbooks state that the optimal size of a therapy group should be approximately 8 people. SBC groups range in size from 8 to 30. Textbooks state that group members should be homogeneous and at the same "stage." SBC groups are extremely heterogeneous, and new people can join at any time. Whenever the groups are surveyed (which is weekly and annually in a more formal manner), the consensus is happiness with the current format and a preference for large heterogeneous groups.

Details of the Adult Interest Group The AIG has dual aims to (1) stop illegal sex acts and (2) enhance noncriminal sexual interests. The AIG meets weekly for 90 minutes. Due to the popularity of the group, the SBC offers two AIG groups: The first is on Monday mornings from 9 to 10:30 a.m., and the second occurs on Tuesday evenings from 6 to 7:30 p.m. Group members are strongly encouraged to arrive on time and to stay for the entire group session. Due to the timing of the groups, the Monday morning group is most popular for patients who are unemployed. The Tuesday evening group is more popular for those who are employed. Contrary to popular belief, most SBC patients do obtain gainful employment.

Although patients are welcome to attend as many or as few groups as they like, they are advised not to attend both Monday and Tuesday groups in the same week because the topics of the week are the same. Importantly, they are reminded and assured that group attendance is entirely voluntary.

A theme of the SBC is respect for informed, voluntary, revocable, consent. Sex crimes are crimes not because they are sexual but because they involve sex without consent. Therefore, it is vital that treatment programs and therapists specifically demonstrate respect for consent.

As stated previously, all SBC groups are voluntary. Sometimes, patients attending their first SBC group state that they are there because they have been ordered to be at group by their probation or parole officer or the court. When that happens, they are told that group attendance is always voluntary, and if they do not want to be there, the SBC will write a note explaining (truthfully) that the person will not benefit from group treatment because attendance would be nonconsensual. It is rare the note ever needs to be written once the person realizes that SBC groups are designed to help them and not to punish them. On one occasion, a patient insisted he was being forced to attend group. The therapist wrote a note on the spot excusing him and handed it to the patient. He read the note and then tore it up, saying that because he was not being forced, he now wanted to attend and preferred his parole officer not see the note. His wish was honored, and he became a regular and enthusiastic group attendee.

Although consensual, the SBC groups do have rules. All SBC groups require no hats, no headphones, no use of cell phones, and no dark glasses. This rule is in place to help group members know they are on an equal footing and are in group to communicate openly and honestly with fellow group members. At the beginning of each session, every person is asked to say their first name. Some new members mimic the pattern of many AA groups and introduce themselves as follows: "Hi, I am [first name], and I am a pedophile." They are discouraged from doing so by other group members, who explain that self-labeling can be self-fulfilling. Instead, they are invited to introduce themselves by their first name as a first step in establishing a new identity as a person who no longer has pedophilia (or other unwanted paraphilia). These steps help to personalize the experience for people who often feel both martialized and stigmatized.

Next, the sign-in sheet is reviewed (Figure 2.1). Group members sequentially read each of the group rules aloud, with the next group member explaining what the rule means. The therapists are careful to ensure that any person who is unable to read is not embarrassed during the process. The sequence of one person reading followed by the next person explaining helps establish a pattern in the group of respectful listening and consideration of what is being said.

The group expectations discussed next are read, explained, and agreed to at the beginning of each group meeting.

Royal Ottawa Hospital
SBC PROGRESS NOTE
(Please print, ink only)

Chart No. ____________________

Name ____________________

Date ____________________

ADDRESSOGRAPH

I AGREE TO THE FOLLOWING (please initial each condition to wich you agree):

— I respect the confidentiality (privacy) of all members in this group.
— I respect the right of all group members to be free from physical and/or verbal intimidation.
— I agree that I will be asked to leave the group if there is a concern that i am under the influence of alcohol or non-prescription drugs.
— I understand that if I disclose sexual activity with a child who is identifiable, therapists or other group members may be legally and ethically obliged to take action to protect the child, including reporting the information to the appropriate authorities.

PLEASE COMPLETE THE FOLLOWING CHART BY CIRCLING THE APPOPRIATE NUMBER TO SHOW HOW YOU HAVE BEEN FEELING OVER THE LAST SEVEN (7) DAYS:

	NONE (0)	A LITTLE (1)	MODERATELY (2)	A LOT (3)	VERY MUCH SO (4)
a. Suicidal	0	1	2	3	4
b. Intrested in legal sex	0	1	2	3	4
c. Intrested in illegal sex	0	1	2	3	4
d. In danger of relapsing	0	1	2	3	4

By signing this document I confirm that I received group psychotherapy from _______ to _______ under the direction of initial beside the therapist(s) in attendance on this date:

☐ P. Fedoroff ☐ Heather Tarnai-Feeley ☐ Other (list names) ____________________

____

____________________ (Patient signature)

____________________ (Therapist signature(s))

Figure 2.1 SBC sign-in sheet.

Group Expectations

Confidentiality Confidentiality is a standard requirement in therapy. It is more complicated in group therapy, especially in groups in which highly personal issues may be discussed. The SBC has chosen to maintain confidentiality from probation and parole (P&P) for issues that do not involve legally mandated reporting or imminent threats. Many other programs require signed reciprocal releases of information between P&P and the program, on the theory that it is essential that all members of the team be able to share information.

However, P&P officers do not (or should not) attempt to do therapy. By guarding the confidentiality of what is said in therapy sessions, the SBC again emphasizes respect for consent and makes it possible for patients to disclose more freely. For example, if a probationer has a condition not to drink alcohol, he is more likely to disclose that he had a "slip" to therapists in the SBC program because he knows the information will not automatically be disclosed to their P&P officer, who may be obliged to charge him for breaching conditions. By knowing the person has been drinking, the SBC can take steps to help the person rather than being kept in the dark until more concerning events have occurred. The SBC's approach demonstrates respect for consent and confidentiality and establishes the principle of respect for boundaries. These issues are all critical for former sex offenders.

Politeness Each patient each week is reminded that although frank and open discussion about anything relevant regarding why they are in group is encouraged, aggression is not. This is in contrast to other programs in which patients are, for example, put on the "hot seat" and accused of lying if they disagree with the police report about what happened (Waldram, 2012). The SBC group rule helps overcome the natural discomfort experienced from being in a "sex group." It also fosters respect for honesty, alternative perspectives, and the right to disagree.

Sobriety This rule is phrased to give the therapists the option of excusing a person from group if they appear to be too drunk or stoned to follow what is going on in group. It is also presented as a way of respecting others in the group who may be in the process of decreasing their drug or alcohol use. Patients like this rule, and it is of interest that in 15 years it has never needed to be enforced. Patients take group seriously, likely because for many, it is the first time their rights are honored and respected. Often, new group members report they do not think they deserve respect due to their crimes. They are reassured that although they are correct to feel badly for the harm they have caused, they have a right to feel proud of the fact that they have changed or at least are in the process of changing.

Reporting Suicidality, Hopelessness, and/or Desperation to the Therapists When the SBC intake form was initially presented to the Royal's documents committee for approval, a question was raised about whether a question regarding current suicidality should be included. A committee member asked, "What if a patient said they were suicidal?" to which the SBC responded, "Wouldn't that be important to know?"

The rule to promptly report thoughts of suicide or self-harm reminds group members is included in the sign-in sheets because they are not read immediately. Therefore group members are reminded they should not rely on the forms to communicate relevant information such as thoughts of self-harm. It also serves to emphasize that if they are feeling hopeless, they should tell a therapist without delay so that help can be offered quickly. In addition, it helps group members to view the group as a source of support and aid. They are reminded that the group is even more critical to attend when they are not doing well. This issue arises often. Because the groups are voluntary, there is a natural tendency to come to group when things are going well and to avoid group when they are not. This is especially true in the Mood and Anxiety group, in which group members with depression sometimes stop coming when they are most depressed, a time when the group can be most beneficial.

Reporting of Concerns About Harm to Children The legal requirement to report any concerns about imminent harm to a child who is still a child and who is identifiable is read aloud every session. It emphasizes that the SBC respects the law and reminds the group that everyone is morally and ethically bound to protect children. See Chapter 6 on pedophilia for a more in-depth discussion of reporting laws.

Weekly Self-Ratings Following the review of the "group rules," all group members are asked to rate how they have been feeling during the past 7 days in terms of suicidality, interest in legal sex, interest in illegal sex, and danger or relapsing (see Figure 2.1). In addition to generating data for research, the process of rating the four statements on the sign-in sheet reminds group members that interests and feelings, by their nature, change from week to week. They are also reminded that the aim of therapy is not only to eliminate harmful paraphilic interests but also to replace them with healthy sexual interests.

On the reverse side of the sign-in sheet is a section for the patient to essentially create their own progress note by commenting on personal concerns and by critiquing the therapy session. Once signed by the patient and the therapist, each individual sign-in sheet is scanned and filed in the patient's electronic clinical record.

This method of generating progress notes contrasts with many group therapy programs in which the therapist constructs a "progress note" for each group member, often by cutting and pasting generic comments such as "participated well." In the SBC, the intake form verifies that the patient was aware of and understood the rules of the group. The sign-in sheets also provide data that can be used for quality assurance and research.

Again, one of the most important characteristics of the SBC is the fact that it is truly a clinical-research clinic. All SBC patients are invited to participate in research and of course are given the option to opt out of research as well. Treatment is presented as a series of informed research projects in which the treatment plan is presented as a hypothesis that the patient is invited to test and report the results. This makes the patient the principal investigator rather than a "guinea pig."

Question of the Day After the formal "sign-in," the therapists provide a "question of the day" for patients to consider. The question of the day is intended to focus the discussion. It tends to be related to events in the news, new research findings, or "trigger" topics to challenge ingrained ideas about the paraphilias and sex offending. Some sample topics are listed in Table 2.1. These topics are only samples of the hundreds of questions of the day that have been presented to group members. Therapists try to link the question of the day to current issues in the news or new research findings. The exact topic is less important than the way group members respond. There is a tendency for group members to meta-analyze the group process and the topics, so it is important for the therapists to reflect the comments back to the commenter: "Yes but how does this relate to how you feel now?" Therapists should resist the temptation to answer questions immediately. It is better to reflect the question back to the group: "What does the group think?"

Table 2.1 A Sample of SBC Adult Interest Group: "Questions of the Day"

No.	Sample Question	Comment
1	Forgiveness	Members are encouraged to leave forgiveness to other people.
2	Responsibility	Members are helped to accept responsibility for behaviors.
3	Goals	Members are assisted in setting and achieving realistic goals.
4	Friendship	Members are assisted in identifying friends and the nature of friendship.
5	Choices	Members are reminded there are always alternative options.
6	Vacation	Often an important issue, especially for unemployed members who cannot take vacation.
7	Honesty	Especially important for members who are establishing new romantic relationships.
8	Conditions	Important for members who may have conditions for probation or parole that they do not understand or believe are unfair.
9	Secrets	Past, present, and future.
10	Reframing	A therapeutic concept that members often quickly grasp in novel ways.
11	Special days	Especially important for members: Father's Day, children's birthdays.
12	Court	Important for members facing court as well as those whose interests could lead to arrest.
13	Change	Extremely important for members who believe or have been told change is not possible.

The impact of a therapist telling a group member with pedophilia that fantasizing about children while masturbating is not a good idea is less than that of the same comment coming from a group member who was convicted of a crime soon after he performed the same action. This is one time when "group think" can be beneficial. It is often helpful to summarize discussion with a comment such as,

> Well, you have gotten a lot of opinions and you need to decide for yourself what is right for you but it is pretty clear the group thinks cutting through the park on the way to the bus stop is not a good idea for you.

The question of the day is presented at the end of the sign-in process but is not addressed until the second half of the group session. First, the group is opened up for a "check-in" by the group members. This is important in order to identify "hot issues," such as a recent police investigation, that will be distracting if not addressed early on. It also gives group members the chance to direct the group to issues that are concerning them at the moment, such as unemployment.

Issues to Avoid

Group members sometimes request sessions in which other group members confess what they did. Others ask if victims of sex abuse can be invited to speak to the group. Some ask for lectures. The SBC avoids these options. Confessions have the problem of inviting exhibitionistic and voyeuristic interests, and there is no way to be sure of their veracity. They also have the problem of focusing group members on the past rather than the future. Concerning inviting victims, group members are reminded that approximately one-third of group members have themselves been sexually abused. SBC therapists avoid lecturing because it undoes the process of group therapy.

Unique Aspects of SBC Groups

As mentioned previously, there are some unique aspects to SBC groups that have evolved during the past 15 years in response to constant patient feedback.

Group Size In part due to necessity, the SBC has ignored textbook recommendations concerning group size. Most SBC patients prefer larger groups. One explanation is that it allows members to be "lost in the crowd." However, SBC groups are designed to ensure every group member speaks at least once, and the therapists are careful to ensure people are following the discussion. From the written comments provided by patients on their sign-in sheets, it is clear that the most talkative patients are not always the ones who are doing the most thinking about what the group is offering. Because attendance is strictly voluntary, the number of group members varies every week but is often as high as 30 people.

Group Composition Textbooks often recommend groups be homogeneous. The only homogeneous aspects of the Adult Interest SBC groups are that everyone speaks English, is at least 18 years old, and has a concern arising from possible sexual interest in children or minors, including people younger than age 18 years in the case of child pornography. So-called deniers are welcomed, as are people at all stages of the criminal justice process, including people who have never offended; people who have not been caught (but have no reporting issues); people who have been arrested (whether they plan to plead guilty or not guilty); people in trial; people awaiting sentence; people serving house arrest sentences or "weekends" in jail; and those who have completed their in-custody sentence and are now on parole or probation, a peace bond, or designated as a long-term sex offender or dangerous offender. The diversity of the group is further enhanced by the inclusion of both male and female patients and patients with all ranges of intellectual ability, from those who are intellectually delayed to those with advanced postgraduate degrees. There are no restrictions on types of comorbid or concurrent medical or psychiatric conditions.

Diversity and Inclusion How does the SBC do it? Diversity is a catalyst for change, which is the aim of all SBC groups. SBC groups do not waste time reviewing the accuracy of a patient's "official" crime(s). The reason is that in the case of sex crimes, the only people who really know what happened are the people who were present at the time of the events in question. In fact, even the people present at the time of the crime do not really know what happened because recollections of sexual encounters are reconstructed and subject to influence by the emotions of self and others and by the effect of retelling what happened. Once a "fact" has been entered in a police memo book, it can take on a life of its own.

Case Report 2.3

On one occasion, a patient was transferred to an in-patient ward from another facility. He was not an SBC patient because the SBC is out-patient only. His clinical record was replete with designations as a "cop killer." He arrived tied to a stretcher wearing a helmet and mask to prevent him from biting or spitting. In his initial presentation, he looked very much like the fictional character Hannibal Lecter (Harris, 1981) and was being accorded the same degree of respect by the officers who delivered him. It took some time to review his clinical record properly. He had been homeless and begged for food outside of a grocery store. One day, a police officer told him to move along, and there was a minor physical altercation in which the patient refused to hand over a bag he was holding. Approximately 1 week later, the police officer was in a fatal motor vehicle accident (MVA) while off duty. The MVA had absolutely nothing to do with the patient. Unfortunately, the events were recorded in the patient's record as "Mr. X assaulted a police officer, who subsequently died." The patient had become a "cop killer" due to a poorly written sentence that was subsequently reproduced at the top of every discharge summary from then on. Clinicians should always be careful about accepting uncorroborated chart notes, especially if they involve allegations of past sexual activities involving "he-said/she-said" scenarios.

In the SBC, people often disagree with the accusations they face or the "facts" listed in their charts. Instead of wasting time deciding what in fact happened, the SBC focuses on the present. The person is told that the SBC is fortunately not tasked with retrying the case. The SBC's job is to help ensure that the patient is never re-accused (falsely or otherwise). It is explained that unfair as it may seem, once a person has been accused of being a sex offender, people will think about them as a sex offender and treat them differently than before, regardless of their degree of innocence. Deniers are quick to agree. But if they do not, one group session in which they meet deniers and admitters convinces them that having "sex assault" on their record changes their job and relationship prospects.

Again, once they accept that the SBC is there to help them and is 100% voluntary, the problems associated with "deniers" disappear. It is also notable that many people who are complete deniers pretrial become admitters after they are released from custody and return for treatment. This is because for safety reasons, no one wants to enter prison as a sex offender. Once they become confident about the confidentiality of the SBC system and the fact that the SBC is designed to help them become successful and healthy members of society, many confess.

Group Identity Many new SBC group members arrive with a behavioral or addictions perspective. As mentioned previously, when it is their turn to say their first name during the initial introduction, they often echo the AA method and say, "Hi my name is X and I am a sex offender." This gives other group members the chance to explain:

> In this group, no one is a sex offender, or at least we hope not. Not everyone in this group has ever committed a sex offense; many are here because they want to be sure they never become sex offenders. Others used to be sex offenders, but in this group, everyone changes to being an ex-sex offender and on-going sex offending is both unnecessary and wrong.

The idea of not self-labeling as a sex offender who is incorrigible and/or incurable is a novel idea for people accustomed to the (now largely abandoned) addictions model, which claims "once an alcoholic always an alcoholic." This is one reason that the SBC does not use an "addictions paradigm" for group therapy. Paraphilias are not addictions. Unlike addictive substances such as alcohol, paraphilic behaviors do not need to be tapered. And unlike addictions, because sexual behaviors are entirely voluntary, there is no evidence that "slips" (i.e. minor or major relapses) are inevitable.

Unlike AA groups, SBC groups always have at least one professional therapist (SBC groups are therapy groups and not support groups). In addition, group members are discouraged from socializing with each other outside of group. They are told that SBC staff do not follow them around so the SBC cannot prevent them from socializing with each other, and in fact the SBC encourages everyone to be friendly and polite to each other. However, although SBC groups are good places to practice being friendly, they are not good places to make friends. The goal of the SBC is for each person to outgrow any need for the SBC. If all their friends are SBC group members, it will mean they will always be tied to the SBC, and it will be more difficult for them to move on to entirely independent, healthy lives.

On this note, the SBC also cautions people to not disclose to others that they belong to the SBC. They are cautioned not to talk about group topics at the bus stop and elsewhere. They can talk about group with their spouses and their probation and parole officers, but only regarding how they are doing—not how other group members are doing. Also, the SBC consistently models a pattern of not talking about people who are not present in the group (e.g., when a group member starts to complain about his parole officer).

Other Differences A unique aspect of SBC groups is the fact that people with intellectual disabilities are treated alongside people with average or above average intelligence and abilities. To the surprise of many, it works. Sex offenders with ordinary intelligence often have characteristics that are referred to as psychopathic, most notably a willingness to use others for their pleasure without regard to the consequences. Those who have been to prison are particularly prone to engage in self-destructive competitions with others. SBC groups provide a microcosm in which psychopathy's usual rules of engagement are suspended. These people learn about the value of sharing experiences honestly and about the importance of consent. As a result, when a new person with psychopathic tendencies joins the group and starts to mock or take advantage of a group member with intellectual disability, one of the more experienced group members with psychopathic characteristics will quietly pull the new one aside and say, "We do not say things like that here, he is one of us."

People with psychopathy rarely allow themselves to be vulnerable or to help others. The SBC groups give them a chance to do both in a safe environment. Similarly, people with intellectual disability often resent being grouped with other disabled people. Provided they are not embarrassed—for example, by being told to read if they are illiterate—they can be comfortable talking about similar problems. Often, it is a person with intellectual disability who says what everyone else is thinking—for example, by remembering and commenting that an excuse offered by a non-intellectually disabled person to explain a questionable act is the same one offered by that person the day before he was arrested.

A concern of the RNR school of thought mentioned previously is that low-risk offenders may become high risk if they have contact in custody. The SBC experience is the reverse: High-risk offenders become lower risk when brought into contact with low-risk offenders. The difference in outcome is that RNR treatment programs are implemented within in-custody programs that by necessity downplays consent, whereas the SBC is an out-patient program that honors and respects consent.

Readers may note that psychopathy is not viewed as a contraindication to treatment in the SBC. The notion that treatment makes people with psychopathy worse has been debunked (Barbaree, 2005). In the same way that opinions about the untreatability of borderline personality disorder, psychopathy, and other severe personality disorders have been replaced (Choi-Kain, Finch, Masland, Jenkins, & Unruh, 2017; Sturmey, Wong, Stockdale, & Olver, 2017), the SBC has replaced the idea that all people with paraphilic disorders are untreatable with the expectation that each person treated in the SBC should aim for the elimination of all problematic sexual interests together with replacement of those interests with non-problematic interests and behaviors.

Members in the SBC groups include both men and women. There are fewer female patients in the SBC, but they represent a growing number. To date, there have never been any problems due to inclusion of both genders (and the occasional transgender person) in the same treatment groups. The increased diversity of perspectives only increases the options for change.

As a side note, the SBC has never treated people for transgender issues per se. This is because the issues for which people with transgender problems seek treatment involve problems with gender and not sex. Similarly, the SBC does not treat people seeking treatment for sexual dysfunctions because problems such as erectile dysfunction typically do not involve paraphilic interests. One possible exception is problems reaching orgasm that can be associated with unconventional interests or behaviors that are resorted to in order to reach orgasm.

Topics of Interest Many group therapy treatment programs for people with sexual interest in children are offered to men while they are incarcerated. The men sign up for therapy often hoping it will help them reduce the time they spend in custody. Since they are removed from their normal living environment, therapists have tended to resort to programs that involve a review of the official record of what happened. One of the most widely used and well-tested treatment paradigms, relapse prevention, is an adaptation of a paradigm used to treat addictions. It is based on the premise that the temptation to relapse increases the closer the person gets to the "triggers" that unleash the maladaptive behaviors (e.g., drinking alcohol). In one of the most well-designed tests of treatment efficacy in sex offenders, RPT was found to be ineffective (Marques, Day, Nelson, Miner, & West, 1991). This, of course, was a disappointment but not a surprise to the SBC because paraphilias are not addictions. In RPT, patients are encouraged to think about their offenses and create an "offense cycle" that delineates the pattern leading to reoffense. Patients then learn alternative behaviors or options to take that will decrease the likelihood of reoffending. RPT borrows from the addiction paradigm by assuming that the basic deviant interest cannot change in the same way that older addiction theories assumed people with alcoholism could never overcome their vulnerability to alcohol.

RPT was replaced by GLM, in which the RPT preoccupation with avoiding triggers was replaced by plans to replace maladaptive behaviors with healthy ones (Ward, Mann, & Gannon, 2007). The premise of GLM therapy is that people will self-actualize and become healthy if they are given a chance and appropriate support.

In the SBC, useful elements of RPT and GLM are incorporated into therapy designed to change problematic sexual interests into healthy ones. Topics of discussion focus on the present and plans for the future.

Resiliency Group

A common misconception is that children (especially boys) who were sexually abused are more likely to become sex offenders when they grow up. In the SBC, approximately 30% of the men have histories of being sexually abused when they were children, which is approximately the same as the general population (Fedoroff & Pinkus, 1996). Nevertheless, sex offenders with a history of personal sex abuse have few therapeutic resources because they are excluded from treatment programs set up for victims of sex abuse. Recognizing this problem, the SBC set up a group for patients with paraphilias who were sexually abused when they were children. The group was not popular. It turned out that patients in the SBC had learned that discussing past abuse simply opened old wounds. Therefore, the SBC changed the group from a past abuse group to a Resiliency group, open to all SBC patients who wanted to increase their sense of resiliency to the stresses of everyday life. This group has proven to be very popular. It is attended by people with a history of personal abuse as well as others with post-traumatic stress disorder and anxiety syndromes from other causes. They are an anxious group, so it is the only SBC group limited to 60 minutes. The sign-in sheet and rules are the same as those for the other groups. The Resiliency group is another example of the way the SBC has responded to the needs of patients based on evidence.

Mood and Anxiety Group

A third SBC group is the Mood and Anxiety group, which is designed to directly address the needs of SBC patients diagnosed with problems related to mood and/or anxiety. The format of this group is similar to that of the AIG except that at the beginning of the group, each person is asked to say their first name and to provide one item from the news (TV, radio, newspaper, or word of mouth) that made them happy. This intervention was originally introduced to slow people down as they raced around the circle saying their first names. However, it turned out to be highly effective in helping people with depression or anxiety to seek and find happy news.

It is rare to complete the introduction section of the group without the entire group breaking into laughter in response to at least one news item.

Although mood and anxiety are the topics on the agenda in the group, because everyone in the group also has a sex-related problem, the group often focuses on issues related to paraphilic problems. In this group, people with paraphilias and/or sex offenses that do not involve children are included. Again, this does not cause any problems because the focus is on current issues of anxiety and depression and not on past offenses. It is remarkable how often people in the group think their problem is unique (e.g., zoophilia) without realizing that several other people in the group have the same problem. Although the specific diagnoses of each individual group member are never disclosed, members are frequently reminded that (1) not everyone in the group has committed a sex crime; (2) not everyone has a sexual interest in children; and (3) everyone in the group once had a sex-related issue of some type but is expected to have entirely stopped committing any crimes and at least started to establish a new, healthy life free of criminal and/or nonconsensual activities.

Social Skills Group

By definition, all people with paraphilic disorders have problems with social skills. However, there are two subgroups of SBC patients in which social skills problems are especially prominent: those with autistic spectrum disorder (ASD) and those with an antisocial personality disorder (ASPD). People with ASD do not understand the rules (they are asocial), whereas people with ASPD do not care about the rules (they are antisocial). Surprisingly, both groups of patients do well in the same group. It is a group that can present challenges to therapists due to the communication problems of the patients who, left to their own devices, would not talk to each other at all.

However, in written feedback, the Social Skills group is the highest (best) rated group by group members out of all the groups offered by the SBC. The reason is that each week, one group member volunteers to present a chosen topic on some aspect of social skills to the group. For most, this is the only time they have ever spoken to a group and been listened to. By tradition, the group always applauds after the presentation, no matter how brief. The mother of a group member who has autism and is barely verbal commented that the group is the one thing in her son's life that he looks forward to every week. He has attended faithfully for more than 3 years. During that time, he has not only done presentations but also significantly altered his behaviors. He has become a respected group member who now has a job outside of the group and who has never reoffended.

Although the Social Skills group was initially designed to meet the needs of SBC patients with severe social deficits due to ASD or ASPD, the group has become popular with patients who do not have ASD or ASPD but who want to work on issues involving their relationships with their probation or parole officers or in establishing healthy romantic relationships.

Pharmacotherapies

There are several reviews of pharmacotherapies for the paraphilias and sex offenders (Fedoroff, 1994, 1995; Fedoroff & Fedoroff, 1992; Bradford & Fedoroff, 2005). Perhaps the most critical recent review of medical treatments for the paraphilias is the guidelines published by the World Federation of Societies of Biological Psychiatry (WFSBP; Thibaut, de la Barra, Gordon, Cosyns, & Bradford, 2010), with more recent guidelines for adolescent sex offenders (Thibaut et al., 2016). The 2010 guidelines have been reviewed and critiqued (Fedoroff, 2011), and new WFSBP guidelines (on which Fedoroff is a coauthor) are now in press.

The WFSBP 2010 guidelines suggest that different medications should be used depending on the "severity" of the person's behavior, by which the WFSBP means the likely consequences that would result if the patient acted on their paraphilic interests. Recommendations begin with "psychotherapy only" for the "lowest risk" patients, selective serotonergic reuptake inhibitors (SSRIs) for non-contact paraphilias such as exhibitionism, SSRIs plus low-dose anti-androgen medications for people with interests that are not "sadistic," higher dose anti-androgens for "moderate to high risk violence," injected gonadotropin-releasing hormone (GnRH) partial agonists for high-risk sadism or poor compliance, and a combination of anti-androgens and GnRH partial agonists for "catastrophic" sexual interests. The stated level of evidence for each of these recommendations is Cochrane system C or D.

There are some problems with the WFSBP recommendations, beginning with confusion between interest in paraphilic acts and sex offending. In addition, the WFSBP pharmacologic recommendations are all based on the idea that risk can be reduced by reducing sex drive. However, there is little or no evidence that sex drive is directly related to sexual offending. The strength of sex drive is not a factor in any actuarial measure of risk of sex offending, and at least one study has found no relationship between free testosterone and proxies of sexual violence (Kingston, Seto, Ahmed, Fedoroff, & Bradford, 2012). Also, there is no discussion of accentuation or facilitation of noncriminal or nonparaphilic sexual acts. Most importantly, in the 2010 guidelines, consent to treatment issues are insufficiently addressed.

The SBC does not follow the 2010 WFSBP guidelines. Rather than focus on suppressing sex drive, the goal of treatment is to enhance healthy sex as a substitution for unhealthy sex acts. Patients are told there is an expectation that they stop any illegal sex acts immediately. Sometimes they object. When they do, they are reminded that if they have not already been arrested, they eventually will be if they continue to break the law. They are also reminded that sexual behaviors are entirely voluntary. They are reminded that contrary to what they may have been told, there is absolutely no evidence that paraphilic interests cannot be changed.

Following a comprehensive assessment, they are presented with all the treatment options, including individual, couple's, family, and group therapies, as well as pharmacotherapies including the full range of psychiatric medications—5-hydroxytryptamine receptor 1A partial agonists, SSRIs, serotonin and norepinephrine reuptake inhibitors, monoamine oxidase inhibitors, mood stabilizers, novel neuroleptics, amphetamines, anti-androgens, GnRHs, and phosphodiesterase type 5 inhibitors. A treatment program is devised based on the patient's consent and the wishes of the patient and the patient's actual or potential consenting sexual partner(s). Importantly, the treatment plan is presented as merely the first intervention from which the SBC team will learn more about the patient's problem(s) so that the treatment can be refined until it is optimal.

Patients are often surprised to hear the situation is not hopeless and that the proposed treatment will be both voluntary and designed to help them, especially when they learn that a treatment goal is for them to have better, consensual sex. Not surprisingly, most become enthusiastic participants in the treatment program, even those who previously had been stigmatized and labeled as being "beyond hope."

Analogies are often helpful to introduce patients to new concepts. A helpful one is language. The following is a typical dialogue between a new SBC patient and the clinician:

PATIENT: Doc. You say I am curable, but no one has ever told me that before.

CLINICIAN: That may be true. But has anyone ever listened to you before?

PATIENT: No. But I have never told anyone before.

CLINICIAN: So, things are different already.

PATIENT: True. So what are you going to do to me?

CLINICIAN: Nothing. That is the point. What is going to happen is going to happen because of you, not me. Have you ever tried to learn a new language?

PATIENT: Well I was born bilingual [French and English], and I have started to learn Russian which is very different, and hard.

CLINICIAN: Perfect. So you already know what the process feels like. First, let me tell you that no one is born bilingual. When you were born, you were born with the ability to speak any human language which is one of the most amazing differences between humans and animals which cannot speak any human language aside from some parrots that can mimic a word or two. The languages you learned to speak as a child are the languages the people who raised you spoke, in your case, your bilingual parents. Most children learn their first language or languages through imitation and practice. Some people think once the "mother tongue" is learned, a critical period has passed, and it is harder to learn anything after that. However, we now know that while the process may change, people can add vocabulary and grammar and accent and understanding to their language as long as they live and can hear and speak. In fact, 60% [the majority] of the world's population speaks more than one language.

Sexual interest is like language. When you were born, you had sex organs and probably had a sex drive, but you had no idea what sex or gender or orientation was, or what your sexual interests might be. For reasons we do not understand, you now have sexual interests that are causing you and other people problems. It is like you have started to speak a language that other people do not understand

and dislike. Treatment is going to involve a process like learning to speak the same language as the language spoken by the people in the society you live.

PATIENT: So, you are saying it is going to be like learning Russian? That is hard.

CLINICIAN: No. I am saying it is going to be like learning to speak English or French again. Right now, for some reason, your sexual interests have become problematic. We are going to make your sexual interests something you enjoy, and which makes your partner[s] happy.

PATIENT: Awesome. So you are saying I am going to start enjoying sex more?

CLINICIAN: Exactly, and so will your partners because people always prefer to do the things they agree to which is another way to say, to which they consent.

PATIENT: So, you are saying I have a choice?

CLINICIAN: I am saying not only do you have a choice, to get better, you must have a choice.

PATIENT: I am gay. Are you saying I can choose to be straight too? I tried that. It does not work.

CLINICIAN: Good point. Remember from the last session; gender is different from orientation which is different from drive which is different from interest. Society is way past the days when people had to change their orientation to fit in. You did not get arrested because you are gay. At least I hope you were not. If you were you need a human rights lawyer, not a psychiatrist. You were arrested because your sexual interests led you to harm another person. To get better, you do not need to become a woman or straight. You only need to change your preferred sexual interests.

PATIENT: This sounds easier than learning Russian!

CLINICIAN: I think it is. I think so because I have seen more people learn consensual sexual interests than I have seen learn Russian as a third language! So let me ask you a question. If you were going to learn a language, do you think we would start by having you forget English or French?

PATIENT: Of course not.

CLINICIAN: Right. So, forget about the past treatment programs that told you to forget your problematic interests. Instead, I want you to practice your new consensual sexual interests. That is easier if you do not try to change your gender or orientation which make it harder and which I do not recommend since there is nothing wrong with your gender or orientation.

PATIENT: I like this. Let's get started. It is going to take a long time right?

CLINICIAN: I am glad you like to plan. You are going to like it more once you hear from other people who have done it successfully and your partner tells you how much better you seem. My experience is that it takes much less time than you think. It depends on how much you already know and how well you practice your new interests. Like a new language, at first, it will feel awkward but keep at it. Before you know it, your dreams will change, and you will find consensual sex is more comfortable and more fulfilling than sex that harms others and yourself.

After a discussion such as this, patients are asked if they need help in making the change. For some, their lives are so damaged that they prefer to "take sex off the table" and elect to go on a course of sex drive-reducing medication with the idea that once their lives are more healthy, they can stop the medication and resume living with a sex drive that they can lawfully direct.

Some readers may be wondering if the success of this treatment approach is just speculation. In the chapters that follow, more information is provided about the paraphilias and why this treatment approach works. The SBC has been operating in its current form for approximately 15 years. In that time, most patients have reported a change in their sexual interests that has been confirmed in multiple ways. Of thousands of SBC patients motivated by paraphilic interests who had committed sex offenses before starting treatment in the SBC, there have been virtually no known reoffenses against children that involved in-person contact by the patient. This is not to say there have not been any, only that official and self-reports have been virtually nil.

Summary of the Literature Since 2008

The following table is intended to summarize some of the published English language research focusing primarily on the past 10 years concerning treatment of paraphilic disorders. It is not intended to be comprehensive but, rather, to provide a jumping off point for more in-depth reading or for alternative views to the ones expressed in the current chapter. Chapters 3–9 provide more specific information about specific paraphilic disorders.

The table organizes the treatment methods that have been researched and found on PsycINFO (from 1967 to 2018). The *paraphilia* column begins with general articles on treatment of the paraphilias followed by a listing of the various paraphilias in alphabetical order. The chart is also organized by age group of the research samples from youngest to oldest.

Paraphilia	Treatment	Age Group	Reference
Treatments for paraphilic disorders in general	Multisystemic therapy for youths with problem sexual behaviors	Male youths	Borduin, Dopp, Borduin, & Munschy (2017)
	Medication: selective serotonin reuptake inhibitors, naltrexone, anti-androgens	Adult males	Berner & Briken (2010)

Paraphilia	Treatment	Age Group	Reference
	Behavioral techniques (reconditioning by electric aversion therapy, olfactory aversion therapy, ammonia aversion therapy, covert sensitization, masturbatory reconditioning, and verbal satiation)	Adult males	Beech & Harkins (2012)
	Cognitive–behavioral therapy Anti-androgenic drugs (cypoterone acetate, medroxyprogesterone, leuprolide, goserelin, and triptorelin) Surgical castration: selective serotonin reuptake inhibitors		
Apotemnophilia	Cognitive–behavioral therapy	35-year-old male	Braam, Visser, Cath, & Hoogendijk (2006)
Asphyxophilia	Behavioral and psycho-educational programs	18-year-old male with autism	Thompson & Beail (2002)
Coprophagia	Sertraline	Adolescent female with hypersexuality, urophagia, and coprophagia	Mendhekar & Duggal (2005)
Ephebophilia	12-step recovery program	44- and 57-year-old males	Nu Ez (2003)
Exhibitionism	Social skills training Covert conditioning principles (whenever urges to expose arise, patient thinks of consequences)	Adolescent males	Green (1987)

Paraphilia	Treatment	Age Group	Reference
	Systematically vary masturbation fantasies. Patient instructed to masturbate while fantasizing to exhibitionism fantasies for 7 days, and then consensual and nonparaphilic fantasies for 7 days. Patient reported more interest in "normal" fantasies than exhibition fantasies. At the same time, he was instructed to use aversive imagery to eliminate the exhibitionistic fantasies prior to ejaculating—the patient imagined a graffiti wall naming him an exhibitionist.		
Exhibitionism	Functional analytic psychotherapy and acceptance and commitment therapy	20-year-old male	Paul, Marx, & Orsillo (1999)
Exhibitionism	Carbamazepine	26-year-old male	Corretti & Baldi (2010)
Exhibitionism	Aversive treatment and reconditioning, focusing on changing cognitions, improving interpersonal and relationship skills, stress management, and relapse prevention	Adult males (average age of 29 years)	Marshall, Eccles, & Barbaree (1991)
Exhibitionism	Fluoxetine and medroxyprogesterone acetate	31-year-old male with intellectual disability	Rea, Dixon, Zettle, & Wright (2017)
Exhibitionism	"Sensate focus" homework to increase comfort with sexual partner	45-year-old male	Metz & Sawyer (2004)

Paraphilia	Treatment	Age Group	Reference
	Structured behavioral exercises focusing on physiological relaxation, sensory experience, and communication between the couple		
Exhibitionism	6-point program for exhibitionism	Adult males	Zechnich (1971)
Exhibitionism	Counseling, short-term psychodynamic therapy, cognitive therapy, behavioral treatment; all sometimes paired with hormonal treatment	Adult males	Snaith (1983)
Exhibitionism	Aversive electric shock	Adult males	Green (1987)
Exhibitionism	Desensitizing the individual to sexual contact with consenting adults (anxiety reduction), reading erotica involving consenting female adults, and engaging in satisfying sexual intercourse with spouse	Adult males	Wickramasekera (1968)
Exhibitionism	Community-based sex offender treatment program involving behavior therapy, family therapy, marital/sexual therapy, and medication. Notably, it was found to be ineffective.	Adult males	Dwyer & Myers (1990)
Exhibitionism	GnRH therapy with leuprolide acetate injections	Adult males	Koo, Ahn, Hong, Lee, & Chung (2014)
Exhibitionism	Anti-androgen therapy with behavioral modification	Elderly male (aged 82 years)	Kenyon (1989)

Paraphilia	Treatment	Age Group	Reference
Fetishism	Risperidone	3½-year-old male with fetish for female legs, feet, and stockings	Zarei & Bidaki (2013)
Fetishism	Mirtazapine	13-year-old male with autism	Coskun & Mukaddes (2008)
Fetishism	Methylphenidate and "cognitive-rational" emotive psychotherapy	14-year-old male with attention-deficit/hyperactivity disorder	Chang & Chow (2011)
Fetishism	Modified avoidance therapy	Two males (aged 16 and 19 years) with underwear fetish	Bond & Evans (1967)
Fetishism	Naltrexone	40-year-old male with fetish for women's underwear	Firoz, Sankar, Ramohan, Kumar, & Raghuram (2014)
Fetishism	Behavioral activation and sensate focused therapy	57-year-old male with podophilia and anxiety	Sarver & Gros (2014)
Fetishism	Anticonvulsant medication for fetishistic disorder due to temporal lobe dysfunction	Adult males	Wise (1985)
Fetishism	GnRH leuprolide acetate injections	Adult male	Koo et al. (2014)
Fetishism	Directive guidance, behavior modification, cognitive-rational emotive approach Behavioral conditioning Psychoanalysis Cognitive and behavioral approaches Anticonvulsant medication (carbamazepine)	Adult male	Lowenstein (2002)

Paraphilia	Treatment	Age Group	Reference
Fetishism	Psychoeducational intervention	Adult male with autism and a baby paraphernalia fetish	Cambridge (2013)
Fetishism	Response-interruption and time-out procedure	Adult male with autism and fetish for women wearing sandals	Dozier, Iwata, & Worsdell (2011)
Formicophilia	Counseling and anti-androgens	28-year-old male	Dewaraja & Money (1986)
Formicophilia	Counseling and behavior therapy	28-year-old male	Dewaraja (1987)
Frotteurism	"Solution-focused" therapy	31-year-old male	Guterman, Martin, & Rudes (2011)
Hypersexuality/ "sex addiction"	Sertraline	Adolescent female with hypersexuality, urophagia, and coprophagia	Mendhekar & Duggal (2005)
Incest (siblings)	Hierarchical realignment in enmeshed families and safety plan	Family	DiGiorgio-Miller (1998)
Incest (siblings)	Education of offense cycle Behavioral therapy	Family	Hargett (1998)
Incest (parent–child)	Two-year Sexual Abuse Treatment program: individual, marriage, family, and group therapy	Family	Scheela & Stern (1994)
Incest (parent–child)	Family therapy	Family	DiGiorgio-Miller (1998)
Incest	Group therapy Aversion therapy Social skills training	Family	Quinsey (1977)
Incest	Offender-oriented treatment Multimodal, family-oriented treatment	Family	Wendy (1992)

Paraphilia	Treatment	Age Group	Reference
Incest	Limitations to the family systems approach when incest occurs	Family	Finkelhor (1986)
Paraphilias	Experiential psychotherapy	Adults	Kleinplatz (2014)
Paraphilic infantilism/ pedophilia	Depo-medroxyprogesterone acetate	Case of a male followed from age 25 to 65 years. He had paraphilic cross-dressing, infantilism, and fondled his 6-year-old son.	Lehne & Money (2000)
Pedophilia	RESPECT system, a 7-step program	Individuals with pedophilic disorder and mental retardation, mental illness, or physical handicap	Keating (2000)
Pedophilia	Satiation therapy	19-year-old male	Hunter, Ram, & Ryback (2008)
Pedophilia	Luteinizing hormone-releasing hormone agonist	38-year-old male	Schiffer, Gizewski, & Kruger (2009)
Pedophilia	Eye movement desensitization and reprocessing trauma treatment with cognitive–behavioral therapy-relapse prevention	Individuals with pedophilic disorder who were sexually abused themselves as children	Ricci, Clayton, & Shapiro (2006)
Pedophilia	Individual therapy, group therapy (12 patients per group) Phenothiazine treatment Surgical castration Hypothalmotomies	Mainly adult males	Travin, Bluestone, Coleman, Cullen, & Melella (1985)

Paraphilia	Treatment	Age Group	Reference
Pedophilia	Surgery: either hypothalamotomy or orchidectomy (removal of testicles)	Mainly adult males	Hughes (2007)
	Pharmacology: medroxy-progesterone acetate, cyproterone acetate, triptorelin, leuprolide acetate, risperidone, sertraline, and anti-convulsants (carbamazepine and clonazepam)		
	Combinations of medication and behavioral therapy Behavioral therapy Group therapy "Masturbation therapy"		
Pedophilia	Address cognitive distortions	Adult males	Marshall, Marshall, & Kingston (2011)
Pedophilia	Chemotherapy (anti-androgens) Psychoanalytic therapy Family-systems approaches Behavioral therapy: aversive imagery (covert sensitization)	Adult males	Lanyon (1986)
Pedophilia	Psychotherapy (i.e., psychodynamic therapy), behavior therapy, punishment (i.e., incarceration and/or behavior modification), neurosurgery, testes castration via surgery, pharmacological castration (i.e., cyproterone acetate, medroxyprogesterone acetate [MPA]) MPA and counseling	Adult males	Berlin & Krout (1986)

Paraphilia	Treatment	Age Group	Reference
Pedophilia	Cognitive–behavioral therapy	Adult males	Johnson (2010)
Pedophilia	Combination of medication and behavioral treatment	Adult males	Erdogan (2010)
Pedophilia	Leuprolide acetate injections	Adult males	Koo et al. (2014)
Pedophilia—child pornography use	Cognitive–behavioral therapy focusing on "sexual self-regulation" skills, and sex drive-reducing medication if necessary	Adult males	Seto & Ahmed, (2014)
Pedophilic disorder	Cognitive–behavioral therapy	Adult males	Von Franque & Briken (2017)
Podophilia	Aversive conditioning	27-year-old male referred for indecent assault	Kunjukrishnan, Pawlak, & Varan (1988)
Podophilia	Behavioral activation and sensate focus therapy	57-year-old male with anxiety	Sarver & Gros (2014)
Public masturbation	Behavioral therapy: positive reinforcement and overcorrection, aversive conditioning, in vivo desensitization, response cost treatment	Males aged 7–52 years with developmental disabilities	Hurley & Sovner (1983)
Public masturbation	Social skills training	Males with developmental disabilities	Lundervold & Young (1992)
Public masturbation	Masturbation training	Males with intellectual disabilities	Gill (2012)
Public masturbation	Competing nonmasturbatory behaviors	4-year-old girl	Ferguson & Rekers (1979)
Public masturbation	Response blocking with guided compliance and reinforcement of incompatible response	7-year-old girl with traumatic brain injury	Dufrene, Watson, & Weaver (2005)

Paraphilia	Treatment	Age Group	Reference
Public masturbation	Lemon juice contingency (at home and school) was effective compared to ignoring and hand spanking.	Boy treated between ages 7 and 8 years	Cook, Altman, Shaw, & Blaylock (1978)
Public masturbation	Play therapy not effective, but behavioral treatment with fading procedure extinguished masturbatory behaviors	9-year-old girl	Janzen & Peacock (1978)
Public masturbation	Operant conditioning using a continuous, fixed interval and aperiodic reinforcement schedule	11-year-old girl	Wagner (1968)
Sadomasochism	Psychotherapy	45-year-old female	Southern (2002)
Sadomasochism	Kink-focused and consensual nonmonogamy-focused therapy	Adults	Sprott, Randall, Davison, Cannon, & Witherspoon (2017)
Sadomasochism	Self-psychology	Adults	Giugliano (2011)
Scopophilia (voyeurism)/ scoptophilia	Cognitive–behavioral therapy	22-year-old male with voyeurism and scopophilia	Stoylen (1985)
Sexual masochism	Target self-regulation beliefs	Not described	Novick & Novick (2012)
Sexual masochism	Rational emotive and cognitive–behavior therapy	Female with history of childhood sexual abuse by a parent	Abrams & Stefan (2012)
Sexual masochism	Cognitive–behavioral therapy and self-regulation skills	35-year-old Iranian male with comorbid disorders	Khodayarifard, Pritz, Alavi, & Abedini (2013)
Sexual masochism	Cognitive–behavioral therapy and dialectical–behavioral therapy	56-year-old male with chronic depression and hypersexuality	King (2014)

Paraphilia	Treatment	Age Group	Reference
Telephone scataologia	Psychodynamic therapy	25-year-old male	Goldberg & Wise (1985)
Telephone scataologia	Psychodynamic therapy and behavioral approaches	Adults	Matek (1988)
Transvestic fetishism	Sertraline	9-year-old boy	Guay (2009)
Transvestic fetishism	Sertraline	9-year-old boy	Guney, Ceylan, & Sener (2011)
Transvestic fetishism	Aversion therapy	18-year-old male	Strzyzewsky & Zierhoffer (1967)
Transvestic fetishism	Strategic marriage therapy	Adult man	Gallo (2016)
Transvestic fetishism	Depo-medroxyprogesterone acetate	Case of a male followed from age 25 to 65 years. Patient had paraphilic cross-dressing, paraphilic infantilism, and fondled his 6-year-old son.	Lehne & Money (2000)
Urophagia	Sertraline	Adolescent female with hypersexuality, urophagia, and coprophagia	Mendhekar & Duggal (2005)
Vampirism	Carbamazepine Fluvoxamine	31-year-old male with multiple psychiatric disorders and substance-related problems	Cro, Peronti, & Bersani (1997)

Paraphilia	Treatment	Age Group	Reference
Voyeurism	Sertraline	16-year-old male	Yalcin, Guney, & Saripinar (2014)
Voyeurism	Cognitive–behavioral therapy	22-year-old male with voyeurism and scopophilia	Stoylen (1985)
Voyeurism	Leuprolide acetate injections	Adult males	Koo et al. (2014)
Voyeurism	Psychoanalysis	Adult males	Blechner (2016)
Books and Book Chapters			

General

Balon, R. (2016). *Practical guide to paraphilia and paraphilic disorders.* Cham, Switzerland: Springer.
Bradford, J. M. W., Fedoroff, P., & Firestone, P. (2008). Sexual violence and the clinician. In R. I. Simon & K. Tardiff (Eds.), *Textbook of violence assessment and management* (pp. 441–460). Arlington, VA: American Psychiatric Publishing.
Laws, D. R., & O'Donohue, W. T. (1997). *Sexual deviance: Theory, assessment, and treatment.* New York, NY: Guilford.
Laws, D. R., & O'Donohue, W. T. (2008). *Sexual deviance: Theory, assessment, and treatment* (2nd ed.). New York, NY: Guilford.
O'Donohue, W. T. (2014). *Case studies in sexual deviance: Toward evidence-based practice.* New York, NY: Routledge/Taylor & Francis.

Exhibitionism/Exhibitionistic Disorder

Becker, J. V. (2000). Exhibitionism. In *Encyclopedia of psychology* (Vol. 3, pp. 288–290). New York, NY: Oxford University Press.

Incest

Horton, A. L., Johnson, B. L., Roundy, L. M., & Williams, D. (1990). *The incest perpetrator: A family member no one wants to treat.* Thousand Oaks, CA: Sage.
Pedophilia/Pedophilic Disorder
Lowenstein, L. F. (1998). *Paedophilia: The sexual abuse of children, its occurrence, diagnosis & treatment.* Knebworth, UK: Able Publishing.
Seto, M. (2008). *Pedophilia and sexual offending against children: Theory, assessment, and intervention.* Washington, DC: American Psychological Association.
Seto, M. (2018). *Pedophilia and sexual offending against children: Theory, assessment, and intervention* (2nd ed.). Washington, DC: American Psychological Association.

References

Abel, G., Huffman, J., Warberg, B., & Holland, C. (1998). Visual reaction time and plethysmography measures of sexual interest in child molesters. *Sex Abuse, 10*, 81–95. https://doi.org/10.1023/A:1022063214826

Abrams, M., & Stefan, S. (2012). Sexual abuse and masochism in women: Etiology and treatment. *Journal of Cognitive and Behavioral Psychotherapies, 12*(2), 231–239.

American Psychiatric Association. (2000). *Diagnostic and Statistical Manual of Mental Disorders* (4th ed., text revision). Washington, DC: Author.

Andrews, D. A., Bonta, J., & Wormith, J. S. (2011). The risk–need–responsivity (RNR) model: Does adding the Good Lives Model contribute to effective crime prevention? *Criminal Justice and Behavior, 38*, 735–755. doi.org/10.1177/0093854811406356

Azoulay, N., Murphy, L., Winder, B., & Fedoroff, J. P. (2019). Circles of Support and Accountability (CoSA): A review of the development of CoSA and its international implementation. *International Review of Psychiatry*.

Barbaree, H. (2005). Psychopathy, treatment behavior, and recidivism: An extended follow-up of Seto and Barbaree. *Journal of Interpersonal Violence, 20*, 1115–1131. https://doi.org/10.1177/0886260505278262

Becker, J. V. (2000). Exhibitionism. In *Encyclopedia of psychology* (Vol. 3, pp. 288–290). New York, NY: Oxford University Press.

Beech, A. R., & Harkins, L. (2012). DSM-IV paraphilia: Descriptions, demographics and treatment interventions. *Aggression and Violent Behavior, 17*(6), 527–539.

Berlin, F. S., & Krout, E. (1986). Pedophilia: Diagnostic concepts, treatment, and ethical considerations. *American Journal of Forensic Psychiatry, 7*(1), 13–30.

Berner, W., & Briken, P. (2010). Therapy options for men with sexual preference disorders/paraphilias and sexual delinquency [in German]. *Forensische Psychiatrie, Psychologie, Kriminologie, 4*(Suppl. 1), S8–S16.

Blechner, M. J. (2016). Psychoanalysis and sexual issues. *Contemporary Psychoanalysis, 52*(4), 502–546.

Bond, I. K., & Evans, D. R. (1967). Avoidance therapy: Its use in two cases of underwear fetishism. *Canadian Medical Association Journal, 96*(16), 1160–1162.

Bonta, J., & Wormith, J. S. (2013). Applying the risk–need–responsivity principles to offender assessment. In L. A. Craig, L. Dixon, & T. A. Gannon (Eds.), *What works in offender rehabilitation: An evidence-based approach to assessment and treatment* (pp. 71–93). Malden, MA: Wiley. https://doi.org/10.1002/9781118320655.ch4

Borduin, C. M., Dopp, A. R., Borduin, B. J., & Munschy, R .J. (2017). Multisystemic therapy for youths with problem sexual behaviours: Empirical, theoretical, and clinical foundations. In D. P. Boer, A. R. Beech, T. Ward, L. A. Craig, M. Rettenberger, L. E. Marshall, & W. L. Marshall (Eds.), *The Wiley handbook on the theories, assessment, and treatment of sexual offending* (pp. 1331–1346). Malden, MA: Wiley-Blackwell.

Braam, A. W., Visser, S., Cath, D. C., & Hoogendijk, W. J. G. (2006). Investigation of the syndrome of apotemnophilia and course of a cognitive–behavioural therapy. *Psychopathology, 39*(1), 32–37.

Bradford, J. M. W., & Fedoroff, P. (2005). The pharmacologic treatment of the juvenile sex offender. In H. Barbaree & W. Marshall (Eds.), *The juvenile sex offender* (2nd ed., pp. 358–382). New York, NY: Guilford.

Bradford, J. M. W., Fedoroff, P., & Firestone, P. (2008). Sexual violence and the clinician. In R. I. Simon & K. Tardiff (Eds.), *Textbook of violence assessment and management* (pp. 441–460). Arlington, VA: American Psychiatric Publishing.

Cambridge, P. (2013). A rights approach to supporting the sexual fetish of a man with learning disability: Method, process and applied learning. *British Journal of Learning Disabilities, 41*(4), 259–265.

Chang, H. L., & Chow, C. C. (2011). The treatment of fetishism in an adolescent with attention deficit hyperactivity disorder. *Chang Gung Medical Journal, 34*(4), 440–443.

Cheng, J. C., Secondary, J., Burke, W. H., Fedoroff, J. P., & Dwyer, R. G. (2015). Neuroimaging and sexual behavior: Identification of regional and functional differences. *Current Psychiatry Reports*, *17*(7), 1–8. doi:10.1007/s11920-015-0593-x

Choi-Kain, L. W., Finch, E. F., Masland, S. R., Jenkins, J. A., & Unruh, B. T. (2017). What works in the treatment of borderline personality disorder. *Current Behavioral Neuroscience Reports*, *4*(1), 21–30. doi:10.1007/s40473-017-0103-z

Cook, J. W., Altman, K., Shaw, J., & Blaylock, M. (1978). Use of contingent lemon juice to eliminate public masturbation by a severely retarded boy. *Behaviour Research and Therapy*, *16*(2), 131–134.

Corretti, G., & Baldi, I. (2010). Oxcarbazepine reduces exhibitionist urges and behaviors in a paraphilic patient. *Archives of Sexual Behavior*, *39*(5), 1025–1026.

Coskun, M., & Mukaddes, N. M. (2008). Mirtazapine treatment in a subject with autistic disorder and fetishism. *Journal of Child and Adolescent Psychopharmacology*, *18*(2), 206–209.

Cro, F., Peronti, M., & Bersani, G. (1997). A case of auto-vampirism in a patient with borderline personality disorder and chronic multiple substance abuse. *Rivisita di Psichiatria*, *32*(4), 165–172.

Dewaraja, R. (1987). Formicophilia, an unusual paraphilia, treated with counseling and behavior therapy. *American Journal of Psychotherapy*, *41*(4), 593–597.

Dewaraja, R., & Money, J. (1986). Transcultural sexology: Formicophilia, a newly named paraphilia in a young Buddhist male. *Journal of Sex & Marital Therapy*, *12*(2), 139–145.

DiGiorgio-Miller, J. (1998). Sibling incest: Treatment of the family and the offender. *Child Welfare: Journal of Policy, Practice, and Program*, *77*(3), 335–346.

Dozier, C. L., Iwata, B. A., & Worsdell, A. S. (2011). Assessment and treatment of foot–shoe fetish displayed by a man with autism. *Journal of Applied Behavior Analysis*, *44*(1), 133–137. doi:10.1901/jaba.2011.44-133

Dufrene, B. A., Watson, T. S., & Weaver, A. (2005). Response blocking with guided compliance and reinforcement for a habilitative replacement behavior: Effects on public masturbation and on-task behavior. *Child & Family Behavior Therapy*, *27*(4), 73–84.

Dwyer, S. M., & Myers, S. (1990). Sex offender treatment: A six-month to ten-year follow-up study. *Annals of Sex Research*, *3*(3), 305–318.

Erdogan, A. (2010). Pedophilia: Clinical features, etiology and treatment [in Turkish]. *Psikiyatride Guncel Yaklasimlar*, *2*(2), 132–160.

Fedoroff, J. P. (1994). Serotonergic drug treatment of deviant sexual interests. *Annals of Sex Research*, *6*, 105–107.

Fedoroff, J. P. (1995). Antiandrogens vs. serotonergic medications in the treatment of sex offenders: A preliminary compliance study. *Canadian Journal of Human Sexuality*, *4*, 111–122.

Fedoroff, J. P. (2003). The paraphilic world. In S. B. Levine (Ed.), *Handbook of clinical sexuality for mental health professionals* (pp. 333–356). New York, NY: Brunner/Routledge.

Fedoroff, J. P. (2008). Treatment of paraphilic sexual disorders. In D. L. Rowland & L. Lacocci (Eds.), *The handbook of sexual and gender identity disorders* (pp. 563–585). Hoboken, NJ: Wiley.

Fedoroff, J. P. (2009). The paraphilias. In M. G. Gelder, N. C. Andereasen, J. J. Lopez-Iber, Jr., & J. R. Beddes (Eds.), *The new Oxford textbook of psychiatry* (2nd ed., pp. 832–842). Oxford, UK: Oxford University Press.

Fedoroff, J. P. (2010). Paraphilic worlds. In S. B. Levine (Ed.), *Handbook of clinical sexuality for mental health professionals* (pp. 401–424). New York, NY: Routledge.

Fedoroff, J. P. (2011, September). The pharmacologic treatment of paraphilic disorders. *AAPL Newsletter*, 21–30.

Fedoroff, J. P. (2016). Managing versus successfully treating paraphilic disorders: The paradigm is changing. In S. B. Levine, C. B. Risen, & S. E. Althof (Eds.), *Handbook of clinical sexuality for mental health professionals* (pp. 345–361). New York, NY: Taylor & Francis.

Fedoroff, J. P., & Fedoroff, I. C. (1992). Buspirone and paraphilic sexual behaviour. *Journal of Offender Rehabilitation*, *18*(3–4), 89–108.

Fedoroff, J. P., Kuban, M., & Bradford, J. M. (2009). Laboratory measurement of penile response in the assessment of sexual interests. In F. Saleh, A. Grudzinskas, Jr., J. Bradford, & D. Brodsky

(Eds.), *Sex offenders: Identification, risk assessment, treatment and legal issues* (pp. 89–100). New York, NY: Oxford University Press.

Fedoroff, J. P., & Marshall, W. L. (2010). Paraphilias. In D. McKay, J. S. Abramowitz, & S. Taylor (Eds.), *Cognitive behavioral therapy for refractory cases* (pp. 369–384). Washington, DC: American Psychological Association.

Fedoroff, J. P., Murphy, L. & Ly, T. (2018). The Royal's Sexual Behaviours Clinic (SBC): Changing perspectives. *Russian Journal of Psychiatry, 2*, 56–62.

Fedoroff, J. P., & Pinkus, S. (1996). The genesis of pedophilia: Testing the abuse to abuser hypothesis. *Journal of Offender Rehabilitation, 23*, 85–101.

Ferguson, L. N., & Rekers, G. A. (1979). Non-aversive intervention in public childhood masturbation: A case study. *Journal of Sex Research, 15*(3), 213–223.

Finkelhor, D. (1986). Sexual abuse: Beyond the family systems approach. *Journal of Psychotherapy & the Family, 2*(2), 53–65.

Firoz, K., Sankar, V. N., Rajmohan, V., Kumar, G. M., & Raghuram, T. M. (2014). Treatment of fetishism with naltrexone: A case report. *Asian Journal of Psychiatry, 8*, 67–68.

Frank, J. D., & Frank, J. B. (1991). *Persuasion and healing: A comparative study of psychotherapy* (3rd ed.). Baltimore, MD: Johns Hopkins University Press.

Gallo, M. (2016). A case study of cross-dressing: Using a strategic therapy lens in couple's counseling. *The Family Journal, 24*(1), 77–84.

Gill, M. (2012). Sex can wait, masturbate: The politics of masturbation training. *Sexualities, 15*(3–4), 472–493.

Giugliano, J. R. (2011). Self-psychological treatment of a sex addict with sadomasochistic behaviours: A case report. *British Journal of Psychotherapy, 27*(4), 352–367.

Goldberg, R. L., & Wise, T. N. (1985). Psychodynamic treatment for telephone scatologia. *American Journal of Psychoanalysis, 45*(3), 291–297.

Green, D. (1987). Adolescent exhibitionists: Theory and therapy. *Journal of Adolescence, 10*(1), 45–56.

Grubin, D. (2010). A trial of voluntary polygraphy testing in 10 English probation areas. *Sex Abuse, 22*, 266–278. doi:10.1177/1079063210369012

Grubin, D., Kamenskov, M., Dwyer, G., & Stephenson, T. (2019). Post-conviction polygraph testing of sex offenders [Epub ahead of print]. *International Review of Psychiatry*. https://doi.org/10.1080/09540261.2018.1561428

Guay, D. R. (2009). Drug treatment of paraphilic and nonparaphilic sexual disorders. *Clinical Therapeutics, 31*(1), 1–31.

Guney, E., Ceylan, M. F., & Sener, S. (2011). Successful treatment of transvestic fetishism with sertralin in a prepubertal child. *Yeni Symposium: Psikiyatri, noroloji ve davranis bilimleri dergisi, 49*(3), 181–184.

Guterman, J. T., Martin, C. V., & Rudes, J. (2011). A solution-focused approach to frotteurism. *Journal of Systemic Therapies, 30*(1), 59–72.

Hanson, R. K., Harris, A. J. R., Helmus, L., & Thornton, D. (2014). High-risk offenders may not be high risk forever. *Journal of Interpersonal Violence, 29*, 2792–2813. https://doi.org/10.1177/0886260514526062

Hanson, R. K., & Morton-Bourgon, K. E. (2005). The characteristics of persistent sexual offenders: A meta-analysis of recidivism studies. *Journal of Consulting and Clinical Psychology, 73*, 1154–1163. doi:10.1037/0022-006X.73.6.1154

Hargett, H. (1998). Reconciling the victim and perpetrator in sibling incest. *Sexual Addiction & Compulsivity, 5*(2), 93–106.

Harris, T. (1981). *Red dragon*. New York, NY: Putnam.

Horton, A. L., Johnson, B. L., Roundy, L. M., & Williams, D. (1990). *The incest perpetrator: A family member no one wants to treat.* Thousand Oaks, CA: Sage.

Hughes, J. R. (2007). Review of medical reports on pedophilia [Commentary]. *Clinical Pediatrics, 46*(8), 667–682.

Hunter, J. A., Ram, N., & Ryback, R. (2008). Use of satiation therapy in the treatment of adolescent-manifest sexual interest in male children: A single-case, repeated measures design. *Clinical Case Studies, 7*(1), 54–74.

Hurley, A. D., & Sovner, R. (1983). Treatment of sexual deviation in mentally retarded persons. *Psychiatric Aspects of Mental Retardation Newsletter, 2*(4), 13–16.

Janzen, W. B., & Peacock, R. (1978). Treatment of public masturbation by behavioral management. *American Journal of Psychotherapy, 32*(2), 300–306.

Johnson, P. R. (2010). Pedophiles: The quest for comprehensive treatment. *Journal on Developmental Disabilities, 16*(1), 103–108.

Keating, T. P. (2000). RESPECT: A 7 step system to treat pedophiles who are mentally retarded, have mental illness, and physical handicaps. *Journal of Psychology & Human Sexuality, 11*(3), 89–114.

Kenyon, E. D. (1989). The management of exhibitionism in the elderly: A case study. *Sexual & Marital Therapy, 4*(1), 93–100.

Khodayarifard, M., Pritz, A., Alavi, S. M., & Abedini, Y. (2013). A case study of cognitive–behavior therapy in Iran: Treatment of sexual masochism along with co-morbid disorders in a collectivist society. *International Journal of Psychotherapy, 17*(1), 53–63.

King, P. R. (2014). Cognitive–behavioral intervention in a case of self-mutilation. *Clinical Case Studies, 13*(2), 181–189.

Kingston, D. A., Seto, M. C., Ahmed, A. G., Fedoroff, J. P., & Bradford, J. M. (2012). The role of central and peripheral hormones in sexual aggression and recidivism in sexual offenders. *Journal of the American Academy of Psychiatry and the Law, 40*, 476–485.

Kirenskaya, A., & Kamenskov, M. (2019). The association between slow cortical potentials preceding antisaccades and disturbances of consciousness in persons with paraphilic sexual behaviour. *International Review of Psychiatry, 31*(2), 149–150.

Kleinplatz, P. (2014). The paraphilias: An experiential approach to "dangerous" desires. In Y. M. Binik & Kathryn S. K. Hall (Eds.), *Principles and practice of sex therapy* (5th ed., pp. 195–218). New York, NY. Guilford.

Knack, N., Murphy, L., Ranger, R., Meston, C., & Fedoroff, J. P. (2015). Assessment of female sexual arousal in forensic populations. *Current Psychiatry Reports, 17*(4), 1–8.

Knack, L., Winder, B., Murphy, L., & Fedoroff, J. P. (2019). Primary and secondary prevention of child abuse. *International Review of Psychiatry* [Epub ahead of print].

Knott, V., Impey, D., Fisher, D., Delpero, E., & Fedoroff, P. (2016). Pedophilic brain potential responses to adult erotic stimuli. *Brain Research, 1632*(1), 127–140.

Komrad, M. (2012). *You need help! A step-by-step plan to convince a loved one to get counseling.* Center City, Minnesota, Hazelden.

Koo, K. C., Ahn, J. H., Hong, S. J., Lee, J. W., & Chung, B. H. (2014). Effects of chemical castration on sex offenders in relation to the kinetics of serum testosterone recovery: Implications for dosing schedule. *Journal of Sexual Medicine, 11*(5), 1316–1324.

Krafft-Ebing, R. von. (1999). *Psychopathia sexualis.* Bloat Books. ISBN:0-9650324-1-8 (Original work published 1886), Burbank, California.

Kukkonen, T. M. (2014). What is the best method of measuring the physiology of female sexual arousal? *Current Sexual Health Reports, 6*(1), 30–37. https://doi.org/10.1007/s11930-013-0010-6

Kunjukrishnan, R., Pawlak, A., & Varan, L. R. (1988). The clinical and forensic psychiatric issues of retifism. *Canadian Journal of Psychiatry, 33*(9), 819–825.

Lanyon, R. I. (1986). Theory and treatment in child molestation. *Journal of Consulting and Clinical Psychology, 34*(2), 176–182.

Laws, D. R. (Ed.). (1989). *Relapse prevention with sex offenders.* New York, NY: Guilford.

Laws, D. R., & O'Donohue, W. T. (1997). *Sexual deviance: Theory, assessment, and treatment.* New York, NY: Guilford.

Laws, D. R., & O'Donohue, W. T. (2008). *Sexual deviance: Theory, assessment, and treatment* (2nd ed.). New York: Guilford.

Lehne, G. K., & Money, J. (2000). The first case of paraphilia treated with Depo-Provera: 40-year outcome. *Journal of Sex Education and Therapy, 25*(4), 213–220. doi:10.1080/01614576.2000.11074353

Lowenstein, L. F. (2002). Fetishes and their associated behavior. *Sexuality and Disability, 20*(2), 135–147.

Lundervold, D. A., & Young, L. G. (1992). Treatment acceptability ratings for sexual offenders: Effects of diagnosis and offense. *Research in Developmental Disabilities, 13*(3), 229–237.

Marlatt, G. A., & Donovan, D. M. (Eds.). (2005). *Relapse prevention: Maintenance strategies in the treatment of addictive behaviors* (2nd ed.). New York, NY: Guilford.

Marques, J. K., Day, D. J., Nelson, C., Miner, M. H., & West, M. A. (1991). *The Sex Offender Treatment and Evaluation Project: Fourth report to the legislature in response to PC2365.* Sacramento, CA: California State Department of Mental Health.

Marshall, W. L., Eccles, A., & Barbaree, H. E. (1991). The treatment of exhibitionists: A focus on sexual deviance versus cognitive and relationship features. *Behaviour Research and Therapy, 29*(2), 129–135.

Marshall, W. L., Marshall, L. E., & Kingston, D. A. (2011). Are the cognitive distortions of child molesters in need of treatment? *Journal of Sexual Aggression, 17*(2), 118–129.

Matek, O. (1988). Obscene phone callers. *Journal of Social Work & Human Sexuality, 7*(1), 113–130.

Mendhekar, D. N., & Duggal, H. S. (2005). Sertraline for Klüver–Bucy syndrome in an adolescent. *European Psychiatry, 20*(4), 355–356.

Metz, M. E., & Sawyer, S. P. (2004). Treating sexual dysfunction in sex offenders: A case example. *Journal of Sex & Marital Therapy, 30*(3), 185–197.

Murphy, L., Bradford, J. B., & Fedoroff, J. P. (2014). Paraphilia and paraphilic disorders. In G. O. Gabbard (Ed.), *Gabbard's treatments of psychiatric disorders* (pp. 669–694). Washington, DC: American Psychiatric Publishing.

Murphy, L., & Fedoroff, J. P. (2017). Assessing people with problematic sexual interests: An overview of the Royal's Sexual Behaviours Clinic and Assessment Laboratory. *Russian Journal of Psychiatry, 5*, 73–79.

Murphy, L., Ranger, R., Fedoroff, J. P., Stewart, H., Dwyer, G., & Burke, W. (2015). Standardization in the use of penile plethysmography testing in assessment of problematic sexual interests. *Journal of Sexual Medicine*, 12(9), 1853–1861.

Murphy, L., Ranger, R., Stewart, H., Dwyer, G., & Fedoroff, J. P. (2015). Assessment of problematic sexual interests with the penile plethysmograph: An overview of assessment laboratories. *Current Psychiatry Reports, 17*(5), 1–5.

Norcross, J. C., VandenBos, G. R., & Freedheim, D. K. (Eds.). (2011). *History of psychotherapy: Continuity and change* (2nd ed.). Washington, DC: American Psychological Association. http://dx.doi.org/10.1037/12353-000

Novick, K. K., & Novick, N. J. (2012). Some suggestions for engaging with the clinical problem of masochism. In D. Holtzman & K. Nancy (Eds.), *The clinical problem of masochism* (pp. 51–75). Lanham, MD: Aronson.

Nu Ez, J. (2003). Outpatient treatment of the sexually compulsive ephebophile. *Sexual Addiction & Compulsivity: The Journal of Treatment and Prevention, 10*(1), 23–51. doi:10.1080/10720160309047

O'Donohue, W. T. (2014). *Case studies in sexual deviance: Toward evidence-based practice.* New York, NY: Routledge.

Paul, R. H., Marx, B. P., & Orsillo, S. M. (1999). Acceptance-based psychotherapy in the treatment of an adjudicated exhibitionist: A case example. *Behavior Therapy, 30*(1), 149–162.

Quinsey, V. L. (1977). The assessment and treatment of child molesters: A review. *Canadian Psychological Review, 18*(3), 204–220.

Rea, J. A., Dixon, M. R., Zettle, R. D., & Wright, K. L. (2017). The development of in vivo measures to assess the impact of sex-drive reducing medications in an offender with an intellectual disability. *Archives of Sexual Behavior, 46*(3), 843–859.

Ricci, R. J., Clayton, C. A., & Shapiro, F. (2006). Some effects of EMDR on previously abused child molesters: Theoretical reviews and preliminary findings. *Journal of Forensic Psychiatry & Psychology, 17*(4), 538–562.

Sarver, N. W., & Gros, D. F. (2014). A modern behavioral treatment to address fetishism and associated functional impairment. *Clinical Case Studies, 13*(4), 336–351.

Scheela, R. A., & Stern, P. N. (1994). Falling apart: A process integral to the remodeling of male incest offenders. *Archives of Psychiatric Nursing*, *8*(2), 91–100.

Schiffer, B., Gizewski, E., & Kruger, T. (2009). Reduced neuronal responsiveness to visual sexual stimuli in a pedophile treated with a long-acting LH-RH agonist. *Journal of Sexual Medicine*, *6*(3), 892–894.

Seto, M. (2008). *Pedophilia and sexual offending against children: Theory, assessment, and intervention*. Washington, DC: American Psychological Association.

Seto, M. (2018). *Pedophilia and sexual offending against children: Theory, assessment, and intervention* (2nd ed.). Washington, DC: American Psychological Association.

Seto, M. C., & Ahmed, A. G. (2014). Treatment and management of child pornography use. *Psychiatric Clinics of North America*, *37*(2), 207–214.

Snaith, R. P. (1983). Exhibitionism: A clinical conundrum. *British Journal of Psychiatry*, *143*, 231–235.

Southern, S. (2002). The tie that binds: Sadomasochism in female addicted trauma survivors. *Sexual Addiction & Compulsivity*, *9*(4), 209–229.

Sprott, R. A., Randall, A., Davison, K., Cannon, N., & Witherspoon, R. G. (2017). Alternative or nontraditional sexualities and therapy: A case report. *Journal of Clinical Psychology*, *73*(8), 929–937.

Stoylen, I. J. (1985). Voyeurism: Treatment by cognitive behavior therapy in a case of scopophilia [in Norwegian]. *Tidsskrift for Norsk Psykologforening*, *22*(10), 561–564.

Strzyzewsky, J., & Zierhoffer, M. (1967). Aversion therapy in a case of fetishism with transvestic component. *Journal of Sex Research*, *3*(2), 163–167.

Sturmey, P., Wong, S. C., Stockdale, K. C., & Olver, M. E. (2017). Violence reduction treatment of psychopathy. In P. Sturmey (Ed.), *The Wiley Handbook of Violence and Aggression*. Malden, MA: Wiley. doi:10.1002/9781119057574.whbva087

Thibaut, F., Bradford, J. W., Briken, P., De La Barra, F., Häßler, F., & Cosyns, P.; on behalf of the WFSBP Task Force on Sexual Disorders. (2016). The World Federation of Societies of Biological Psychiatry (WFSBP) guidelines for the treatment of adolescent sexual offenders with paraphilic disorders. *The World Journal of Biological Psychiatry*, *17*(1), 2–38. doi:10.3109/15622975.2015.1085598

Thibaut, F., de la Barra, F., Gordon, H., Cosyns, P., & Bradford, J. (2010). The World Federation of Societies of Biological Psychiatry (WFSBP) guidelines for the biological treatment of paraphilias. *The World Journal of Biological Psychiatry*, *11*, 604–655. doi:10.3109/15622971003671628

Thompson, A. R., & Beail, N. (2002). The treatment of auto-erotic asphyxiation in a man with severe intellectual disabilities: The effectiveness of a behavioural and educational programme. *Journal of Applied Research in Intellectual Disabilities*, *15*(1), 36–47.

Toates, F. (2009). An integrative theoretical framework for understanding sexual motivation, arousal, and behavior. *Journal of Sex Research*, *46*, 168–193. https://www.jstor.org/stable/20620413

Travin, S., Bluestone, H., Coleman, E., Cullen, K., & Melella, J. (1985). Pedophilia: An update on theory and practice. *Psychiatric Quarterly*, *57*(2), 89–103.

Vazquez, G. H., Holtzman, J. N., Lolich, M., Ketter, T. A., & Baldessarini, R. J. (2015). Recurrence rates in bipolar disorder: Systematic comparison of long-term prospective, naturalistic studies versus randomized controlled trials. *European Neuropsychopharmacology*, *25*, 1501–1512. doi:10.1016/j.euroneuro.2015.07.013

von Franque, F., & Briken, P. (2017). Psychotherapeutic treatment of pedophilic disorder [in German]. *Verhaltenstherapie & Verhaltensmedizin*, *38*(1), 26–41.

Wagner, M. K. (1968). A case of public masturbation treated by operant conditioning. *Child Psychology and Psychiatry and Allied Disciplines*, *9*(1), 61–65.

Waldram, J. B. (2012). *Hound Pound narrative: Sexual offender habilitation and the anthology of therapeutic intervention*. Berkeley, CA: University of California Press. ISBN:9780520272569

Ward, T. (2002). Good lives and the rehabilitation of offenders: Promises and problems. *Aggression and Violent Behavior*, *7*, 513–528. doi:10.1016/S1359-1789(01)00076-3

Ward, T., & Brown, M. (2004). The Good Lives model and conceptual issues in offender rehabilitation. *Psychology, Crime & Law*, *10*(3), 243–257. doi:10.1080/10683160410001662744

Ward, T., Mann, R. E., & Gannon, T. A. (2007). The good lives model of offender rehabilitation: Clinical implications. *Aggression and Violent Behavior, 12*, 87–107. http://dx.doi.org/10.1016/j.avb.2006.03.004

Wendy, C. (1992). Incest perpetrators: Their assessment and treatment. *Psychiatric Clinics of North America, 15*(3), 689–701.

Wickramasekera, I. (1968). The application of learning theory to the treatment of a case of sexual exhibitionism. *Psychotherapy, 5*(2), 108–112.

Wilson, R. J., Cortini, F., & McWhinnie, A. J. (2009). Circles of support and accountability: A Canadian national replication of outcome findings. *Sexual Abuse, 21*(4), 412–430. doi:10.1177/1079063209347724

Wise, T. N. (1985). Fetishism—Etiology and treatment: A review from multiple perspectives. *Comprehensive Psychiatry, 26*(3), 249–257.

Yalcin, O., Guney, E., & Saripinar, E. G. (2014). Dramatic improvement with sertraline in a male adolescent with voyeurism. *Bulletin of Clinical Psychopharmacology, 24*(3), 292–294.

Yatham, L. N., Kennedy, S. H., Parikh, S. V., Schaffer, A., Bond, D. J., Frey, B. N., . . . Berk, M. (2018). Canadian Network for Mood and Anxiety Treatments (CANMAT) and International Society for Bipolar Disorders (ISBD) 2018 guidelines for the management of patients with bipolar disorder. *Bipolar Disorders, 20*, 97–170. doi:10.1111/bdi.12609

Zarei, M., & Bidaki, R. (2013). Female foot fetishism disorder in childhood. *Journal of Research in Medical Sciences, 18*(2), 170.

Zechnich, R. (1971). Exhibitionism: Genesis, dynamics and treatment. *Psychiatric Quarterly, 45*(1), 70–75.

3
Exhibitionistic Disorder

If modesty disappeared, so would exhibitionism.

—Mason Cooley

Introduction

The most recent online *International Classification of Diseases* (ICD-11 beta draft; World Health Organization, 2017) defines exhibitionistic disorder as follows:

> Exhibitionistic disorder is characterized by a sustained, focused and intense pattern of sexual arousal—as manifested by persistent sexual thoughts, fantasies, urges, or behaviors—that involves exposing one's genitals to an unsuspecting individual in public places, usually without inviting or intending closer contact. In addition, in order for exhibitionistic disorder to be diagnosed, the individual must have acted on these thoughts, fantasies or urges or be markedly distressed by them. Exhibitionistic disorder specifically excludes consensual exhibitionistic behaviors that occur with the consent of the person or persons involved as well as socially sanctioned forms of exhibitionism. (Downloaded January 1, 2017)

The Fifth edition of the *Diagnostic and Statistical Manual of Mental Disorders* (DSM-5; American Psychiatric Association [APA], 2013) defines exhibitionistic disorder as follows:

A. Over a period of at least 6 months, recurrent and intense sexual arousal from the exposure of one's genitals to an unsuspecting person, as manifested by fantasies, urges, or behaviors.
B. The individual has acted on these sexual urges with a nonconsenting person, or the sexual urges or fantasies cause clinically significant distress or impairment in social, occupational, or other important areas of functioning (p. 689).

Subspecifications include whether the person is aroused by exposing to prepubertal children or physically mature adults or both.

Also specified in the DSM-5 criteria is the person's living situation (whether there is an opportunity to expose to nonconsenting people) and whether the condition is in "full remission," which means the person has not exposed, is not distressed, and has had the opportunity to expose for at least 5 years (APA, 2013, p. 689).

Readers will note obvious similarities between the ICD and DSM-5 definitions. The ICD requires the person to expose to an "unsuspecting" person, and the DSM-5 specifies "nonconsenting." The ICD excludes "sanctioned" forms of exposing from the definition, whereas the DSM specifies if the person exposes to children and allows for the possibility that exhibitionism can go into "full remission."

Variations

The Sexual Behaviours Clinic (SBC) categorizes people with presumed exhibitionistic disorder differently. Rather than limiting the diagnosis to the person's observed acts, the SBC includes an investigation of the motivation for the act(s). There are three groups with common but distinct motivations for exposing to strangers.

Classic Exhibitionists

This group consists of people who are sexually aroused by the act or fantasy of exposing to nonconsenting victims with no expectation or wish to engage in actual in-person sexual contact with the person. This of course excludes consensual situations such as strippers in bars, who disrobe to patrons who pay to watch, and nudists who enjoy going to nude beaches where they may be seen by strangers but in a socially sanctioned venue.

For men, exposing to women with no expectation of further sexual contact is easy to do because the majority of women do not pursue sex with exhibitionists who expose to them without their consent. For women, it is more difficult because men are more likely to respond to female exhibitionists by attempting to reciprocate. Therefore, women with exhibitionism tend to expose in situations in which they can avoid the possibility of the episode progressing to actual contact, such as by exposing from a car while they are driving or exposing to strangers via webcams.

Public Masturbators

The second type are people those aroused by engaging in sexual acts such as masturbating in public places but with no wish to be seen. The SBC classifies this group as "public masturbators." A common example is a man who parks his car in a public parking lot and then masturbates while watching unsuspecting and therefore nonconsenting women walk past his car. This group is motivated by the idea of "getting away with something," and the sexual arousal comes from the risk of being caught. Of course, members of this group often take the risk too far and do get caught. Because they are exposing in public, they are often mistaken for classic exhibitionists (described previously). In general, public masturbators tend to respond well to treatment and have a lower risk of reoffending (providing they truly are not the first type). Unfortunately, true exhibitionists often claim to be public masturbators when they are caught, so it is important for the assessor to carefully explore the motivations for the act(s) rather than simply making a diagnosis based on the police report.

Opportunistic Masturbators

The third type consists of people who expose with the primary intent of having sex with the person to whom they are exposing. The most common members of this group are men who expose in men's washrooms or gyms or parks with the hope of connecting with another man for an anonymous sexual encounter. These people can be arrested and falsely labeled as exhibitionistic even though they technically meet the DSM and ICD criteria. They are very different from the first two types and are best understood as members of a subculture that can come into conflict with the law by accident. As a side note, they are often also mistakenly labeled as gay even though their motivation is purely sexual. A subgroup consists of men who prefer to limit their contact with men to sexual contact only, with no romantic affiliations in order to avoid self-labelling as gay due to guilt.

Other Variations

Of course, there are always further variations on the theme.

Case Report 3.1

One man would take Polaroid pictures of his penis. He would then check into a motel and slip a Polaroid picture of his penis, face down, under each door in the hallway. He would watch from the door of his room to see the Polaroids pulled into the rooms by the people behind the doors. He said he rarely had to wait long. After one or two of the Polaroids had been zipped under the door, he would close the door to his room and masturbate while fantasizing that attractive women were gazing at pictures of his penis and were masturbating like he was. An interesting addendum to this man's pattern of behavior is that he always left his motel room door unlocked. In this way, he could imagine that aroused women could find their way to him. He admitted he was also aroused by the fantasy that angry husbands might also burst through the door to punish him. This combination of irrational thoughts made him both anxious and aroused, which is a state that many people with paraphilias attempt to achieve.

Case Report 3.2

A man was arrested after his ex-girlfriend discovered he had secretly taken pictures of her naked and while they had sex. He would post the pictures online to various sites on which people consensually exchanged sexual images. On assessment, he explained that he had low self-esteem and was aroused by the idea that people would be jealous when they saw him with his girlfriend. Treatment in his case was simple because he responded well to education about the fact that what he did was nonconsensual.

Hypothesized Etiologies

Learned Behaviors

Many women report at least one incident of a man exposing his genitals to them without consent (Riordan, 1999). It is remarkable that most men with exhibitionism attempt to justify their behavior as simple, healthy nudity. When asked what the response to their "spontaneous nudity" has been to date, they typically confess that women are not impressed. Nevertheless, these men continue to engage in the behaviors, thinking no one is harmed. Often, they present a behavioral learning explanation involving maladaptive learning. In one case report (Fedoroff, 2010), a man claimed that he had been masturbating in a park. He said a beautiful and sexy woman saw him and could not resist herself. He said they spontaneously engaged in such a satisfying sexual encounter that he could not help but continue to masturbate in parks with the hope of re-creating the event (but not with the same woman).

Of course, the fact that the man had been masturbating in the park in the first place suggests he had a vulnerability to exhibitionism before the event with the woman happened (if in fact it ever happened at all). Parenthetically, it is typical for people with exhibitionism to have no interest in progressing from exposing to more intimate forms of sexual activity, especially with the same person.

A common question, reviewed by Morin and Levenson (2008), involves whether people with exhibitionism have sex drives that are too strong (Kafka, 2003, 2010) and/or have too little ability to inhibit their behaviors in response to sexually arousing situations (Taylor, 1947).

Hypersexuality

The evidence that exhibitionism is the result of so-called hypersexuality is meager. People with exhibitionism do not masturbate more than others, and exhibitionistic acts typically are not the result of sexual deprivation. In the SBC, people with exhibitionism are asked what they think is the cause of their problem. The most common answer from people with exhibitionism is "Doctor, I have a lack of willpower." This is because they think that all adults, or at least all *male* adults, must constantly resist the urge to disrobe when they see a sexually attractive stranger. They are surprised and relieved when they are informed they are wrong. Often, they are moved to tears when told their problem is not a lack of "intestinal fortitude or lack of willpower" but, rather, an interest in an activity that is easy to do but for which most people have no interest in engaging.

Courtship Disorders

A third explanation is based on the hypothesis that people with exhibitionism do not follow normal courtship behaviors (Freund, 1990). The idea that exhibitionism represents a "short-circuit" in normal courtship behavior has enjoyed phenomenal longevity since it was first proposed under the rubric of "courtship disorder" (Freund & Blanchard, 1986). The notion of so-called courtship disorders is that people are "programmed" to follow a standard sequence of behaviors in the process of mating. The major stages, in order, are (1) seeing or noticing a potential mate, (2) establishing a close enough relationship with the person to allow touching, (3) progressing to kissing, followed by (4) disrobing and then (5) intercourse.Freund suggested that people who deviate from this sequence of courtship behaviors can be understood as having what he called a "courtship disorder." The paraphilias corresponding to each stage except kissing are as follows: voyeurism corresponds with seeing, frotteurism corresponds with touching, exhibitionism corresponds with disrobing, and coercive paraphilic disorder corresponds with sexual intercourse. It is interesting that a paraphilia for kissing has not been reported. This may be because kissing is commonly regarded as romantic as opposed to sexual. For example, many men who have sex with men who are not gay avoid kissing; as do many sex workers.

Courtship disorders are theorized to be the result of either "getting stuck" on one stage (e.g., voyeurism) or "skipping" a step (e.g., exhibitionism, frotteurism, or coercive paraphilic disorder). It is notable that people who proceed through the courtship stages quickly but in the "correct" order are generally regarded as less deviant than people who skip stages. There is also a gender bias. For example, when President-elect Donald Trump bragged that women allowed him to "grab them by the pussy," few questioned his claim that women allowed him to do so, presumably because he was rich and famous. Questions only arose about whether it was ethical for him to take advantage of his status to do so, or whether it was advantageous for him to brag about it.

"Courtship disorders" have a heuristic appeal but little evidence to support the concept. In fact, the best evidence provided in their support is that they often occur together (Freund & Blanchard, 1986), a finding replicated in the SBC. But if courtship disorders are the result of "skipping" or "getting stuck" on a phase of courtship, shouldn't each of the courtship disorders be *less* likely to occur together? More importantly, courtship disorders are based on the premises that people are "programmed" and "can get stuck" or can unintentionally "skip" stages of mating. There is no evidence to support any of these three premises.

On one occasion, the author discussed the concept of courtship disorders with John Money. Money said he did not believe in courtship disorders as defined by Freund, commenting, "Name one paraphilia that is not a courtship disorder. All paraphilias by definition interfere with mating." Following a lecture by Freund on his concept of courtship disorders, Fedoroff told Freund about Money's comment. In response, Freund thought for a moment and then answered, "Dr. Money is right" (personal communication).

Counterfeit Deviance

Another explanation is that some people display exhibitionistic behaviors because they have intellectual disabilities or acquired intellectual deficits that contribute to so-called counterfeit deviance (Hingsburger, Griffiths, & Quinsey, 1991; Kelly, G., & Simpson, G. (2011). The premise of counterfeit deviance is that some people with intellectual disabilities may engage in apparently paraphilic acts (e.g. exhibitionism) due to impaired cognition leading to impaired social skills. In one published example (Fedoroff, 2010), a man with intellectual disability who lived in a group home was reported because he often exited his room naked. On assessment, it was discovered that he had lived in all-male group living situations in which nudity was permitted (e.g., while walking from the multiperson shared bedroom to the communal shower). The problem was solved by purchasing a housecoat for him.

Prevalence

Theories about the prevalence, nature, and etiology of all the "courtship disorders" are complicated by important variations. The DSM-5 claims that "the highest possible prevalence for exhibitionistic disorder in the male population is 2%–4%" (APA, 2013, p. 690). However, another study reported a slightly higher prevalence rate of 4.3% for males (Långström & Seto, 2006).

There are two main problems in estimating prevalence rates of this disorder. The first is that people with exhibitionistic disorder rarely seek treatment until they are arrested. This means that what is known about exhibitionism is based almost solely on studies of people in the criminal justice system.

The second problem is that exhibitionistic acts are rarely reported by the victims (Riordan, 1999). This is especially true for victims of women with exhibitionistic disorder. In one previously published case involving a self-referred woman who exposed from her living room to men passing by on the street, she accurately pointed out that any man who reported her was in more danger of arrest (for voyeurism) than she was for exhibitionism (Fedoroff, 2010).

The low reporting rate for men and women, combined with the ease of committing an act of exhibitionism, means that most people with this disorder have many victims before they are arrested. In one unreplicated study, 142 people with exhibitionism claimed to have an average of more than 500 victims each (Abel & Rouleau, 1990). This makes estimates of the prevalence of exhibitionism based on surveys of victims difficult to interpret.

Recidivism Rates

As indicated previously, people with exhibitionism often report multiple acts of exhibitionism involving multiple people before they come to clinical attention, usually following an arrest. The literature to date indicates that people with exhibitionism have rates of recidivism as high as 48–71% based on one compilation of recidivism studies (Marshall, Law, & Barbaree, 1990). Fortunately, improved treatment strategies have significantly reduced the rate of recidivism (see the next section).

Assessment and Treatment Recommendations

Approaches to the assessment and treatment of people with exhibitionism disorder have been published elsewhere (Morin & Levinson, 2008; Murphy, Bradford, & Fedoroff, 2014; see also Chapter 2, this book).

It Is Not a Lack of Willpower

The first task in the first appointment with a person presenting with exhibitionistic behaviors is to unequivocally tell the person to stop exhibiting. This recommendation is often greeted with surprise or open opposition. The person may say they have already tried to stop and failed. They may say they have had this problem all their life and often will say they just cannot control their behaviors due to a lack of willpower. The person must be told that if they truly have exhibitionism, their problem is not lack of willpower but, rather, a sexual interest in doing something that is illegal.

It Is Not an Addiction

Some people with exhibitionism will claim they have a "sex addiction" or "hypersexuality." This is code for communication that they have adopted a selective version of Alcoholics Anonymous or Sexaholics Anonymous that supports their claims that (1) they are helpless to their "addiction," (2) will need to "taper" their illegal behaviors, (3) will inevitably have "slips," and (4) will always be exhibitionists.

Here, the therapist should respectfully explain that there is no evidence that exhibitionism is an addiction. It should be explained that an addiction is a dependence on an external substance to which the addict has built a tolerance and who will have characteristic withdrawal symptoms when they stop using it. In contrast, exhibitionism is a well-described paraphilia in which a person achieves persistent sexual arousal from exposing to nonconsensual strangers. Although they may believe they have no control over what turns them on, they absolutely have complete control over when and where they choose to pull their zippers down. Recalcitrant and skeptical people with exhibitionism can be reminded they are not exposing now and have not done so the entire time they were sitting in the waiting room for their appointment.

The therapist should explain that the therapist has no question the person with exhibitionism is troubled by exhibitionistic urges but that getting better requires stopping the problematic behavior to see what happens.

The next step is to conduct a comprehensive assessment (as described in Chapter 2, this book). It is important to determine which of the three main variant types of exhibitionism is affecting the person (discussed previously). It is also important to establish a comprehensive differential diagnosis and to systematically diagnose all the person's mental health and physical problems. Of course, all these problems need to be dealt with either in-person or through referral to the appropriate specialist.

In the SBC, voluntary phallometric testing is conducted that includes audiotapes describing scenarios maximally arousing to each of the three types of exhibitionism described previously. The purpose of phallometry is never to determine guilt or innocence but, rather, to provide a baseline against which treatment efficacy can be measured. If there are clinical concerns, phallometric response to audiotapes consistent with other courtship disorders can also be measured. In the SBC, the concept of courtship disorders is employed as a useful heuristic rather than as a diagnosis per se. It can also lead to useful discussions about the concept of consent, which involves not only "yes" or "no" but also revocable consent to the order and duration of the phases of courtship.

In the SBC, most new patients with exhibitionism are referred to the Social Skills program (see Chapter 2, this book). It is important to emphasize that the problem is not sex or lack of willpower. It must be explained that the problem is their sexual interest in committing an illegal act.

Consideration can be given to pharmacologic treatments, but there are no definitive studies showing medications can cure exhibitionism. However, sometimes pharmacologic treatment of anxiety disorder, mood disorder, attention-deficit disorder, and psychotic disorders is extremely helpful in improving the person's ability to make rational decisions about whether to act on their exhibitionistic interests in an illegal manner. Fortunately, for people with so-called courtship disorders, there are multiple alternatives to illegal acts, including use of internet websites, chat sites, and fantasy. In the SBC, some people with exhibitionism have found that exposing in front of their webcam on sites frequented by consenting viewers meets their needs. Others use so-called swingers (or lifestyle) clubs in which sexual activity in front of others is satisfactory. Of course, people with exhibitionism are aroused by the fantasy of exposing to an unsuspecting person, so nudist sites and swingers/lifestyle clubs initially seem uninteresting. One woman with exhibitionism successfully treated in the SBC overcame this problem by blindfolding herself while disrobing in a swing club. In this way, she was able to imagine the people who saw her were like the strangers to whom she had previously exposed without their consent. She was also aroused by the idea that men she subsequently encountered while walking down the street may have seen her naked when she was in the club. Another person with voyeurism was able to satisfy his interest in spying on unsuspecting women by "spying" on women in a club in which sex was permitted by watching from a distance.

For people who claim they absolutely cannot control their exhibitionism due to sexual arousal, it is sometimes helpful to temporarily suppress their sex drive with anti-androgen medication and/or a gonadotropin-releasing hormone. In the SBC, patients are told that sex drive suppression is purely voluntarily and should be temporary. The aim of treatment is to improve the person's sex life, not eliminate it.

Prognosis

For people with exhibitionism, the most important intervention is to explain that although nudity is normal, it can be traumatizing to nonconsenting victims. They should be told that up to 30% of the population has been sexually assaulted. Because they expose to strangers, they have no way of knowing whether the person they expose to has post-traumatic disorder (PTSD) from a previous sexual assault. PTSD is a widely known and understood diagnosis by most exhibitionists. Once they learn that their practice of exposing to a stranger may trigger flashbacks and other harm to the person, most exhibitionists are horrified and lose their interest in exposing.

The idea of cautioning people with exhibitionism that they may cause trauma to people with PTSD has only been used in the SBC for approximately 5 years. However, since the practice was instituted, with one known exception, the known reoffense rate for patients with exhibitionism has declined to virtually zero.

Review of the Literature

The following table summarizes the literature that has been published on "exhibitionism" from 2008 to 2018 based on PsycINFO and PubMed searches.

Summary	Reference
Etiology	
This author proposes that exhibitionistic acts could be motivated by gaining control over interpersonal engagements.	Tuch (2008)
Case example of the development of exhibitionism. The author found support for "countershame" and components of courtship disorder.	Raley (2011)
Discusses the risk factors for the development of exhibitionism before age 18 years.	Swindell et al. (2011)
Insights into Exhibitionism	
Found six personality types associated with exhibitionists. Discussion of motivations.	Hanafy, Clervoy, & Brenot (2016)
Speculates on the ratio of individuals who use technology as a means of exhibitionism and whether sending sexually explicit pictures can indicate exhibitionism.	Kaylor, Jeglic, & Collins (2016)
Escalation to Contact Offense	
Examined 106 individuals suspected of exhibitionism and their recidivism rates and subsequent sexual offenses.	Bader, Schoeneman-Morris, Scalora, & Casady (2008)
Literature review on exhibitionism in 12 peer-reviewed studies. The most supported risk factor of exhibitionism and escalation to contact offenses was antisocial features. Five to 10% of exhibitionists escalated.	McNally & Fremouw (2014)
Diagnosis	
DSM Modifications	
Review of the empirical literature on exhibitionism, voyeurism, and frotteurism between 1980 and 2008 and suggested criteria changes for the DSM-5.	Långström (2010)
Compares exhibitionism, voyeurism, and "intruders."	Hopkins, Green, Carnes, & Campling (2016)
Possible Variations	
Review of autism spectrum disorder and its relations to sexual behaviors, including exhibitionism (consists of 42 articles).	Beddows & Brooks (2016)

Summary	Reference
Case study of exhibitionistic behavior in a 42-year-old man who used exposing behavior as a way of coping with trauma-related emotions.	Petri-Kelvasa & Shulte-Herbruggen (2017)
Case study of 11-year-old boy with cerebral X-linked adrenoleukodystrophy who displayed exhibitionistic behaviors.	Zheng, Lin, Ye, & Shi (2017)
Male with acquired brain injury used sex worker to reduce and extinguish problematic sexual behaviors (including exhibitionism).	Glenn & Grahame (2011)
Case study of a 67-year-old man with Parkinson's disease and exhibitionism treated with L-dopa and bromocriptine.	Pinggera et al. (2009)
Case study of patient convicted for exhibitionism with previously undiagnosed Huntington's disease.	Mondon et al. (2008)
Treatment	
Case study of using Prozac and Provera to treat 31-year-old man with exhibitionism with an intellectual disability.	Rea, Dixon, Zettle, & Wright (2017)
Case study of 26-year-old male treated with oxcarbazepine. After increasing the dose of oxcarbazepine, his exhibitionistic urges reduced.	Corretti & Baldi (2010)
Book Chapters	
Ball, C. J., & Seghorn, T. K. (2011). Diagnosis and treatment of exhibitionism and other sexual compulsive disorders. In B. K. Schwartz (Ed.), *Handbook for sex offender treatment* (pp. 1–17). Kingston, NJ: Civic Research Institute.	
Balon, R. (2016). Exhibitionistic disorder. In R. Balon (Ed.), *Practical guide to paraphilia and paraphilic disorders* (pp. 77–91). Cham, Switzerland: Springer.	
Hocken, K., & Thorne, K. (2012). Voyeurism, exhibitionism and other non-contact sexual offences. In B. Winder & P. Banyward (Eds.), *A psychologist's casebook of crime: From arson to voyeurism* (pp. 243–262). London: Palgrave Macmillan.	
Krueger, R. B., & Kaplan, M. S. (2016). Noncontact paraphilic sexual offenses. In A. Phenix (Ed.), Sexual offending: Predisposing antecedents, assessments and management (pp. 79–102). New York, NY: Springer.	
Levenson, J. S. (2014). Exhibitionism: A case study. In W. T. O'Donohue (Ed.), *Case studies in sexual deviance: Toward evidence-based practice* (pp. 149–167). New York, NY: Routledge/Taylor & Francis.	

Summary	Reference
Morin, J. W., & Levenson, J. S. (2008). Exhibitionism: Assessment and treatment. In D. R. Laws (Ed.), *Sexual deviance: Theory, assessment, and treatment* (pp. 76–107). New York, NY: Guilford.	
Murphy, W. D., & Page, I. J. (2008). Exhibitionism: Psychopathology and theory. In D. R. Laws & W. T. O'Donohue (Eds.), *Sexual deviance: Theory, assessment, and treatment* (pp. 61–75). New York, NY: Guilford.	

References

Abel, G. G., & Rouleau, J. L. (1990). The nature and extent of sexual assault. In W. L. Marshall, D. R. Laws, & H. E. Barbaree (Eds.), *Handbook of sexual assault: Issues, theories, and treatment of the offender* (pp. 9–22). New York, NY: Springer.

American Psychiatric Association. (2013). *Diagnostic and statistical manual of mental disorders* (5th ed.). Arlington, VA: American Psychiatric Publishing.

Bader, S. M., Schoeneman-Morris, K. A., Scalora, M. J., & Casady, T. K. (2008). Exhibitionism: Findings from a Midwestern police contact sample. *International Journal of Offender Therapy and Comparative Criminology, 52*(3), 270–279.

Ball, C. J., & Seghorn, T. K. (2011). Diagnosis and treatment of exhibitionism and other sexual compulsive disorders. In B. K. Schwartz (Ed.), *Handbook for sex offender treatment* (pp. 1–17). Kingston, NJ: Civic Research Institute.

Balon, R. (2016). Exhibitionistic disorder. In R. Balon (Ed.), *Practical guide to paraphilia and paraphilic disorders* (pp. 77–91). Cham, Switzerland: Springer.

Beddows, N., & Brooks, R. (2016). Inappropriate sexual behaviour in adolescents with autism spectrum disorder: What education is recommended and why. *Early Intervention in Psychiatry, 10*(4), 282–289.

Corretti, G., & Baldi, I. (2010). Oxcarbazepine reduces exhibitionist urges and behaviors in a paraphilic patient. *Archives of Sexual Behavior, 39*(5), 1025–1026.

Fedoroff, J. P. (2010). Paraphilic worlds. In S. B. Levine (Ed.), *Handbook of clinical sexuality for mental health professionals* (pp. 401–424). New York, NY: Routledge.

Freund, K. (1990). Courtship disorder. In W. L. Marshall, D. R. Laws, & H. E. Barbaree (Eds.), *Handbook of sexual assault: Issues, theories, and treatment of the offender* (pp. 195–207). New York, NY: Springer.

Freund, K., & Blanchard, R. (1986). The concept of courtship disorder. *Journal of Sex & Marital Therapy*, 12, 79–92.

Hanafy, I., Clervoy, L., & Brenot, P. (2016). Exhibitionists, so much inhibition . . . . *Sexologies, 25*(4), e61–e63

Hingsburger, D., Griffiths, D., & Quinsey, V. (1991). Detecting counterfeit deviance. *Habilitative Mental Healthcare, 9*, 51–54.

Hocken, K., & Thorne, K. (2012). Voyeurism, exhibitionism and other non-contact sexual offences. In B. Winder & P. Banyward (Eds.), *A psychologist's casebook of crime: From arson to voyeurism*. London: Palgrave Macmillan.

Hopkins, T. A., Green, B. A., Carnes, P. J., & Campling, S. (2016). Varieties of intrusion: Exhibitionism and voyeurism. *Sexual Addiction Compulsivity, 23*(1), 4–33.

Kafka, M. P. (2003). Sex offending and sexual appetite: The clinical and theoretical relevance of hypersexual desire. *International Journal of Offender Therapy and Comparative Criminology, 47*(4), 439–451.

Kafka, M. P. (2010). Hypersexual disorder: A proposed diagnosis for DSM-V. *Archives of Sexual Behavior, 39*, 377–400.

Kaylor, L., Jeglic, E. L., & Collins, C. (2016). Examining the impact of technology on exhibitionistic behavior. *Deviant Behavior, 37*(10), 1152–1162.

Kelly, G., & Simpson, G. (2011). Remediating serious inappropriate sexual behavior in a male with severe acquired brain injury. *Sexuality and Disability, 29*(4), 313–327.

Krueger, R. B., & Kaplan, M. S. (2016). Noncontact paraphilic sexual offenses. In A. Phenix (Ed.), *Sexual offending: Predisposing antecedents, assessments and management* (pp. 79–102). New York, NY: Springer.

Långström, N. (2010). The DSM diagnostic criteria for exhibitionism, voyeurism, and frotteurism. *Archives of Sexual Behavior, 39*(2), 317–324.

Långström, N., & Seto, M. C. (2006). Exhibitionistic and voyeuristic behavior in a Swedish national population survey. *Archives of Sexual Behavior, 35*(4). 427–435. doi:10.1007/s10508-006-9042-6

Levenson, J. S. (2014). Exhibitionism: A case study. In W. T. O'Donohue (Ed.), *Case studies in sexual deviance: Toward evidence-based practice* (pp. 149–167). New York, NY: Routledge/Taylor & Francis.

Marshall, W. L., Law, D. R., & Barbaree, H. E. (1990). *Handbook of sexual assault: Issues, theories, and treatment of the offender*. New York, NY: Springer.

McNally, M. R., & Fremouw, W. J. (2014). Examining risk of escalation: A critical review of the exhibitionistic behavior literature. *Aggression and Violent Behavior, 19*(5), 474–485.

Mondon, K., Beaufils, E., Marqué, A., de Toffol, B., Constans, T., & Hommet, C. (2008). A case report of exhibitionist behaviour revealing unsuspected Huntington's disease: A pitfall in forensic medicine. *Journal of Forensic and Legal Medicine, 15*(7), 467–468.

Morin, J. W., & Levenson, J. S. (2008). Exhibitionism: Assessment and treatment. In D. R. Laws (Ed.), *Sexual deviance: Theory, assessment, and treatment* (pp. 76–107). New York, NY: Guilford.

Murphy, L., Bradford, J. B., & Fedoroff, J. P. (2014). Paraphilia and paraphilic disorders. In G. O. Gabbard (Ed.), *Gabbard's treatments of psychiatric disorders* (pp. 669–694). Washington, DC: American Psychiatric Publishing.

Murphy, W. D., & Page, I. J. (2008). Exhibitionism: Psychopathology and theory. In D. R. Laws & W. T. O'Donohue (Eds.), *Sexual deviance: Theory, assessment, and treatment* (pp. 61–75). New York, NY: Guilford.

Petri-Kelvasa, M., & Schulte-Herbruggen, O. (2017). Disinhibited exposing behavior, hypersexuality, and erectile dysfunction as a consequence of posttraumatic stress in a 42-year-old male patient. *Archives of Sexual Behavior, 46*(7), 2197–2205.

Pinggera, G. M., Pichler, R., Rehder, P., Kerschbaumer, A., Buttazzoni, A., Zangerl, F., & Mitterberger, M. (2009). Penile strangulation in a patient with Parkinson's disease: A case report. *Cases Journal, 2*(1), 9379.

Raley, J. A. (2011). Etiology of exhibitionism in adolescence: A case example of countershame theory. *Adolescent Psychiatry, 1*(2), 179–183.

Rea, J. A., Dixon, M. R., Zettle, R. D., & Wright, K. L. (2017). The development of in vivo measures to assess the impact of sex-drive reducing medications in an offender with an intellectual disability. *Archives of Sexual Behavior, 46*(3), 843–859.

Riordan, S. (1999). Indecent exposure: The impact upon the victim's fear of sexual crime. *Journal of Forensic Psychiatry, 10*(2), 309–316. doi:10.1080/09585189908403684

Swindell, S., Stroebel, S. S., O'Keefe, S. L., Beard, K. W., Robinett, S. R., & Kommor, M. J. (2011). Correlates of exhibition-like experiences in childhood and adolescence: A model for development of exhibitionism in heterosexual males. *Sexual Addiction & Compulsivity, 18*(3), 135–156.

Taylor, F. H. (1947). Observations on some cases of exhibitionism. *Journal of Mental Science, 93*(392), 631–638.

Tuch, R. H. (2008). Unravelling the riddle of exhibitionism: A lesson in the power tactics of perverse interpersonal relationships. *International Journal of Psychoanalysis, 89*(1), 143–160.

World Health Organization. (2017). *International classification of diseases*. Geneva, Switzerland: Author. Retrieved from http://apps.who.int/classifications/icd11/browse/f/en#/http%3a%2f%2fid.who.int%2ficd%2fentity%2f141881468

Zheng, F., Lin, Z., Ye, X., & Shi, X. (2017). Unusual brain images of a boy with adolescent cerebral X-linked adrenoleukodystrophy presenting with exhibitionism: A CARE-compliant case report. *Medicine, 96*(51), e9481.

4
Fetishistic Disorders

> A fetish is a story masquerading as an object.
>
> —Robert Stoller (1985)

Introduction

The term *fetish* was originally used to describe inanimate objects that had religious or spiritual significance. By the early 20th century, the term was also used to describe the condition of being sexually aroused by a specific inanimate object or class of objects (Bullough, 1995). Since then, fetishism has expanded to include reference to a sexual interest in animate objects (e.g., body parts) and/or specific sexual activities (e.g., sex in dangerous places) or a combination of both an object and activity (e.g., transvestic fetishism). This is problematic because virtually any paraphilia can be called a fetish (i.e., "people with pedophilia have fetishes for children" or "people with sadism have a fetish for humiliation"), leading to diagnostic confusion. This chapter deals with fetishes as defined by the Fifth edition of the *Diagnostic and Statistical Manual of Mental Disorders* (DSM-5; American Psychiatric Association [APA], 2013).

The DSM-5 defines *fetishistic disorder* as a condition consisting of "recurrent, and intense sexual arousal from either the use of nonliving objects or a highly specific focus on nongenital body part(s), as manifested by fantasies, urges, or behaviors" (APA, 2013, p. 700). The B criteria state the fetish must cause "clinically significant distress or impairment in social, occupational, or other important areas of functioning," and the C criteria specify that the fetish objects must not be limited to "articles of clothing used in cross-dressing . . . or devices specifically designed for the purpose of tactile genital stimulation (e.g. vibrators)" (p. 700). The DSM-5 states that fetishes can develop prior to adolescence and occur "nearly exclusively in males".

The 10th revision of the *International Classification of Diseases* (ICD-10; World Health Organization, 2004) has a similar definition of fetishism (F65.0):

> Reliance on some non-living object as a stimulus for sexual arousal and sexual gratification. Many fetishes are extensions of the human body, such as articles of clothing or footwear. Other common examples are characterized by some particular texture

such as rubber, plastic, or leather. Fetish objects vary in their importance to the individual: in some cases, they serve simply to enhance sexual excitement achieved in ordinary ways (e.g. having the partner wear a particular garment).

Diagnostic Guidelines

Fetishism should be diagnosed only if the fetish is the most important source of sexual stimulation or essential for satisfactory sexual response.

Fetishistic fantasies are common, but they do not amount to a disorder unless they lead to rituals that are so compelling and unacceptable as to interfere with sexual intercourse and cause the individual distress.

Fetishism is limited almost exclusively to males.

The ICD-11 will likely delete fetishism from its list of diseases (Krueger et al., 2017) because fetishes do not inherently involve nonconsent or harm to self or others, and in fact, inclusion of fetishism may lead to unintended stigmatization (Reiersøl & Skeid, 2006). The same arguments have been made concerning fetishistic transvestism (F65.1) and sadomasochism (F65.5).

This situation highlights how the intent of the classification system affects what is deemed important. The DSM is intended primarily to diagnose psychiatric disorders and to "ascertain" variants that are preclinical. The ICD is intended primarily to facilitate epidemiologic surveys of diseases.

Medicine is replete with syndromes that are variants of normal (e.g., Makowicz, Poniatowska, & Lusawa, 2013). Identifying, classifying, and naming both normal and pathologic variations is worthwhile because it helps more accurately identify conditions. Some normal variations may be associated with concurrent conditions or identify vulnerabilities or protections against diseases or disorders. The best classification systems are ones that are comprehensive but also based on an accurate understanding of what is being classified. For example, the classification of the orbits of the planets proposed by Copernicus is better than that of Ptolemy because Copernicus based his classification on a system in which the sun and not the earth was the center of the solar system (see Chapter 1, this book). In other words, provided the system is based on true premises, the more comprehensive the classification system, the better. How the system is used and for what purpose is another matter. For example, although it is true that being diagnosed as having a fetish may cause that person to feel "stigmatized," in the Sexual Behaviours Clinic (SBC), people with fetishes typically express relief to discover their fetish is a well-described condition that not only is known but that has a name. Whether the fetish requires treatment and what type of treatment should be tried is another matter.

Variations

The literature on fetishes is confusing because the word "fetish" is used in so many ways. People talk about having a "fetish" for anything about which they are preoccupied, including nonsexual objects, activities, and ideas. What we know about fetishes derives from studies of people who were arrested for sex crimes and who also happen to have fetishes that they disclosed or from surveys of people with self-identified fetishes who have never committed a crime. The third, and smallest, group consists of people with fetishes who sought assessment or treatment on their own (or at the insistence of their sexual partner or partners).

In her blog, Greta Christina (2010) writes about a new fetish for hairbrushes she personally acquired. In the article, she speculates that her interest in hairbrushes developed due to her use of sadomasochistic pornography during masturbation. Of interest are several comments from other women who also describe acquired fetishistic interests.

Theories of Etiology

Everyone can describe features they find maximally sexually arousing. For example, people self-identify as being "leg men" or "preferring blondes." Many of these preferences are culturally determined or acquired from experience. For example, until recently, there was sufficient interest by men in the United Kingdom to support the "Mackintosh Society," which is a rubber fetishist club based on Mackintosh rain coats that are virtually unknown in North America. Recent reports indicate that membership in both leather bars and the Mackintosh Society has decreased due to changing fashion interests. Men and women in Japan have founded interest groups based on a variety of fetishistic interests, including *oshouji* (writing on a woman's body), *omorashi* (full bladder), and arousal from watching women lick doorknobs (Griffiths, n.d.). These "fetishes" involve acts or situations rather than objects.

Fetishes and Phobias

More traditional fetishes involve sexual interest in feet, shoes, gloves, rubber, leather, panties (soiled or clean), hair, fur, and so on. Why these items? One explanation is that fetishes are analogous to phobias. Any item or situation can become a phobic stimulus through pairing of a traumatic or anxiety-inducing situation and the item or situation. The theory is that people have genes that predispose to phobias involving things that might be dangerous, such as darkness, heights, snakes, or insects. By analogy, items that are prone to become fetishized tend to be those with specific odors or textures.

Transitional Objects and Behavior

Another idea is that fetishes represent sexualized transitional objects. Most people can remember having a favorite blanket or doll when they were a child. That item becomes the thing that the child reaches for when upset or anxious. It can become a "transitional object" that the child relies on for comfort when the child's parents are not around (Winnicott, 1953). In some cases, the transitional object becomes associated with sexual arousal and is eroticized (see Chapter 8, this book).

Most theories about fetishes involve the behavioral perspective (e.g., Abel, Coffey, & Osborn, 2008). It is of interest that the one animal model of paraphilias involves a learned "leather fetish" in rats (Pfaus, Kippin, & Centeno, 2001).

Fetishes and the Disease Perspective

An important aspect of transvestic fetishism is its association in some cases with brain pathology. Epstein (1973) described a man with boot and raincoat fetishism and four men with variants of transvestic fetishism, all of whom had demonstrated brain pathology, focused primarily in the left temporal lobe. There is also a case report of a man with temporal lobe epilepsy who also had a safety pin fetish that was cured following an anterior temporal lobectomy (Mitchell, Falconer, & Hill, 1954).

Case Report 4.1

A young man was referred to a clinic in Saskatchewan, Canada, due to a "sexual problem." He had a lengthy history of substance use and gang-related criminal activities. On his first visit, he wanted assurance of confidentiality. He had a scrapbook with him in which he proudly displayed newspaper articles documenting, as he put it, "being arrested by a SWAT team in every province in Canada." He was proud of his criminal past but had a secret. He explained that he had been "perfectly normal" sexually until he was in a single-vehicle accident in which he drove his motorcycle into a tree. He claimed it was accidental and not a suicide attempt. He dramatically described waking up in the hospital:

> I was lying on my back with a brace on my neck so I could hardly move. Then a nurse walked into the room and I could hear her nylons rubbing together. I have never been so turned on and I could not even see the nurse. It was the sound of her nylons. Since then, nylons are all I think about when I think about sex. I want to wear them and even know their colors but I like any color. Before, if I knew a guy liked nylons I would beat him up. Now I am one of them!

Treatment in this case involved educating him about the likelihood that his new fetish may be secondary to his head trauma. He had a closed head injury, and the exact nature of his brain injury was not localized. Once he knew his fetish could be due to head injury, he lost interest in treatment of his fetish, which he had come to enjoy. A few months later, a call was received from the closed head injury program where he went for treatment of his head injury. The caller expressed concern about the fact that the patient had rented a van and was arranging for men at the head injury center to visit with prostitutes who were in the van. When he was confronted, he said, "Doctor, can you blame me? I identified a need!"

The patient's observation was correct that survivors of head injury (and other neurologic pathology) often have unmet sexual wishes that are ignored by treatment providers. It is notable that this patient reported that after his head injury he was unable to reach orgasm unless he was wearing nylons. Fedoroff, Peyser, Franz, and Folstein (1994) conducted a study on a series of men and women with Huntington's disease. They found that novel paraphilias emerged following the onset of inhibited orgasm. The proposed explanation, supported by patient interviews, is that men who have difficulty reaching orgasm often resort to paraphilic fantasies or behaviors in an attempt to facilitate orgasm.

Assessment and Treatment Recommendations

The most important aspect in the assessment and treatment of sexual fetishes is to determine why the person is seeking treatment. As indicated previously, there is nothing intrinsically wrong with sexual fetishes per se, so it is important to learn what caused the person to seek help now. Sometimes it is an event such as being caught using the fetish object or having their collection of fetish objects found. Sometimes it is the realization by the person's sexual partner that the fetish is more important for sexual arousal than the person. Occasionally, the preoccupation with the fetish becomes too much of a distraction to be ignored.

Case Report 4.2

One day, a middle-aged man in a tailored business suit arrived for his appointment precisely on time. In the waiting room, he tapped on his pocket watch. He was nervous but was also anxious to discuss his problem. He explained that he had a shoe fetish that began when he was a young boy. The fetish had been persistent, but he had managed to keep it secret. He had been successful in business and was now married and had children. Asked why he had sought help for his "problem" now, he took a deep breath and explained:

> Doctor, my fetish is for men's shoes. Leather shoes. I am straight and have no interest in men but men's leather shoes are extremely sexually arousing to me. I do not care if they are new or used, as long as they are leather and are men's shoes. I have an ordinary interest in women's shoes, especially high heels, but it is only in relation to the woman wearing them. For my fetish, it is the shoes alone. In fact, seeing a man in them is a turn off, I am just aroused by the shoes. But you asked me, why now? Why have I come to you now? The answer is because I can no longer afford my fetish. I have bought so many pairs of shoes that I had to rent a very large storage locker to hold them. The locker is now stuffed with shoes, most are in boxes that have never been opened. But I just cannot keep buying shoes and I cannot afford to rent another locker!

This person is instructive on several levels. First, he presents as a classic shoe fetishist. He recalled onset of the interest when he was a child, even before it was associated with identified sexual feelings. The fetish object typically has a characteristic feel and/or smell. Leather fulfills both of these fetishistic tactile and olfactory criteria. Although fetish objects are often gendered (e.g., lingerie and shoes), they often do not associate with the gender or orientation of the person with the fetish. For example, this man was heterosexual, but his sexual fetish was directed toward men's shoes. Similarly, most people with transvestic fetishism are aroused by women's clothes but gender identify as male and have a heterosexual orientation.

The man in this case said he could no longer afford his fetish and that was true, not so much because he did not have enough money but because it was costing his relationship due to increasing difficulties keeping his fetish secret from his wife. An added issue that he did not immediately disclose was the onset of some problems maintaining an erection during intercourse with his wife. People with fetishes sometimes rely more on their fetish for arousal during times when they have sexual dysfunctions.

Treatment began by reminding the man that he was in control of his own finances. When he said he could not possibly stop buying shoes, he was advised to cut up the credit card with which he used to secretly charge his purchases. Next, therapy focused on helping him dissociate the sexual arousal of his fetish from the anxiety-reducing aspects of his fetish. This proved to be a very effective strategy, likely due to the fact that much of his shoe hoarding resembled an anxiety-related obsessive–compulsive disorder (OCD). He was encouraged to keep track of when he felt the urge to buy shoes, and he soon noticed this happened when he was under stress at work or in relations with his wife. Due to his anxiety and OCD-like symptoms, he was offered and accepted a treatment trial with a selective serotonin reuptake inhibitor (SSRI), which greatly improved his symptoms. Readers will note that none of these interventions directly targeted his sexual fetish. As his anxiety and OCD symptoms remitted, his concerns about his fetish decreased. He was asked if he wanted to include his wife in the treatment, which caused him to literally gasp. His entire relationship with his wife had centered around what he thought was his successful ability to hide his fetish from her. However, when asked if he would have come for treatment if he had not been married, he laughed and said "of course not." He now realized it was his relationship with his wife, and not his finances or his fetish, that had motivated him to seek help.

At his next appointment, his wife was at his side. They were holding hands. Of course, the therapist had no idea what she knew, so he began by explaining the rules of confidentiality. The patient interrupted to say, "I told her everything." His wife confirmed he had told her about his shoe fetish and the storage shed and secret credit card. She said she had been aware of missing money and had worried he was having an affair. The shoes were a relief, but she wondered, because he had a shoe fetish, whether he also had other unconventional sexual interests. Those were not her words. She asked, "Is he a pervert?" She had heard that people with fetishes often were "perverts" who could deteriorate and become sex offenders.

Treatment involved educating her about the fact that studies on alleged sexual deterioration and an association between fetishes and sex crimes all had significant flaws. Most people with fetishes are remarkably true to their single fetish. For example, her husband had no special interest in boots, sneakers, sandals, women's shoes, or even feet. The remainder of therapy focused on improving communication between her and her husband and rebuilding the trust that had been threatened by his wife's suspicion he was having an affair with another woman. In the context of substantial improvement in the couple's relationship, both marital and sexual, the shoes "lost their power." This loss of dependence in the fetish when it became an interest known to his wife is typical. John Money stated, "Paraphilias are like mushrooms, they grow well in the dark" (personal communication, 1996–2001). Fortunately, the reverse is also true.

Krafft-Ebing and Rebman (1906) described a man (Case 72) who had erectile dysfunction when he was with women that he overcame with masochistic fantasies and a shoe/boot fetish. He "cured" himself of the fetish by a self-devised behavioral reconditioning program in which he kissed "an elegant boot" every day while asking himself why he was so aroused by the boot. With time, he stopped having erections when he thought of shoes and was able to have intercourse, although he occasionally still had masochistic fantasies.

Fetish as an Aid to Treatment

Case Report 4.3

A somewhat disheveled middle-aged man called to book an appointment in the SBC clinic. He was clearly anxious when he was seen the next day. In response to questions, he said he was self-referred and had never been charged or convicted of any sex offenses. He was single and had never been in a romantic relationship. He was working on a PhD, but it had taken too long for him to complete so his committee had told him to discontinue his studies. He was "between jobs." Asked why he had come to the SBC, with some trepidation he admitted, "I masturbate . . . while I watch people hanging. I know that is wrong. I can't stop doing it." He offered assurances he had never acted on his sexual fantasy with a person or an animal. He was offered treatment.

As part of the assessment, he was examined with phallometry, which confirmed arousal from scenarios involving people (women more than men) being hanged to death. On further discussion, it was discovered that his primary source of arousal was not the idea of harm to the victims or death or strangulation. His arousal derived from the characteristic twitching of the toes seen in people who are being asphyxiated. On further testing, it was established that he had a foot fetish and a "tickle fetish," both of which he had not been fully aware of.

He was told to stop viewing hangings (which he found easily on the Internet). He found it difficult to masturbate without viewing hanging videos, so it was suggested he instead seek out foot fetish videos (also easily accessible on the Internet). He found this reasonably satisfactory, but when he discovered a website devoted to women being tickled, he was ecstatic, especially when the camera focused on the women's feet. He was able to completely replace his worrisome hanging fantasies with materials that most would not even recognize as pornographic.

Case Report 4.3 highlights several aspects of paraphilia treatment. The first is that people do self-refer, and the SBC has noticed this is an increasing trend. The second is that people are often frightened to disclose their sexual interests even when they have not committed any crimes. Third is the way phallometry can be used not to determine guilt or innocence but, rather, to more fully explore sexual arousal patterns. Finally, Case Report 4.3 illustrates how nonharmful sexual fetishes (in this case, feet and tickling) can assist in modifying and eventually completely replacing worrisome sexual interest such as hanging. For the man in Case

Table 4.1 Summary of the Literature on the Efficacy of Treatments of Fetishes

Treatment	*N*	Results	Comment	References
Masturbatory satiation	1	Almost complete cure (confirmed with phallometry)	Pantyhose fetish	Marshall & Lippens (1977)
Covert sensitization	1	Complete elimination of fetish	Shoe fetish (retifism)	Kunjukrishnan, Pawlak, & Varan (1988)
Behavioral + cognitive–behavioral therapy	76	70 had favorable results	Multiple paraphilias	Lowenstein (1997)
Buspirone	1	Complete remission; remitted when medication stopped	Transvestic fetishism	Fedoroff (1988)
Buspirone	1	Complete remission	Atypical paraphilia	Fedoroff & Fedoroff (1992)

Report 4.3, treatment at this stage is now focused on helping him establish healthy friendships and relationships with women. He has recently started dating for the first time in his life and reports he never thought he would be able to do so. It is expected he will continue to do well.

Prognosis

Table 4.1 summarizes the brief literature concerning the efficacy of various treatments of fetishes. Review of the table, although based almost entirely on case reports, indicates that fetishes respond well to treatment.

One review of published cases (Fedoroff, 1994) of various paraphilias with SSRIs found that all but two papers reported successful results. The two negative papers were notable for the fact that they reported on treatments with SSRIs using doses usually used to treat OCD. Unfortunately, at those doses, inhibited orgasm is a frequent occurrence. Fedoroff noted that people with fetishes (and other paraphilias) tend to revert back to their paraphilic fantasies in order to achieve orgasm. It has been the SBC's experience that SSRIs are more effective in treating fetishes, and other paraphilias, when they are used at doses that are low enough to not cause inhibited orgasm.

Sexual fetishes are very much an understudied aspect of human sexuality. They provide a means to investigate unconventional sexual interests (paraphilias) that typically are not criminal. Unfortunately, because they are rarely associated with crime, people with fetishes are less often seen in clinics such as the SBC. The SBC is currently recruiting for a study comparing the neuroimaging of men with pedophilia to men with fetishes, and it is hoped the results of that study will be available in the future.

In the meantime, people who have sexual fetishes should be assured that they can look forward to satisfying and fulfilling sexual lives. In fact, their fetish may enhance their sexuality by providing a reliable source of sexual arousal. If the fetish interferes with a person's life due to concerns about stigma, education about the benign nature of most fetishes is helpful. If the fetish interferes because it causes relationship problems, couple's therapy is helpful. If the fetish interferes due to replacement of other healthy sexual acts, assessment in a clinic such as the SBC is in order because multiple treatments based on behavioral, pharmacologic, and/or psychotherapeutic interventions are effective.

Review of the Literature

The following table summarizes the literature that has been published on "fetishism" or "fetishistic disorder" from 2008 to 2018 based on PsycINFO and PubMed searches.

Summary	Reference
Etiology	
Fetishism may develop during childhood. Fetishism seems to be associated with altered temporal lobe function.	Masuda, Ishitobi, Tanaka, & Akiyoshi (2014)
Case study of a 41-year-old man whose fetish with wearing women's underwear seemed to coexist with his methamphetamine use. When he used more methamphetamine, his fetish/cross-dressing symptoms increased.	Mehdizadeh-Zareanari, Ghafarinezhad, & Soltani (2013)
Investigated whether critical period exists for the acquisition of "sexual preferences." The authors believe that their findings support a critical period of 1½–5 years of age for acquiring sexual preferences.	Enguist, Aronsson, Ghirlanda, Jansson, & Jannini (2011)
Author suggests that circumstances (including trauma) can create and support fetishes.	Weisel-Barth (2013)
Author suggests that fetishes develop from the acquisition of "errors in locating erotic targets in the environment."	Lawrence (2009b)
A literature review of erotic target location errors, their etiology, and suggestions for the DSM-5.	Lawrence (2009b)
Case study of a woman in her 20s with depression who was sexually aroused by diapers.	Cernovsky & Bureau (2016)
Examined smoking fetish videos on YouTube.	Kim, Paek, & Lynn (2010)

Summary	Reference
Case study of a 32-year-old man with fetishism and kleptomania.	Oncu, Turkcan, Canbek, Yessilbursa, & Uygur (2009)
Discusses the possibility that transvestic fetishism and male-to-female transsexualism could be "outgrowths of autogynephilia."	Lawrence (2009c)
Case histories of individuals with deviant sexual interests and the development of these sexual interests, which are believed to have stemmed from early childhood.	Abel, Coffey, & Osborn (2008)
Literature review of infantilism, diaperism, and pedophilia.	Doshi, Zanzrukiya, & Kumar (2018)
Explored whether the enjoyment of adult baby/ diaper lover behavior was related to relationships with their parents, attachment style, negative mood, and gender.	Zamboni (2017)
Case study of a 22-year-old man with Williams syndrome and a glove fetish who assaulted women to get their gloves.	Noguchi & Kato (2010)
Interview of a former escort woman and stripper catering to men with fetishes. The most frequent requests (involving fetishes) were foot or shoe fetish, selling her underwear, and selling her underwear after urinating in it.	Cernovsky (2016)
Mixed methods study found that individuals with a fetish do not require the object to be present to enjoy sexual activities and it is not required for sexual arousal, but it is preferred for the fetish object to be present.	Rees & Garcia (2017a)
Mixed methods study found that having solitary fetish activity was just as satisfying as engaging in partner fetish activity.	Rees & Garcia (2017b)
Escalation to Contact Offense	
Case review of 47-year-old man whose fetish developed to sadism. It was found that he had gliotic scars in his frontal lobe and right hippocampus.	Nedopil et al. (2008)
Diagnosis	
DSM Criticisms	
History and definition of sexual fetishism in the DSM, and its relation to partialism.	Kafka (2010)

Summary	Reference
Treatment	
Case study of a 57-year-old man using behavioral activation and sensate-focused therapy to treat foot fetishism and co-occurring anxiety symptoms.	Sarver & Gros (2014)
Case study of a 40-year-old man who had a fetish toward women's underwear and was treated with naltrexone. Fetishism remitted.	Firoz, Sankar, Rajmohan, Kumar, & Raghuram (2014)
Case study of a man with a mild learning disability and autism, who had a fetish with baby paraphernalia and was treated with a psycho-educational intervention.	Cambridge (2013)
Case study of 13-year-old male with autistic disorder and fetishism. His fetish was successfully treated using mirtazapine 15 mg daily.	Coskun & Mukaddes (2008)
Case study of 14-year-old male with attention-deficit/hyperactivity disorder and fetishistic behavior who was treated with methylphenidate and cognitive-rational emotive psychotherapy.	Chang & Chow (2011)
Case study of a man with autism who had a fetish for women wearing sandals. It was found that a response-interruption/time-out procedure eliminated the behavior.	Dozier, Iwata, & Worsdell (2011)
Case study of a 3½-year-old male displaying arousal from seeing female legs, feet, and stockings. He was diagnosed with fetishism of these objects and treated with risperidone. His fetish symptoms remitted when he was 6½ years old.	Zarei & Bidaki (2013)
Books and Book Chapters	
Bass, A. (2018). *Fetishism, psychoanalysis, and philosophy: The iridescent thing.* New York, NY: Routledge/Taylor & Francis.	
Darcangelo, S., Hollings, A., & Paladino, G. (2008). Fetishism: Assessment and treatment. In D. R. Laws & W. T. O'Donohue (Eds.), *Sexual deviance: Theory, assessment, and treatment* (2nd ed., pp. 119–130). New York, NY: Guilford.	
Hinman, M. (2013). Understanding clients with alternative expressions of sexuality using music. In S. Loue (Ed.), *Expressive therapies for sexual issues: A social work perspective* (pp. 137–155). New York, NY: Springer.	

References

American Psychiatric Association. (2013). *Diagnostic and statistical manual of mental disorders* (5th ed.). Arlington, VA: American Psychiatric Publishing.

Bass, A. (2018). *Fetishism, psychoanalysis, and philosophy: The iridescent thing*. New York, NY: Routledge/Taylor & Francis.

Bullough, V. L. (1995). *Science in the bedroom: A history of sex research*. New York, NY: Basic Books.

Cambridge, P. (2013). A rights approach to supporting the sexual fetish of a man with learning disability: Method, process and applied learning. *British Journal of Learning Disabilities, 41*(4), 259–265.

Cernovsky, Z., & Bureau, Y. (2016). Lady with erotic preference for diapers. *Mental Illness, 8*(2), 6687.

Cernovsky, Z. Z. (2016). Fetishistic preferences of clients as ranked by a sex worker. *Journal of Sex & Marital Therapy, 42*(6), 481–483.

Chang, H. L., & Chow, C. C. (2011). The treatment of fetishism in an adolescent with attention deficit hyperactivity disorder. *Chang Gung Medical Journal, 34*(4), 440–443.

Coskun, M., & Mukaddes, N. M. (2008). Mirtazapine treatment in a subject with autistic disorder and fetishism. *Journal of Child and Adolescent Psychopharmacology, 18*(2), 206–209.

Christina, Greta. (2010). https://the-orbit.net/greta/2010/02/23/the-learn/ (retrieved July 21, 2019).

Darcangelo, S., Hollings, A., & Paladino, G. (2008). Fetishism: Assessment and treatment. In D. R. Laws & W. T. O'Donohue (Eds.), *Sexual deviance: Theory, assessment, and treatment* (2nd ed., pp. 119–130). New York, NY: Guilford.

Doshi, S. M., Zanzrukiya, K., & Kumar, L. (2018). Paraphilic infantilism, diaperism and pedophilia: A review. *Journal of Forensic and Legal Medicine, 56*, 12–15. doi:10.1016/j.jflm.2018.02.026

Dozier, C. L., Iwata, B. A., & Worsdell, A. S. (2011). Assessment and treatment of foot-shoe fetish displayed by a man with autism. *Journal of Applied Behavior Analysis, 44*(1), 133–137. doi:10.1901/jaba.2011.44-133

Enguist, M., Aronsson, H., Ghirlanda, S., Jansson, L., & Jannini, E. A. (2011). Exposure to mother's pregnancy and lactation in infancy is associated with sexual attraction to pregnancy and lactation in adulthood. *Journal of Sexual Medicine, 8*(1), 140–147. doi:10.111/j.1743-6109.2010.02065.x

Epstein, S. (1973). The self-concept revisited: Or a theory of a theory. *American Psychologist*, 28, 404–416.

Fedoroff, J. P. (1988). Buspirone hydrochloride in the treatment of transvestic fetishism. *Journal of Clinical Psychiatry, 49*, 408–409.

Fedoroff, J. P. (1994). Serotonergic drug treatment of deviant sexual interests. *Annals of Sex Research, 6*, 105–107.

Fedoroff, J. P., & Fedoroff, I. C. (1992). Buspirone and paraphilic sexual behaviour. *Journal of Offender Rehabilitation, 18*(3–4), 89–108.

Fedoroff, J. P., Peyser, C., Franz, M. L., & Folstein, S. E. (1994). Sexual disorders in Huntington's disease. *Journal of Neuropsychiatry and Clinical Neurosciences, 6*, 147–153.

Firoz, K., Sankar, V. N., Rajmohan, V., Kumar, G. M., & Raghuram, T. M. (2014). Treatment of fetishism with naltrexone: A case report. *Asian Journal of Psychiatry, 8*, 67–68. Retrieved October 7, 2018, from http://gretachristina.typepad.com/greta_christinas_weblog/2010/02/the-learn.html

Griffiths, M. (n.d.). About Dr. Mark Griffiths [Blog]. Retrieved May 7, 2017, from https://drmarkgriffiths.wordpress.com/about

Hinman, M. (2013). Understanding clients with alternative expressions of sexuality using music. In S. Loue (Ed.), *Expressive therapies for sexual issues: A social work perspective* (pp. 137–155). New York, NY: Springer.

Kafka, M. P. (2010). The DSM diagnostic criteria for fetishism. *Archives of Sexual Behavior, 39*(2), 357–362.

Kim, K., Paek, H. J., & Lynn, J. (2010). A content analysis of smoking fetish videos on YouTube: Regulatory implications for tobacco control. *Health Communication, 25*(2), 97–106.

Krafft-Ebing, R., & Rebman, F. J. (1906). *Psychopathia sexualis: With especial reference to the antipathic sexual instinct; A medico-forensic study*. New York, NY: Rebman.

Krueger, R. B., Reed, G. M., First, M. B., Marais, A., Kismodi, E., & Briken, P. (2017). Proposals for paraphilic disorders in the International Classification of Diseases and Related Health Problems, Eleventh Revision (ICD-11). *Archives of Sexual Behavior, 46*, 1529–1545. https://doi.org/10.1007/s10508-017-0944-2

Kunjukrishnan, R., Pawlak, A., & Varan, I. R. (1988). The clinical and forensic psychiatric issues of retifism. *Canadian Journal of Psychiatry, 33*, 819–825.

Lawrence, A. A. (2009a). Anatomic autoandrophilia in an adult male. *Archives of Sexual Behavior, 38*(6), 1050–1056.

Lawrence, A. A. (2009b). Erotic target location errors: An underappreciated paraphilic dimension. *Journal of Sex Research, 46*(2–3), 194–215.

Lawrence, A. A. (2009c). Transgenderism in nonhomosexual males as a paraphilic phenomenon: Implications for case conceptualization and treatment. *Sexual and Relationship Therapy, 24*(2), 188–206.

Lowenstein, L. F. (1997). Fetishes: General and specific. *Psychotherapy in Private Practice, 16*(4), 53–65.

Makowicz, G., Poniatowska, R., & Lusawa, M. (2013). Variants of cerebral arteries. *Polish Journal of Radiology, 78*(3), 42–47. doi:10.12659/PJR.889403

Marshall, W. W., & Lippens, K. (1977). The clinical value of boredom: A procedure for reducing inappropriate sexual interests. *Journal of Nervous and Mental Disease, 165*, 283–287.

Masuda, K., Ishitobi, Y., Tanaka, Y., & Akiyoshi, J. (2014). Underwear fetishism induced by bilaterally decreased cerebral blood flow in the temporo-occipital lobe. *BMJ Case Reports*, bcr2014206019. doi:10.1136/bcr-2014-206019

Mehdizadeh-Zareanari, A., Ghafarinezhad, A., & Soltani, H. (2013). Fetishism due to methamphetamine (glass) abuse: A case report. *Addiction & Health, 5*(1–2), 73–76.

Mitchell, W., Falconer, M., & Hill, D. (1954). Epilepsy with fetishism relieved by temporal lobectomy. *Lancet, 264*(6839), 626–630. doi:10.1016/s0140-6736(54)90404-3

Nedopil, N., Blumcke, I., Bock, H., Bogerts, B., Born, C., & Stubner, S. (2008). Sadistic fetishism—Deadly passion: Forensic psychiatric assessment of sex offenders. *Der Nervenarzt, 79*(11), 1249–1262.

Noguchi, M., & Kato, S. (2010). A case of Williams syndrome with glove fetishism. *Psychiatry and Clinical Neurosciences, 64*(6), 663.

Oncu, F., Turkcan, S., Canbek, O., Yessilbursa, D., & Uygur, N. (2009). Fetishism and kleptomania: A case report in forensic psychiatry. *Noropsikiyatri Arsivi, 46*(3), 125–128.

Pfaus, J., Kippin, T., & Centeno, S. (2001). Conditioning and sexual behavior: A review. *Hormones and Behavior, 40*, 291–321. doi:10.1006/hbeh.2001.1686

Rees, G., & Garcia, J. R. (2017a). All I need is shoe: An investigation into the obligatory aspect of sexual object fetishism. *International Journal of Sexual Health, 29*(4), 303–312.

Rees, G., & Garcia, J. R. (2017b). An investigation into the solitary and interpersonal aspects of sexual object fetishism: A mixed-methods approach. *Psychology & Sexuality, 8*(4), 252–267.

Reiersø, O., & Skeid, S. (2006). The ICD Diagnoses of Fetishism and Sadomasochism. *Journal of Homosexuality, 50*(2-3), 243–262. doi:10.1300/J082v50n02_12

Sarver, N. W., & Gros, D. F. (2014). A modern behavioral treatment to address fetishism and associated functional impairment. *Clinical Case Studies, 13*(4), 336–351.

Stoller, R. (1985). *Observing the Erotic Imagination*. New Haven: Yale University Press.

Weisel-Barth, J. (2013). The fetish in Nicole Krauss' *Great House* and in clinical practice. *Psychoanalytic Dialogues, 23*(2), 180–196.

Winnicott, D. (1953). Transitional objects and transitional phenomena. *International Journal of Psychoanalysis, 34*, 89–97.

World Health Organization. (2004). *International classification of diseases* (10th revision, 2nd ed.). Geneva, Switzerland: Author.

Zamboni, B. D. (2017). Characteristics of subgroups in the adult baby/diaper lover community. *Journal of Sexual Medicine, 14*(11), 1421–1429.

Zarei, M., & Bidaki, R. (2013). Female foot fetishism disorder in childhood. *Journal of Research in Medical Sciences, 18*(2), 170.

5
Frotteuristic Disorder

Grab 'em by the pussy. You can do anything.
—Donald J. Trump (2005, as cited in Fahrenthold, 2016)

Introduction

The Fifth edition of the *Diagnostic and Statistical Manual of Mental Disorders* (DSM-5; American Psychiatric Association [APA], 2013) defines *frotteuristic disorder* as a condition consisting of "recurrent, and intense sexual arousal from touching or rubbing against a nonconsenting person, as manifested by fantasies, urges, or behaviors" (p. 691). The B criteria state the individual has "acted on the urges with a nonconsenting person or the sexual urges or fantasies cause clinically significant distress or impairment in social, occupational, or other important areas of functioning" (p. 691). The disorder can be specified as "in a controlled environment" if "opportunities to rub against a nonconsenting person are restricted" and as "in full remission" if there are no Category A or B signs or symptoms "for at least 5 years while in an uncontrolled environment" (p. 692).

The 10th revision of the *International Classification of Diseases* (World Health Organization, 2004) describes frotteurism as "rubbing up against people for sexual stimulation in a crowded public place," under the category of "Other disorders of sexual preference" (F65.8).

Diagnostic Guidelines

The DSM-5 states that frotteuristic acts may be committed by up to 30% of adult males in the general population (APA, 2013, p. 692). It also states that there is no minimum age at which the diagnosis can be assigned to a person and that the characteristics of frotteurism may "by definition" change over time (p. 693).

Differential Diagnosis

The DSM-5's suggested differential diagnoses is surprisingly brief, listing as possibilities only conduct disorder, antisocial personality disorder, and substance use disorders (p. 693).

In fact, patients often present with the complaint of feeling "compelled" to touch, especially when they know it is wrong. This combination of symptoms suggests a variant of obsessive–compulsive disorder (OCD) in which thoughts arise unbidden, leading to a perceived need to act.

Lesch–Nyhan Syndrome

Perhaps the quintessential example of a condition in which a person experiences an irresistible urge to act against their own wishes is Lesch–Nyhan syndrome. This is a rare X-linked genetic condition resulting in a deficiency of the enzyme hypoxanthine–guanine phosphoribosyltransferase (Puig et al., 2001). Individuals with this condition can tell when an urge to self-harm is coming on and will ask to be tied up or otherwise incapacitated to keep from biting their own fingers or lips. Some voluntarily elect to have their teeth removed to prevent more serious self-injury. People with this condition clearly state they do not want to harm themselves (they do not have borderline personality disorder or suicidal ideation) but feel overwhelmed by a perceived need. It is important to note that the urge to touch or self-mutilate, in this condition, is not sexually motivated.

Obsessive–Compulsive Disorder

A much more common condition associated with acting on unwanted wishes is OCD. People with OCD often experience obsessions that can involve sex-related themes, which can progress to actions. Again, it is important to investigate whether the actions are sexually motivated. Clinicians should be careful to distinguish between obsessions that involve (ego-dystonic) sexual themes and sexual preoccupations that are sexually motivated (true paraphilias). Some important differences are as follows: Sexual obsessions are always unwanted and actively avoided by the person; sexual preoccupations are enjoyed and sought after by the person; and sexual obsessions inhibit sexual arousal, whereas sexual preoccupations do the opposite. People with sexual obsessions have guilt about the idea of acting on their obsessions due to the harm that will be caused, whereas people with sexual preoccupations may have guilt about the sexual nature of their fantasies but less about the consequences of acting on their fantasies.

Smith–Magenis Syndrome

A third condition associated with frequent touching involves people with intellectual disabilities (ID). Some people with ID have a habit of seeking to shake hands repeatedly. Others try to hug, such as people with the genetic condition Smith–Magenis syndrome, caused by a deletion on chromosome 17 (Smith, Dykens, & Greenberg, 1998). In addition to nonconsensual touching, this syndrome is associated with polyembolokoilamania, which is a (nonsexual) compulsion to self-insert objects into bodily orifices, including the rectum and vagina (Ingves, Lau, Fedoroff, & Levine, 2014).

Williams Syndrome

Another genetic syndrome is Williams Syndrome, caused by micro gene deletions on chromosome. This syndrome is characterized by so-called cocktail party demeanor, in which the person is overly friendly and physically affectionate with strangers (Dykens & Rosner, 1999). People with this condition often have more advanced linguistic abilities, which can result in an overestimation of their intellectual abilities, leading to a misunderstanding of the person's intent and ability to understand how their behaviors will be perceived.

Epigenetic Syndromes

There are several epigenetic syndromes, including the so-called happy puppet syndrome (Angelman's syndrome), which is associated with happy demeanor and hand flapping, and Prader–Willi syndrome (also caused by deletions on chromosome 15 but from the paternal chromosome). People with Prader–Willi syndrome are of particular interest because they demonstrate "compulsions" to eat due to lack of satiety and to oversleep, likely secondary to sleep apnea, as well as hypogonadism. They may engage in "skin picking." People with either Angelman's syndrome or Prader–Willi syndrome can be mistakenly diagnosed as engaging in frotteuristic behaviors (Angelman, 1965; D. Clark, Boer, & Webb, 1995; Watson, Miodrag, Richards, & Fedoroff, 2012).

Counterfeit Deviance

In most cases, people with ID resort to physical behaviors because they have difficulty expressing themselves verbally. Some suffer from experiences in institutions in which they were treated like children and hugged or kissed without their consent. When they re-enact these acts with others, they may be falsely labeled as frotteuristic. This phenomenon has been described as "counterfeit deviance" (Griffiths, Quinsey, & Hingsburger, 1989).

Of course, touching does not make the diagnosis of frotteuristic disorder. The two crucial elements are that the touching is sexually motivated and that the touching is nonconsensual. Unfortunately, DSM-5 does not emphasize the fact that people with true frotteurism are aroused not only by touching but also by the fact that the touching is nonconsensual.

Case Report 5.1

A woman called the office. She was crying. She explained that her fiancé had called her from jail. They had moved in together soon after meeting each other online. He had been "between jobs" and drank a bit too much but was "otherwise charming." He had left that morning neatly dressed in a suit and tie on his way to a job interview downtown. Unfortunately, he had been detained by the transit authority and subsequently arrested. A woman had accused him of standing behind her and intentionally rubbing against her. It was crowded on the train and at first she thought the contact was accidental, but he had persisted, and she realized he had an erection.

An appointment for her fiancé was made, and the next day he arrived 15 minutes late, having been granted bail. He admitted annoyance at his predicament but claimed he had done nothing wrong, "at least not yesterday." With further qu.estioning, he admitted to engaging in similar acts when the opportunity arose, for years. Asked how he had come to be arrested on this occasion, he said he made a mistake when he had slipped the woman his business card with his cell number on it together with an "invitation" that he declined to characterize further. He admitted most women never called, but he claimed that enough did to convince him it was a good way to meet women—"cheaper than nightclubs."

The man in Case Report 5.1 would meet DSM-5 criteria for frotteuristic disorder because he acted on sexual urges with a nonconsenting person and had engaged in similar acts for years. However, a diagnosis of antisocial personality disorder (ASPD) was also considered likely. The ASPD diagnosis was confirmed when further investigation revealed a history of conduct disordered behaviors as a child and he revealed he had more than one "fiancé" on whom he relied for financial support. Of course, most people with frotteurism do not have ASPD, and most do not attempt to have follow-up contact with their victims.

Case Report 5.2

A man presented to the Sexual Behaviours Clinic (SBC) on referral from his family doctor, who wrote simply, "My patient says he heard about your clinic and is asking for a referral, not sure why."

When seen, the man also had some difficulty explaining his problem. He started by saying he was happily married and loved his wife. In response to questions, he said he was not facing any charges, and his wife was unaware of his appointment. In fact, he said he wife was unaware of the problem.

With some assurance about confidentiality, he explained. For as long as he could remember, he had been sexually aroused by feet, especially the idea of a woman whose left foot had a second toe that was longer than her third toe and a right foot in which the toe lengths were opposite. His wife had exactly the type of feet that he found maximally arousing, with the "perfect left–right foot–toe lengths." He was ashamed of this interest and had never told his wife. The reason he had come to the clinic was because he had adopted a habit of waiting until his wife fell asleep before slipping under the covers to fondle his wife's feet while he masturbated. Sometimes he would rub his penis against her toes but avoided this practice because he often ejaculated prematurely in such a stimulating situation. He said he had engaged in the same activity for as long as he had been married but was worried he might get caught and was concerned his wife would think he was a "pervert."

In interview, the man in Case Report 5.2 admitted that a large part of his arousal derived from being able to act on his fetishistic interest with no concern about disapproval from his wife. On reflection, he expanded his opinion to admit he was more aroused by the fact that his wife was unaware of his interest and acts than if she had consented. It was the idea of getting away with something forbidden that most aroused him. Diagnoses for the man in Case Report 5.2 included both a foot fetish (see Chapter 4, this book) and frotteuristic disorder.

In terms of paraphilic diagnosis, there is a clear difference between the man in Case Report 5.1 and the man in Case Report 5.2. For the man in Case Report 5.1, his frotteuristic acts were motivated by the narcissistic belief that women enjoyed his unsolicited attention, as is common in men with antisocial personality disorder. Although his act of grinding his pelvis against the buttocks of an unsuspecting woman on a crowded train car seems pathognomonic of frotteurism, the fact that he acted due to the opportunity and with the intent of subsequent contact with his victim makes his problem fundamentally different from that of the man in Case Report 5.2. For the man in Case Report 5.2, the nonconsent (unawareness) by the woman of what he was doing added to his arousal.

In the SBC clinic, the diagnosis of frotteuristic disorder is reserved for people for whom nonconsensual contact is the key sexually arousing element. By these criteria, the prevalence is likely less than the DSM-5 estimate of 30%. A further important distinction is made between people who are aroused by the idea of sexual relations with a person who actively does not consent and those who are aroused by the idea of sexual relations with a person who does not consent because they are unaware of the act.

The term frotteurism is derived from the French word *frotteur*, meaning "one who rubs." It is classically conceptualized as a man who rubs his genitals against the backside of an unsuspecting woman while both are clothed, usually in a crowded situation that permits the man to get close to the woman without arousing suspicion. However, clinicians often include other forms of physical contact (primarily by hands) under the term *toucherism*. Again, the key characteristic of both of these forms of nonconsensual touching is that they can be done surreptitiously. For example, conditions involving an attempt to kiss victims without consent have not been described, even though kissing is a common act in courtship. This may be because it is difficult to kiss surreptitiously (occasionally this happens when the victim is asleep or drugged or dead), but as noted previously, it may be because kissing on the lips is more associated with romance than sex.

Two of the best reviews of frotteurism and toucherism commented on the fact that most of the literature involves case reports (Krueger & Kaplan, 2008; Lussier & Piche, 2008). They listed clinical samples of psychiatric patients or people with a history of paraphilia-related behaviors, indicating a frequency of between 10% and 22% (both less than the prevalence reported in the DSM-5). A more recent literature review (Johnson, Ostermeyer, Sikes, Nelsen, & Coverdale, 2014) was critical of the quality of the currently available prevalence studies. This review reported possible prevalence rates of between 7.9% and 35% based of local samples.

Lussier and Piche (2008) also addressed the frequent question of whether people with frotteurism "escalate" to rape, and they concluded on the basis of the evidence at that time that such an escalation "appears to characterize only a small proportion of sex offenders" (p. 137).

Assessment and Treatment Recommendations

Krueger and Kaplan (2008) reviewed the literature and suggested a variety of assessment techniques, including careful clinical interviews, penile plethysmography, viewing time, psychological testing, and polygraphy. Their treatment recommendations included cognitive–behavioral treatment and 12-step programs. They strongly advocated for group treatment as "the most effective" (p. 157) but did not exclude individual psychotherapy, particularly for concurrent conditions such as erectile dysfunction and "frank phobia of sexual intercourse" (p. 157). These authors also reviewed the use of a variety of medications but without specific reference to studies on the pharmacologic treatment of paraphilias.

In the SBC, individuals diagnosed with frotteurism are offered group therapy in which the wrongfulness and harmfulness of their actions are pointed out by other patients. Importantly, they learn that their actions are voluntary and learn how to avoid high-risk situations. As indicated previously, patients are offered a treatment trial with a full range of medications. In the SBC, many men with frotteurism voluntarily elect to take anti-androgen medications while they reorganize their lives. This is because people with frotteurism often self-perceive their problem as being one of so-called hypersexuality. Often, however, the "hypersexuality" turns out to be sexual frustration combined with social skills incompetence.

There is a misconception that only people with impaired social skills and/or intellectual disability engage in frotteuristic acts. In fact, many people with frotteuristic disorder have normal or above average intelligence. Opportunistic frotteurs (such as the man in Case Report 5.1) simply take advantage of people in vulnerable situations. They may be in adult consenting relationships and, as indicated, simply take advantage of a chance opportunity, thinking they will get away with it, the victim will not realize what happened, and everyone will go home happy. A second type of frotteurs comprises people who intentionally seek out situations to commit frotteuristic acts—for example, intentionally taking crowded subways and standing next to victims they find sexually arousing. A third type may engage in frotteuristic acts with the specific intention of rubbing up against or touching a victim due to sexual arousal specifically from engaging in anonymous sex with an unsuspecting and therefore nonconsenting victim. Although each type of person with frotteurism presents different needs, it is important to remind each that their acts are fully voluntary. Treatment should start with completely stopping the behavior to help discover why the person was engaging in the criminal behavior in the first place. As indicated in Chapter 3, the most important intervention is helping the person realize their frotteuristic acts can be traumatizing for their victims. As Kreuger and Kaplan (2008) noted, this can be done most effectively in group therapy.

Prognosis

There is virtually no literature concerning the efficacy of treatment(s) for frotteuristic disorders. In the SBC, prognosis is affected by concurrent disorders, ability of the person to accept the harmfulness of their behaviors, and the motivation(s) for the behaviors in the first place. Of the so-called courtship disorders (voyeurism, exhibitionism, frotteurism, and paraphilic rape), frotteurism is the paraphilia most dependent on surreptitious physical contact. This means that interventions that make it more difficult to be in physical contact with potential victims can be very effective.

Case Report 5.3

A woman with schizophrenia was referred to the SBC due to repeated incidents of attempting to rub up against other women and sometimes men. Her *modus operandi* was to victimize people riding alone with her on the elevator in her apartment in an attempt to reach orgasm either from contact with the victim or from fantasies about the act later when she was masturbating. She was sent for assessment after being released from jail following her most recent offense involving rubbing up against one of her neighbors in the condominium complex in which she was residing.

During the assessment, it was established that her frotteuristic acts were not due to hallucinations or delusions. When asked, she also reported difficulty reaching orgasm since she had started a new antipsychotic medication. She was diagnosed with frotteuristic disorder and female orgasmic disorder secondary to medication. As per routine, she was told she must stop her criminal activities immediately. Because her crimes all occurred on elevators, she was advised to use the stairs. "Doctor, I cannot do that", she said. When the doctor started to explain how sexual behaviors are voluntary, she interrupted, "Doctor, you do not understand. My apartment is on the 25th floor!" A call to the woman's parole officer confirmed that the "system" had found her accommodation on one of the highest buildings in the city and that she had been ordered not to change her living arrangements without notification. The first, and ultimately most effective, intervention in this case was obtaining permission to move her to a ground floor apartment. Her medications were also carefully altered so she could masturbate to orgasm, and she was encouraged to change her fantasies to consensual ones. This was something she was able to do after she was reminded that lesbian fantasies were perfectly fine and she was assured she did not have to fantasize about men unless she wanted to do so. In every case of habitual frotteuristic behaviors, it is important to interrupt the pattern and deal with the symptoms that result when the pattern is interrupted. In this case, the woman's life improved and her risk of reoffense decreased dramatically. To date, she has not reoffended since she was moved. Importantly, her interest in frotteuristic activities disappeared when she was "given permission" to use lesbian fantasies by assuring her they are normal.

Review of the Literature

The following table summarizes the literature that has been published on "frotteur*," "frotteurism," or "frotteuristic disorder" from 2008 to 2018 based on PsycINFO and PubMed searches.

Summary	Reference
Etiology	
Review of the history of the term "frotteuristic disorder."	Janssen (2018)
Characteristics of Frotteuristic Behaviors	
In this systematic review, the authors found that the prevalence of frotteurism is between 7.9% and 9.7%.	Johnson, Ostermeyer, Sikes, Nelsen, & Coverdale (2014)
Frotteurism and exhibitionism occur most often in public transportation, with the majority of victims being females.	S. Clark, Jeglic, Calkins, & Tatar (2016)
Case study of a man with bipolar disorder and multiple paraphilic behaviors, including frotteurism.	Kamalzadeh, Alavi, & Salehi (2015)
Comparison of psychopathological profiles for nonhomicidal sex offenders and homicidal sex offenders. A higher percentage of homicidal sex offenders tend to engage in paraphilic behaviors (including frotteurism) compared to nonhomicidal sex offenders.	Chan & Beauregard (2016)
Case study of 12-year-old boy who displayed impulsive "hypersexual" frotteuristic behaviors.	Patra et al. (2013)
Case study of patient with depression and compulsive frotteuristic behaviors.	Kalra (2013)
Diagnosis	
DSM Criticisms	
A literature review for exhibitionism, voyeurism, and frotteurism from 1980 to 2008. Långström suggested that empirical support for these paraphilic disorders is limited.	Långström (2010)
Variations	
Case study of differential diagnosis of frotteurism and "hypersexual" behavior with depression.	Bhatia, Jhanje, Srivastava, & Kumar (2010)

Summary	Reference
Assessment	
Investigated the gender biases of clinicians when examining atypical sexual interests as a mental disorder. When five vignettes were presented to 546 mental health professionals, it was found that professionals were less likely to pathologize female subjects but that females were more likely to be stigmatized (for exhibitionistic, frotteuristic, sexually sadistic, and pedophilic behavior).	Fuss, Briken, & Klein (2018)
Treatment	
Case example of treating frotteurism with solution-focused therapy.	Guterman, Martin, & Rudes (2011)
Use of dopaminergic treatment for a patient with Parkinson's disease and frotteuristic behavior.	Wilson (2010)
Book Chapters	
Balon, R. (2016). Frotteuristic disorder. In R. Balon (Ed.), *Practical guide to paraphilia and paraphilic disorders* (pp. 93–106). Cham, Switzerland: Springer.	
Krueger, R. B., & Kaplan, M. S. (2008). Frotteurism: Assessment and treatment. In D. R. Laws & W. T. O'Donohue (Eds.), *Sexual deviance: Theory, assessment, and treatment* (2nd ed., pp. 150–163). New York, NY: Guilford.	
Lussier, P., & Piche, L. (2008). Frotteurism: Psychopathology and theory. In D. R. Laws & W. T. O'Donohue (Eds.), *Sexual deviance: Theory, assessment, and treatment* (2nd ed., pp. 131–149). New York, NY: Guilford.	
McAnulty, R. (2017). Frotteurism. In B. A. Sharpless (Ed.), *Unusual and rare psychological disorders: A handbook for clinical practice and research* (pp. 136–148). New York, NY: Oxford University Press.	

References

Angelman, H. (1965). "Puppet" children: A report of three cases. *Developmental Medicine and Child Neurology, 7*, 681–688.

American Psychiatric Association. (2013). *Diagnostic and statistical manual of mental disorders* (5th ed.). Arlington, VA: American Psychiatric Publishing.

Balon, R. (2016). Frotteuristic disorder. In R. Balon (Ed.), *Practical guide to paraphilia and paraphilic disorders* (pp. 93–106). Cham, Switzerland: Springer.

Bhatia, M., Jhanjee, A., & Srivastava, S. (2011). An uncommon case of hypersexual behaviorur and frotteurism. *Medicine, Science and the Law*. doi/pdf/10.1258/msl.2010.010103

Chan, H. C., & Beauregard, E. (2016). Non-homicidal and homicidal sexual offenders: Prevalence of maladaptive personality traits and paraphilic behaviors. *Journal of Interpersonal Violence, 31*(13), 2259–2290.

Clark, D. J., Boer, H., & Webb, T. (1995). General and behavioural aspects of PWS: A review. *Mental Health Research, 8*(195), 38–49.

Clark, S. K., Jeglic, E. L., Calkins, C., & Tatar, J. R. (2016). More than a nuisance: The prevalence and consequences of frotteurism and exhibitionism. *Sexual Abuse, 28*(1), 3–19.

Dykens, E. M., & Rosner, B. A. (1999). Refining behavioral phenotypes: Personality-motivation in Williams and Prader–Willi syndromes. *American Journal on Mental Retardation, 104*(2), 158–169. doi:10.1352/0895-8017(1999)104<0158:RBPPIW

Fahrenthold, D. A. (2016, October 7). Trump recorded having extremely lewd conversation about women in 2005. *The Washington Post.*

Fuss, J., Briken, P., & Klein, V. (2018). Gender bias in clinicians' pathologization of atypical sexuality: A randomized controlled trial with mental health professionals. *Scientific Reports, 8*(1), 3715.

Griffiths, D. M., Quinsey, V. L., & Hingsburger, D. (1989). *Changing inappropriate sexual behaviour: A community based approach for persons with developmental disabilities.* Baltimore, MD: Brookes.

Guterman, J. T., Martin, C. V., & Rudes, J. (2011). A solution-focused approach to frotteurism. *Journal of Systemic Therapies, 30*(1), 59–72.

Ingves, M. V., Lau, T., Fedoroff, J. P., & Levine, S. (2014). A man with urethral polyembolokoilamania successfully treated with electroconvulsive therapy. *Archives of Sexual Behavior, 43*(6), 1203–1207.

Janssen, D. F. (2018). "Frotteuristic disorder": Etymological and historical note. *Archives of Sexual Behavior, 47*(4), 821–824.

Johnson, R. S., Ostermeyer, B., Sikes, K. A., Nelsen, A. J., & Coverdale, J. H. (2014). Prevalence and treatment of frotteurism in the community: A systematic review. *Journal of the American Academy of Psychiatry and the Law Online, 42*(4), 478–483.

Kalra, G. (2013). The depressive façade in a case of compulsive sex behavior with frottage. *Indian Journal of Psychiatry, 55*(2), 183.

Kamalzadeh, L., Alavi, K., & Salehi, M. (2015). Comorbidity of bipolar disorder and multiple paraphilias: A case report. *Iranian Journal of Psychiatry and Clinical Psychology, 121*(1), 69–74.

Krueger, R. B., & Kaplan, M. S. (2008). Frotteurism: Assessment and treatment. In D. R. Laws & W. T. O'Donohue (Eds.), *Sexual deviance: Theory, assessment, and treatment* (2nd ed., pp. 150–163). New York, NY: Guilford.

Långström, N. (2010). The DSM diagnostic criteria for exhibitionism, voyeurism, and frotteurism. *Archives of Sexual Behavior, 39*(2), 317–324.

Lussier, P., & Piche, L. (2008). Frotteurism: Psychopathology and theory. In D. R. Laws & W. T. O'Donohue (Eds.), *Sexual deviance: Theory, assessment, and treatment* (2nd ed., pp. 131–149). New York, NY: Guilford.

McAnulty, R. (2017). Frotteurism. In B. A. Sharpless (Ed.), *Unusual and rare psychological disorders: A handbook for clinical practice and research* (pp. 136–148). New York, NY: Oxford University Press.

Patra, A. P., Bharadwaj, B., Shaha, K. K., Das, S., Rayamane, A. P., & Tripathi, C. S. (2013). Impulsive frotteurism: A case report. *Medicine, Science and the Law, 53*(4), 235–238.

Puig, J. G., Torres, R. J., Mateos, F. A., Ramos, T. H., Arcas, J. M., Buno, A. S., & O'Neill, P. (2001). The spectrum of hypoxanthine–guanine phosphoribosyltransferase (HPRT) deficiency: Clinical experience based on 22 patients from 18 Spanish families. *Medicine (Baltimore), 80,* 102.

Smith, A. C., Dykens, E., & Greenberg, F. (1998). Behavioral phenotype of Smith–Magenis syndrome (del 17p11.2). *American Journal of Medical Genetics, 81*(2), 179–185.

Watson, S., Miodrag, N., Richards, D., & Fedoroff, J. P. (2012). Sexual genes Part 1: Sexuality and Down, Williams, and Prader–Willi syndromes. *Intellectual and Developmental Disabilities, 50,* 155–168.

Wilson, A. (2010). Disinhibition and narrative in the paraphilias. *Progress in Neuro-Psychopharmacology and Biological Psychiatry, 34*(2), 431–431.

World Health Organization. (2004). *ICD-10: International statistical classification of diseases and related health problems: tenth revision, 2nd ed.* World Health Organization. https://apps.who.int/iris/handle/10665/42980

6
Pedophilic Disorder

> I mean, I have the feeling that something in my mind is poisoning everything else.
>
> —Humbert in *Lolita* (Nabokov, 155, p. 360)

Introduction

The Fifth edition of the *Diagnostic and Statistical Manual of Mental Disorders* (DSM-5; American Psychiatric Association [APA], 2013a) defines "pedophilic disorder" as a condition lasting at least 6 months, consisting of "recurrent, intense sexual arousing fantasies, sexual urges, or behaviors" involving sexual activity with a prepubescent child or children (generally aged 13 years or younger) (p. 697). The B criteria state the individual has "acted on these sexual urges, or the sexual urges or fantasies cause marked distress or interpersonal difficulty" (p. 697). The C criteria focus on age discrepancy and state that the person with pedophilia must be older than age 15 years and at least 5 years older than the child or children in Criterion A. The definition further states that the definition of pedophilia does not apply in the case of an individual in late adolescence involved in an ongoing sexual relationship with a minor as young as age 12 years (p. 697). There are six specifiers: "exclusive type," "nonexclusive type," "sexually attracted to males," "sexually attracted to females," "sexually attracted to both," and "limited to incest" (p. 698).

The 10th revision of the *International Classification of Diseases* (ICD-10; World Health Organization, 1992) defines pedophilia simply as "a sexual preference for children, boys or girls or both, usually of pre-pubertal or early pubertal age" (F 65.4).

Diagnostic Guidelines

The DSM-5 guidelines for diagnosis of pedophilia are unchanged from the DSM-IV-TR (APA, 2000). This may explain why the DSM-5 diagnostic criteria are so confusing. For example, the text of the DSM refers to people who have committed sex crimes with children as having pedophilic disorder. This is untrue, however, because many sex offenders against children do not have pedophilia (Fedoroff, 2016). The text also states that having multiple victims "is sufficient but not necessary for diagnosis" (p. 698). The text cautions against making the diagnosis if the sexual interest in children is "merely transient" (p. 698). People with recurrent sexual interests in children who have chosen not to commit in-person sex crimes were referred to as people with a "pedophilic sexual *orientation*" in the first edition of the DSM-5 (p. 698). The APA subsequently issued a statement indicating that referring to pedophilia as an orientation was a "typo" and the word should have been "interest."

Is Pedophilia an Orientation?

Although referring to pedophilia as an orientation has been rejected by the APA, the question remains, does it make sense to refer to a paraphilia as an orientation? The answer depends in part on what is meant by "orientation." John Money was on the side of blending gender, orientation, and sexual interest (Goldie, 2015). He was preoccupied with nomenclature and taxonomy. The walls of his office were lined with dictionaries. However, his magnum opus, *Lovemaps* (Money, 1986), merged the concepts of gender, orientation, and interest into a single taxon: "lovemaps." Since then, some authors have advocated for the notion of classifying paraphilias as orientations. Seto (2012) attempted to marshal the evidence and arguments to support the amalgamation of orientation and paraphilias. Seto's suggestion has been reviewed and challenged by others (Cantor, 2012; Fedoroff, 2018a). Those who argue that pedophilia is an orientation like homosexuality appear to conflate persistence with orientation. However, the DSM-5 statement that pedophilia appears to be a lifelong condition (APA, 2013a, p. 699) has been proposed for deletion from the DSM-5 due to insufficient evidence. A second confusion is the unverified and unchallenged acceptance of the idea that orientation is genetic and thus unchangeable. Both parts of this premise are questionable because to date, a gene or genes for orientation have not been identified in any replicated study. Furthermore, there are many genetic conditions (e.g., phenylketonuria or diabetes) whose expressions are modifiable by diet or medications.

Case Report 6.1

A priest was arrested for allegedly sexually abusing several of the male choirboys in his church. During his intake assessment, he was ashamed and angry. He explained that as a child, before he was aware of sex, he had "crushes" on men. As he grew up, he increasingly worried he might be "gay," which he defined as a man who has sex with men. To avoid that problem, he chose a life of celibacy and joined the Catholic church. He admitted that being celibate did not end his conflict. He convinced himself that he would not be gay if he only had sexual interactions with choirboys because that would mean he was not having sex with men. He justified his sexual activities sex with boys as permissible because he thought it might keep them from pursuing sex with girls (a sin) and would allow him to "get closer" to the boys as a teacher. When it was suggested to him that he likely had pedophilia, he reluctantly admitted that was a possibility but added, "Like people who are gay."

Case Report 6.1 illustrates how confusing definitions can result in confused thinking. In fact, the priest was gay. He attempted to avoid accepting the identity of being a man with a homosexual orientation by creating a false definition—that is, men are gay if (and only if) they have sex with men. Next, he elected to enter a profession that not only allowed but also encouraged abandonment of sexual activity by promoting celibacy. The priesthood also gave him a "respectable" explanation for why he did not have a girlfriend or wife.

Unfortunately, his problem was not homosexuality, which is a normal, nonpathologic variant of human nature. His problem was pedophilia, which is defined as a recurrent, intense sexual interest in people who are unable to give consent (i.e., children). When arrested, he was shameful for having committed a crime but also for the possibility that he was gay. In the Sexual Behaviours Clinic (SBC), it is not uncommon for accused to admit pedophilia but strenuously deny the idea that they might be gay. Successful treatment begins with education about the fact that homosexuality is healthy and that recovery from pedophilia does not and should not require a change in orientation. This step is important because it helps the person focus on what actually needs to change. It also helps to disabuse the person from the idea that pedophilic interests cannot be modified. It may also explain why programs that do not explicitly distinguish between orientation and interest report failures in any attempts to modify sexual interest.

Pedophilia is a paraphilia and therefore, according to the DSM-5 and ICD-10, is defined by sexual interest. Orientation, at least in the SBC, is defined by romantic interest. This is consistent with the view that men who have sex with men are not necessarily gay. Similarly, men who have sex with women are not necessarily straight. Furthermore, men who lose their sex drive do not lose their orientation.

Homosexuality does not involve sexual interest in non-consensual acts. It therefore is never the focus of treatment. In addition, because homosexuality is defined by the gender of romantic interest instead of sexual interest, it tends to be less changeable than sexual interest, even if that were a legitimate treatment aim (which it is not). Some men with pedophilia latch onto the idea that they are gay for one of two reasons. Some fail to appreciate the difference between a romantic interest (orientation) and a sexual interest in non-consensual acts (pedophilia or other paraphilias involving non-consent). They hope that society will change its attitude toward pedophilia in the same way that some societies have changed their attitudes toward homosexuality or toward people who are transgender (which is another example of a condition with no defining criminal interests).

A second reason that men with pedophilia may attempt to identify with homosexuality is because treatments for homosexuality have rightly been debunked. They think that if treatment for homosexuality is illegitimate, then treatment for pedophilia will become illegitimate too. Some take this logical error to the next step, arguing that because treatment for homosexuality is wrong, treatment for both homosexuality and pedophilia must also be both unethical and ineffective.

This is an important but common mistake. The fact is, orientation is not necessarily immutable. For women in particular, there is evidence that people may change the gender of the people with whom they have romantic interests (L. Diamond, 2016, 2018). Modern mental health practices take the view that it is wrong to "treat" a person who wants to change their orientation because they are ashamed of being gay or lesbian. Increasing numbers of US states have legislated against so-called reparative therapy, which is sometimes erroneously referred to as "conversion therapy." This has been viewed as a positive development by advocates of the right to have any orientation. This may be a mistake. The SBC's view is that legislators have (almost) no business in therapists' offices. It is a slippery slope from laws forbidding therapy aimed at changing orientation to laws interfering with legitimate therapeutic interests, such as the wish of a bisexual woman to enhance her sexual interest in her husband.

To be clear, the SBC in no way advocates so-called reparative therapy, which is based on instilling and increasing sexual shame. However, the SBC is not against assisting consenting patients to enhance their orientations, gender identities, sex drives, or sexual interests anyway they wish as long as it enhances consensual (i.e., lawful) sex. As stated previously, the difficulty of changing varies (in descending order of greater difficulty) as follows: genotype, gender identity, orientation, interest, and drive. In each case, the SBC approach is to enhance interest in the desired direction rather than by attempting to shame or otherwise disrespect the patient's current state. In fact, it is legitimate for people who have pedophilic interests to identify as pedophilic provided they are able to guarantee they will not act on their unlawful sexual interests. When patients say they do not want to change their pedophilic interests because they know they would never act on their interests by engaging in sex with a child (a claim made by self-identified "virtuous" pedophiles), the SBC policy is to caution against relying solely on their willpower. Instead, the SBC advocates education about the fact that most SBC patients with pedophilia report a change in their sexual interests and also the fact that most people who acquire a sexual interest in consenting adults report they are more sexually satisfied than when they had pedophilia. In other words, when people insist on adopting the identity of being a person with an unchangeable pedophilic "orientation" as, for example, "virtuous pedophiles" do, it is important to ensure they are not doing so because of the mistaken belief that their pedophilic interests are unchangeable and because they are electing celibacy, as did the priest in Case Report 6.1.

It is important to note that celibacy is a legitimate human variation and a legitimate solution to many sexual problems, including low sexual desire, erectile dysfunction, gender dysphorias, paraphilic disorders, and marital discord. It is hoped, however, that those who adopt celibacy do so because it is a free choice and not due to the mistaken belief that it is the best they can do or because "sex is bad."

Reporting Requirements

There is widespread confusion about the ethical responsibility of clinicians to report sex offenses against children to authorities. Rules vary by jurisdiction, and readers should consult their local jurisdiction. However, the guiding principles of reporting rules are as follows:

1. Protection of children and vulnerable persons
2. Protection of clinicians from breaching confidentiality

Most jurisdictions accept the fact that many people who have experienced sexual abuse prefer to avoid resorting to the criminal justice system, which in most cases focuses on public denunciation and on punishment rather than on rehabilitation of the offender. Therefore, in most places, required reporting is only for situations in which there is a child who is still a child, who is in imminent danger, and who is identifiable. These are easy rules to live with and in fact assist in therapy.

In the SBC, each potential patient is given a sheet with the reporting rules clearly described. If the patient discloses a situation meeting the requirements for reporting, they are advised they have done the right thing. Typically, the call to the appropriate Children's Aid Society (CAS) is made in the presence of the patient, and the patient is invited to explain to the CAS worker what the concern is in their own words. Often, the agency receiving the call is impressed by the self-reporting, and the response is more measured than in situations in which the offender is first arrested by police.

By including the patient in the process, the reporting process becomes therapeutic. In the jurisdiction in which the SBC is located, possession of child pornography is not a reportable offense unless the patients have created the pornography themselves. Clinicians should view reporting legislation in the way it was intended—as their protection when they act ethically. As a side note, some clinicians and agencies prefer to use a term other than *child pornography*, arguing that the term somehow depathologizes the material. The term is used here because this the term used in the legislation.

Variations

As stated previously, the DSM-5 criteria for pedophilic disorder are the only ones that are identical to the criteria listed in the DSM-IV-TR (APA, 1994). They therefore read as even more outdated that the other paraphilic disorders listed in the DSM-5. The first problem is that individuals diagnosed with pedophilic disorder must be at least age 16 years old and at least 5 years older than the children in whom they are sexually interested (APA, 2013a, p. 697). Furthermore, the DSM-5 prohibits diagnosing a person in "late adolescence in an on-going sexual relationship with a 12 or 13-year-old" (p. 697). Why? Presumably, the reason for these idiosyncratic prohibitions is because same-age sexual interest is normal and begins (at the latest) during puberty. Typically, the age of the sexual partner of interest increases as the age of the youth increases. The DSM-5 criteria appears to acknowledge that sexual interests change as people age.

Another peculiarity of the DSM-5 diagnostic criteria is the specifier "limited to incest" (APA, 2013a, p. 698). Why is this qualifier limited to pedophilia and not the other paraphilic disorders? Some patients report sexual arousal based on incest themes that are independent of the age of the person and/or that exclude children. A pornographic videotape series in the 1970s titled "Taboo" involved only adult actors and actresses but focused on incest themes and was very popular among people who were not pedophilic. This of course is not surprising because the concept and definition of incest are independent of age. It is important to remember that patients may report a sexual interest in incestuous acts not because of a sexual interest in a brother or sister but, rather, despite it. For example, in the SBC, patients who report sexual fantasies involving themes of incest often do not have children or siblings. In other cases, it is precisely because of the fact that the person is related and therefore "ineligible" that the person reports incestuous fantasies.

Pedophilic Obsessive–Compulsive Disorder

A common diagnostic dilemma is a person with depression who presents with the chief complaint of "sexual thoughts about children." People who watch classic movies will be familiar with the hollywood trope of portraying people with mental illness wearing Napoleon hats. In current times, it is now rare to see anyone on a psychiatric ward wearing a Napoleon hat or even knowing who Napoleon was. Later, Napoleon hats were replaced with tin foil caps (to keep radio waves out). Those ideas were in turn replaced with ideas of being possessed by Satan. In each time period, people with changes in self-esteem due to depression adopted an identity that, at the time, was considered to be the "worst you could be." In the past, Napoleon was the worst person you could be (at least if you lived in England). In modern times, the idea of being Napoleon has been replaced by the idea of being a sex offender.

People with severe depression who present with ego-dystonic thoughts of having sex with their children, or other children, often suffer primarily from depression. They differ from people with true pedophilia because they are not sexually aroused by the idea of sex with children but, rather, are troubled by a change in self-attitude that causes them to believe they are the worst person they could be: a sex offender. When their depression is treated, their sexual thoughts about children (their own or otherwise) disappear. Clues to this possibility include the presence of symptoms of depression (current and past), an absence of pedophilic fantasies prior to the onset of depression, and a lack of sexual enjoyment from the pedophilic fantasies. Instead, people with this syndrome present in a similar manner to people with obsessional depressions in which thoughts arise unbidden and are ego-dystonic. Commonly, the person will disclose that the pedophilic thoughts interfere with their normal sexual interests and function.

Hebephilia

An important variant of pedophilia that was unsuccessfully championed as a new DSM-5 paraphilic diagnosis by one of the Chairs of the DSM-5 Paraphilias subgroup, Ray Blanchard, is *hebephilia* and/or *pedohebephilia.* Hebephilia has been defined as intense, persistent sexual interest in pubescent children, who in turn are defined as "roughly age 11–14" (Blanchard et al., 2009). There is an obvious problem with this diagnosis. People in this age group may be prepubescent, peripubescent, pubescent, or adult in terms of physiologic and anatomic maturity. Unlike pedophilia, which is a condition characterized by sexual arousal toward sexually immature children, hebephilia includes arousal toward males or females who may potentially be physically indistinguishable from adults. Males in this age range are potentially capable of fathering children, and females in this age range are potentially capable of bearing children.

A consequence of widening the age range for pedophilia (generally younger than age 13years) to pedohebephilia (generally younger than age 15 years) is that it makes the diagnosis less specific. This makes the possibility of false-positive diagnoses greater and in turn makes demonstration of treatment efficacy more difficult. This is analogous to what would happen if the diagnosis of bacterial pneumonia was changed to simply having a cough. More people would be diagnosed with pneumonia, including people who do not have pneumonia, and "pneumonia" would include both bacterial and viral pneumonia. Treatment efficacy based on antibiotics would decrease, not because antibiotics are less effective but because they do not work for coughs that are not caused by bacterial infections. Similarly, if treatment studies include men who already have sexual interest in people as old as 15 years, it will be more difficult to demonstrate a significant change from interest in children only to a sexual interest in adults only.

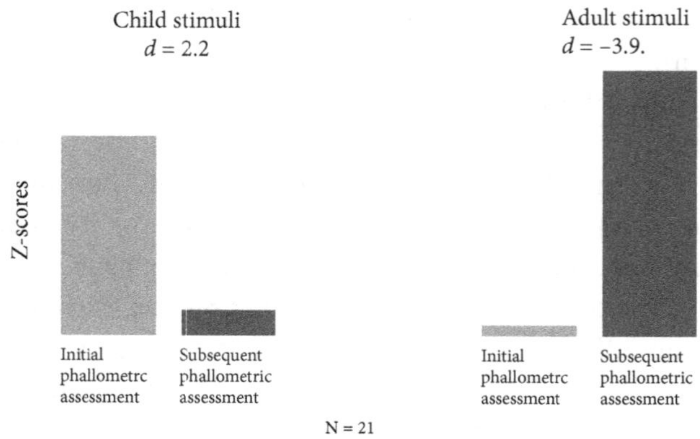

Figure 6.1 Retrospective pre- and post-phallometric test results for men initially diagnosed with pedophilia. Initial and follow-up phallometric *z* scores for 21 men showing a decrease in pedophilic arousal and an increase in non-pedophilic arousal in the lab.

Source: Adapted with permission from Müller, K., Curry, S., Ranger, R., Briken, P., Bradford, J., & Fedoroff, J. P. (2014). Changes in sexual arousal as measured by penile plethysmography in men with pedophilic sexual interest. Journal of Sexual Medicine, 11(5), 1221–1229.

In 2014, an article was published describing a retrospective study of men diagnosed with pedophilia who had phallometric tests that were consistent with a diagnosis of pedophilia (they had greater increases in penile circumference when presented with child stimuli than they did to adult stimuli). On repeat testing at least 6 months later, approximately 20 men responded more to adult stimuli than to child stimuli (Müller et al., 2014). For men who showed changes, the effect sizes were large for both the decrease in response to child stimuli (d = 2.2) and the increase in response to adult stimuli (d = −3.9) (Figure 6.1). That article generated multiple criticisms to which the SBC responded (Fedoroff et al., 2015; Fedoroff, Curry, Ranger, & Bradford, 2016).

The criticisms can be summarized as concern that Money's paradigm based on the idea of immutable lovemaps had been challenged. Specifically, critics have questioned whether the men were really pedophilic, whether the testing was accurate (either the first testing or the second testing or both), whether the men had managed to both suppress their responses to child stimuli and artificially enhance their responses to adult stimuli, and the statistical methods used to analyze change.

Of course, retrospective studies rarely prove anything. Of more interest is how upsetting the study seems to have been, especially to commentators not directly involved in the treatment of people with pedophilia. One might expect that any evidence that pedophilia can be treated successfully would be welcomed, but for some this has not been the case. One argument is that there is insufficient proof to definitively state that sexual interests can change. This is an argument that is difficult to support given that interests of all kinds change more or less constantly. In fact, there is little or no evidence that sexual interests cannot change and that they are somehow permanently fixed. These arguments (and more) were recently discussed in invited reviews (Cantor & Fedoroff, 2018; Fedoroff, 2018). In contrast, there is evidence that telling people with pedophilia that pedophilia is untreatable decreases the efficacy of treatment (Tozdan & Briken, 2017; Tozdan et al., 2018).

Of course, the solution to the question of whether phallometric testing can reliably measure change in sexual interest will rely on independent, prospective studies (one of which is funded and currently underway in the SBC). But the vigorous attacks on the idea that the pedophilic interests can change, in both editorials and letters to the editor in scientific journals and nonscientific journals and social media, are remarkable. Remember, critics who claim pedophilic interests cannot change are essentially claiming they have never seen a person with pedophilic interests change, ever. Otherwise, they would have to admit change is possible but perhaps say it is rare. This is the nature of the scientific process. A single black swan proves not all swans are white, even if an existing paradigm that insists all swans are white predicts that no black swans should exist.

But the problem is worse for defenders of the Money paradigm because not only are there many people with pedophilia who say their pedophilic interests have changed (black swans) but also their reports are supported by their change in behaviors, which is supported by their change in offense patterns (they stop reoffending), and their adult sexual partners. Claims that anyone who says his sexual interests have changed must be lying, are difficult to believe in the case of people who have sought treatment on their own. Why would they say they are better if they are not? Furthermore, if for some reason they are not actually better, why do they not act like people who still have pedophilic interests?

Finally, defenders of Money's immutable paraphilia paradigm claim that telling people with pedophilia there is hope they will get better somehow makes them more dangerous. This approach makes no sense, and there is no evidence to support its efficacy (Tozdan & Briken, 2015). In fact, if the people who claim pedophilic interests are unchangeable are as unsuccessful in treating people with pedophilia as they claim to be, that evidence could be used against their claims that telling people they are incurable does no harm.

As a final point on this topic, some critics say (without evidence) that accepting a patient's claim that they no longer have pedophilic interests somehow interferes with their ability to avoid situations in which they might be accused of reoffending. In fact, the SBC avoids creating an atmosphere in which patients think there is any benefit in misleading the therapists. They are reminded that the therapists make the same amount of money regardless of whether or not SBC patients tell the truth. However, because it is the SBCs job to help its patients become lawful citizens who engage only in consensual sexual activities that are enjoyable, it only makes sense to tell the truth if they are not getting better. All SBC patients with criminal histories are also instructed that anyone who has been accused or convicted of committing a sex offense will be assumed to be guilty by authorities if they are ever accused. Therefore, they are taught how to avoid and not just how to not reoffend; they also learn how to avoid acting in ways that could lead to them being falsely accused. It turns out that people who believe they can get better respond extremely well to interventions designed to help them avoid children.

Prevalence

According to the DSM-5 (APA, 2013a), the "highest possible prevalence for pedophilic disorder in the male population is approximately 3%–5%" (p. 698). The reason for this peculiar phraseology is likely due to the fact that it is based on anonymous surveys in which people (usually students of psychology) were asked if they ever sexually fantasized about children. It is presumed that not all men who answer "yes" to these questions have these interests for at least 6 months and that not everyone who answers "yes" to these questions is telling the truth (Seto, 2008b).

However, the more important question is how many people were lying when they said "no." A more recent anonymous survey included almost 2,000 Swedish older male high school students between the ages of 17 and 20 years (Seto, Hermann, et al., 2015). In the Swedish sample, 4.2% reported having seen child pornography. Of students in this survey, 4.2% indicated they would be "likely" to have sex with a child younger than age 10 years, 5.8% with a child aged 10–12 years, and 33.8% with a child aged 12–14 years. It is of interest that only 2.6% admitted they had ever had sex with a male. Furthermore, epidemiologic studies to date have not investigated the question of how many people once had pedophilic interests and grew out of them or the question of how many did not have pedophilic interests but later acquired them.

Child Pornography

One clue to the actual prevalence of pedophilia is the apparent ubiquity of child pornography on the Internet. One frequently quoted figure is that the production and distribution of child pornography is a multi-billion-dollar industry. However, actual data to support this claim have never been published in peer-reviewed sources.

In the SBC, in the past 15 years there has been only one patient who claimed to have sold child pornography for money. A second patient considered selling pictures of his daughter but changed his mind and turned himself in. It is notable that in that case, Canada's department of immigration chose to deport him to a country in which he had no supports "for the protection of the community" (but obviously not the community to which he was deported).

The likelihood that child pornography is a multi-billion-dollar industry is made less likely due to the fact that most patients in the SBC with pedophilia say they know that their likelihood of arrest is increased if they provide their credit card numbers, which makes tracing of their identities easier. Although many SBC patients admit seeking child pornography and posting or reposting child pornography in order to make contact with other people who have pedophilic interests, to date no SBC patients have said they ever paid for child pornography. Ironically, many say they exchanged child pornography in order to assure the person with whom they were corresponding that they were not themselves a law enforcement official. Child pornography has become a way to prove one's bone fides as a person with pedophilic interests to other people with pedophilic interests. In fact, many people who access child pornography on the Internet do not have a sexual interest in children and therefore do not have pedophilia. They may access the materials by accident, out of curiosity, or due to interest in collecting "weird" pictures. A more important question than whether the person has accessed child pornography is whether they have ever masturbated while viewing child pornography or while recalling child pornography images. A change in pornographic themes that are arousing to SBC patients is another way in which need for therapy and progress in therapy can be monitored. In the SBC, patients are advised that viewing child pornography is not only illegal and immoral but also may impede their progress in therapy, which has the goal of changing their sexual interests from children to adults.

Do Child Pornography Offenders Progress?

The relationship between child pornography and in-person sexual assault is complex (Ly, Murphy, & Fedoroff, 2016; Murphy, Ranger, & Fedoroff, 2014). Of course, the production of child pornography is abusive to children. People arrested for possession of child pornography often fail to appreciate this fact. They think that because the images already exist, the harm is in the past and their choice to look at the images is of no importance. They say they do not support the "industry" because they do not pay for the images or videos. An effective therapeutic intervention is to ask the offender how they would feel if their pictures were released on the Internet for the pleasure of other people to look at? This is a particularly effective intervention because people arrested for child pornography offenses are keenly concerned about public disclosure about who they are and where they live.

Beginning with Berl Kutchinsky (1971) in the 1970s when pornography became available in Europe and continuing with a series of studies by Milton Diamond and colleagues (Diamond, 2009; Diamond & Uchiyama, 1999), there is considerable evidence that increased availability of pornography is associated with decreased rates of sex crimes (with the exception, of course, of child pornography-related crimes). This observation does not justify or excuse child pornography because children are harmed. However, it does open questions about whether child pornography that is animated (and therefore not involving children) is harmful. Clinicians and researchers who believe that sexual interests, once formed, are immutable presumably would not be concerned about animated child pornography because it should not influence the interests of adults and might provide an alternative outlet for people with pedophilia to satisfy their sexual interests (by masturbating while viewing child pornography). Although this may be true, the SBC discourages use of any child pornography based on the view that it may encourage or sustain pedophilic sexual interests. Instead, the SBC advises patients to abstain completely from using any form of child pornography for any reason and encourages them to use fantasy about adults and/or use of legal adult pornography when they masturbate to facilitate the establishment of healthy associations between sexual feelings and adult men and/or women. Importantly, patients are reminded that arousal from men or women or any combination thereof is equally acceptable as long as it promotes sexual interest in adults.

There is also a concern that the availability of child pornography, animated or not, creates a societal tolerance for child abuse. Instead, the SBC again encourages people with pedophilia to avoid any depictions of children and to substitute adult pornography to establish and enhance an association of sexual arousal with adults. Sometimes, offenders are forbidden from accessing any pornography by the courts due to the misinformed belief that all pornography is the same. The SBC recommends that offenders be allowed to use the Internet while they are on probation or parole so they can learn to use it lawfully while they are still under supervision.

Sometimes patients claim they developed a sexual interest in child pornography because they became bored with adult pornography. Existing evidence suggests that although people may become bored from viewing the same picture or video repeatedly, themes of sexual arousal remain remarkably consistent. This is why pornographic video companies have been able to sell millions of videos with only minor variations in theme but with constantly changing performers. In the case of a man arrested for possession of child pornography who claimed he got bored with adult pornography, he was asked why his child pornography consisted of images of girls only. His spontaneous response, "I do not like guys", helped him realize his interest in girls was sexually motivated and not simply due to boredom.

Assessment and Treatment Recommendations

Great effort has gone into developing ways to discover the true sexual interests of people with pedophilia. This is because it is assumed by some commentators that people with sexual interest in children always lie when they say they are no longer sexually interested in children (Blanchard, 2010). Twenty years ago, most referrals to the SBC were pretrial. At that time, many offenders against children claimed they were innocent. Over time, that has changed so that now legal referrals are primarily court-ordered and presentence, meaning the offender has already been found guilty. Therefore, most current SBC referrals admit their sexual interests, including illegal ones. They are encouraged to do so, not only by staff but also by other patients in group therapy sessions.

Phallometric Testing

Phallometric testing is a painless procedure that involves changes in penis volume in response to standardized visual and/or auditory stimuli. In the SBC, this is done by measuring change in the electronic resistance in a ring that the patient places over the shaft of his penis. As the penis becomes erect, the penile circumference changes. By measuring changes in penile circumference while the patient looks at pictures of males and females across a variety of ages or listens to audiotaped sexual scenarios, it is possible to infer sexual interest profiles (Fedoroff, Kuban, & Bradford, 2009).

Anytime that phallometric testing is conducted, it is explained that it is not a lie detector test and not intended to determine guilt or innocence. Instead, it is meant to provide assistance to the patient and his doctor in planning the treatment and to objectively measure their progress in treatment. Phallometric testing, like any other procedures conducted in the SBC, is only done with the consent of the patient.

Sensitivity and Specificity

The SBC has published estimates of the sensitivity and specificity of its phallometric assessments for pedophilia (Murphy, Ranger, Stewart, Dwyer, & Fedoroff, 2015). Comparing men with sex crimes against children to men with no known paraphilic interests, the sensitivity of SBC phallometrics was found to be 75.5% and the specificity was 73.5% (Bradford, Pawlak, & Curry, 1997). These results are similar to the estimates published by other clinics (Fedoroff et al., 2009). It is notable that there are no published measures of test–retest reliability of phallometry. This issue is important to consider when assessing the study by Müller et al. (2014; see Figure 6.1). It is possible that the large effect sizes found in that study were simply due to variance in the test. However, it is difficult to completely dismiss the large effect sizes when combined with the fact that the men who showed changes did so in terms of both decreasing changes in penile circumference when presented with pictures of children and, more importantly, increasing changes in penile circumference in response to pictures of adults. Although it can be argued that the men in this study were statistical outliers, they nevertheless were outliers showing a response pattern inconsistent with the notion that sexual interest is forever immutable.

Occasionally, patients ask for independent validation of their phallometric test results. When this happens, they are reassured that determinations of guilt (or innocence) are never made solely on the basis of phallometric test results. If they insist that something was wrong with the test, they are offered a retest (on the understanding that both test results will still be in the SBC files), referral to another lab, or testing via visual reaction time. Generally, in the SBC, test–retest results remain remarkably similar.

Visual reaction tests are based on the observation that people tend to look longer at slides depicting models in whom they are sexually interested. One commercially available test battery has the advantage of using only clothed models (Abel, Jordan, Hand, Holland, & Phipps, 2001). Work is now underway to compare and standardize assessment of sexual interest internationally (Demidova et al., 2019; Murphy et al., 2019).

Treatment

Approaches to treatment are reviewed in Chapter 2. The most recent review of treatment for paraphilic disorders in general and pedophilia in particular is the open access review article by the World Federation of Societies of Biological Psychiatry (WFSBP; Thibaut, de la Barra, Gordon, Cosyns, & Bradford, 2010). As indicated previously, the SBC does not strictly follow the 2010 WFSBP guidelines because they do not sufficiently emphasize consent. The SBC never "forces" or coerces treatment, not only because it is unethical but also because it decreases treatment efficacy. The SBC also avoids hierarchical treatment models in which more intensive treatments are "saved" for people who "fail" less intensive interventions. Instead, the full range of possible treatments together with risks and benefits are presented to the patient along with an explanation that there is no way to know for sure which treatment is needed until it has been tried. In this context, many patients voluntarily elect to start with gonadotropin-releasing hormone analogs in addition to individual and group psychotherapy.

This treatment approach is also contrary to the risk–need–responsivity (RNR) model (Andrews, Bonta, & Wormith, 2011). The RNR model subscribes to the notion that less severe problems require less intervention. The SBC takes the view that it is not the severity of the current problem(s) but, rather, the severity of potential failure that is paramount. This means that the SBC starts with the requirement of complete cessation of illegal acts, together with immediate care of any identifiable victims who cannot seek treatment themselves. This is important not only to minimize harm but also to communicate that sexual behaviors are voluntary and therefore immediately modifiable. This policy also helps empower patients to take responsibility for their own actions and for their recovery. In addition, it provides an opportunity to reframe treatment not as a "punishment" but, rather, as a combined effort to help the patients lawfully improve their lives and the lives of their significant others and members of the community. This starts with ensuring the welfare of any victims who are too young or vulnerable to seek help on their own by reporting concerns to the appropriate Family and Children's Aid Society agency.

As described in Chapter 2, treatment options are presented as a series of experiments in which working hypotheses are tested. Patients with pedophilia are reminded that sex crimes are due to voluntary acts over which they have control.

They are assured that reporting failure in their efforts to change their pedophilic interests to non-pedophilic interests will never be held against them. Instead, information about failure of the treatment to work is used to modify the treatment to conduct the next "experiment" and improve the quality of their treatment. In this way, lying becomes counterproductive. Is it ethical to "experiment" with treatment? The answer is that all treatment is experimental in the sense that some treatments work better for different people in different situations. Luckily, since sexual behaviors are not involuntary, it is not only possible but more expeditious to assess every intervention for its efficacy and modify accordingly. Accepting the possibility that sexual interest can be changed permits to beginning of work to not only improve current treatment efficacy but to prevent child abuse (Knack et al., 2019).

Prognosis

The DSM-5 is silent about the prognosis of pedophilia and pedophilic disorder (APA, 2013a, p. 699). It also mistakenly refers to pedophilia as an "orientation" possibly due to "neurodevelopmental perturbation in utero" (p. 699). The APA (2013b) has issued a formal statement that the word "orientation" should be replaced with "interest" in the DSM-5 diagnostic criteria for pedophilia, masochism, and sadism.

The fact is that most children and adolescents with sexual interests in same-aged peers lose interest in children when they become adults. This is why the DSM-5 sensibly prohibits diagnosing pedophilia in anyone younger than age 16 years and further comments, "the course of pedophilic disorder may fluctuate, increase, or decrease with age" (APA, 2013a, p. 699).

Other reviews of the treatment of pedophilic disorder tend to confuse or conflate orientation with interest (e.g., Camilleri & Quinsey, 2008), therefore concluding that because orientation is (or should be) untreatable, pedophilia must be also:

> Few sexologists believe that modifying homosexual orientation via current technologies is possible (this is not to argue that such a goal is desirable). It is more than a little surprising that no one applies this central conclusion from the literature on the treatment of homosexuality (now moribund) to the treatment of pedophilia; pedophilia is doubtless a different condition, but nevertheless also an anomaly of sexual preference. (p. 202)

Seto (2009) made a similar argument. Discussing treatment options, he wrote, "The underlining assumption is that pedophilia is a stable sexual preference that is unlikely to change, just as there is little, if any evidence that heterosexual or homosexual orientation can be changed" (p. 398). Seto (2018b) appears to have changed his opinion. Responding to a claim that he thinks "pedophilia cannot change," he wrote, "I did not say this anywhere in the Target Article or in any of my other writings about pedophilia."

The fact is that unlike homosexuality (an orientation), which has maintained the same population prevalence in every population in which it is studied, pedophilic disorder appears to have shown a consistent decrease. This statement is based on multiple studies that indicate a decrease in arrests and convictions for sex offenses against children (Finkelhor & Jones, 2004; Hanson, Harris, Letourneau, Helmus, & Thornton, 2018; Sheilds, Tonmyr, & Hovdestad, 2016). This has happened during a time when the number of potential victims has increased, awareness of child sexual abuse has increased, and reporting has become mandatory for professionals and easier for victims and their parents. While not all sex offenders againt children have pedophilia, it is hard to explain the drop in sex crimes against children without some decrease either in the prevalence of pedophilia or the likelihood of people with pedophilia acting on their sexual interests in a criminal manner.

Summary of SBC Treatment of People with Pedophilic Disorder

As in the case of all paraphilias in which sexual activity involves non-consent if acted upon, treatment begins with the requirement that illegal acts stop completely and immediately. Comorbid and concurrent psychiatric and medical problems are treated vigorously. Patients with pedophilia are reassured that the goal of treatment is to change their sexual interests so they can enjoy a satisfying and fulfilling sex life that is consensual and better than their former illegal sex life. This assurance is particularly easy to make because people with "exclusive" pedophilia are rare and most already have at least some sexual interest in adults. In the SBC, the incidence of hands-on sexual reoffenses against children has been virtually unknown during the past 15 years.

The claim that pedophilic sexual interests cannot be modified is based on a confusion between orientation and interest and on (at best) unreplicated correlational studies. The paradigm of immutable sexual interests does not explain clinical observations or epidemiologic data, including crime reporting. In contrast, a paradigm based on the premise that paraphilic interests are plastic is compatible with current neurologic paradigms of plasticity, clinical observations, and crime reporting. There is also evidence that the claims that "pedophilic interests are unchangeable" and the claim that "pedophilic interests can change" are not equivalent (Fedoroff, 2018) because telling people with pedophilia they cannot change may be an unfounded but self-fulfilling prophesy (Tozdan et al., 2018).

Review of the Literature

The following table summarizes the literature that has been published on "pedophilia" and "pedophilic disorder" from 2008 to 2018 based on using PsycINFO and PubMed searches. The keywords "child sex offender" and "child molester" were not used, with the goal of concentrating on the clinical rather than legal research perspectives. Articles that did not specify pedophilia as a variable (i.e., only examined child sex offenders without distinguishing whether the sample had pedophilia or pedophilic disorder) were also excluded from this summary.

Summary	Reference
Prevalence	
Internet studies suggesting that the prevalence of pedophilia, viewing child pornography, or having an interest in engaging in sexual acts with children ranges from 2% to 10% (most studies report an average of approximately 3% or 4%).	Alanko, Salo, Mokros, & Santtila (2013); Dombert et al. (2016); Santtila et al. (2015); Seto, Hermann, et al. (2015); Wurtele, Simons, & Moreno (2014)
Stigma and Its Effects on People with Pedophilia	
Having pedophilia increases personal distress independent of offense history. *Comment*: Most people with pedophilia do not want to remain pedophilic.	Jahnke, Schmidt, Geradt, & Hoyer (2015); Konrad, Haag, Scherner, Amelung, & Beier (2017); Walter & Pridmore (2012)
Jahnke discusses the potential harm of stigmatizing people with pedophilia and how mental health professionals can improve care for this population. Describes a 10-minute online intervention.	Jahnke (2018); Jahnke, Philipp, & Hoyer (2015)
Etiology	
Articles and studies that consider whether there is a genetic component to developing pedophilic disorder. To date, no significant differences have been found in genetic polymorphisms (concerning behavioral control, addictive behaviors, and sexual dysfunctions) between pedophiles and non-pedophiles, nor between sex offenders and controls.	Alanko et al. (2013); Alanko, Gunst, Mokros, & Santtila (2016); Berryessa (2014); Jakubczyk et al. (2017)
Articles discussing whether pedophilia is a sexual orientation and/or a so-called chronophilia. Fedoroff (2018) disagrees with conceptualizing pedophilic interest as similar to homosexual orientation.	Fedoroff (2018); Grundmann, Krupp, Scherner, Amelung, & Beier (2016, 2017); Hsu & Bailey (2017); Janssen (2015); Seto (2012, 2017); Tozdan & Briken (2017); Tousseul (2018); Walton & Duff (2017)

Summary	Reference
Articles proposing that prenatal or early childhood environment influences the development of pedophilic disorder. *Comment*: These studies are far from definitive, and even if this is true, it does not prove immutability of pedophilic sexual interests.	Bao & Swaab (2010); Dyshniku, Murray, Fazio, Lykins, & Cantor (2015)
Articles suggesting that those with intellectual disability or "low IQ" are more likely to have pedophilia. *Comment*: These correlational studies ignore the fact that most known cases of people with pedophilia do not have intellectual disability.	Rice, Harris, Lang, & Chaplin (2008); Garcia (2009); Kruger & Schiffer (2011); Lamy, Delavenne, & Thibaut (2016)
Studies and articles examining the abused–abuser hypothesis—that is, whether having childhood sexual abuse is related to pedophilic disorder and/or sexual offending against children in later life. Most articles published within the past 10 years imply that childhood sexual abuse is associated with later offending. Fedoroff and Pinkus (1996) found no support for any of the three versions of the abuse to abuser hypothesis. The studies listed here fail to distinguish correlation from causality.	Connolly & Woollons (2008); Fazio (2018); Fedoroff & Pinkus (1996); Garrett (2010); Houssier, Duchet, Chagnon, Robert, & Marty (2011); Ibiloglu, Atli, Oto, & Ozkan (2018); Nunes, Hermann, Malcom, & Lavoie (2013); Witztum, Daie, & Rosler (2012)
Studies examining reported age of onset of masturbation and the development of sexual interest in children.	Tozdan & Briken (2015b); Wurtele, Simons, & Parker (2018)
An unreplicated study suggesting the internet may create pedophilic interest in those who had no prior sexual interest in children.	Wood (2013)b
High self-control reduces the likelihood of engaging in pedophilic interests. *Comment*: It is important to note that sexual activity is a voluntary and not reflexive or addictive behavior.	Babchishin, Seto, Fazel, & Långström (2019); Bailey, Bernhard, & Hsu (2016); K. Jordan et al. (2018); Massau, Kärgel et al. (2017); Mitchell & Galupo (2016, 2018); Ristow et al. (2018); Schiffer & Vonlaufen (2011)

Summary	Reference
Exploring Characteristics of Those Who Have Pedophilia	
General reviews of characteristics in child sex offenders.	Capra, Forresi, & Caffo (2014); Heitzman, Lew-Starowicz, Pacholski, & Lew-Starowicz (2014); Jumper, Babula, & Casbon (2012); Łucka, & Dziemian (2014)
Studies examining the criminal history and antisocial personality characteristics of sex offenders with child victims compared to those with adult victims. In general, offenders with child victims appear to have fewer antisocial and sadistic personality traits compared to sex offenders with adult victims.	Aho (2013); Cohen & Galynker (2012); Cohen, Grebchenko, Steinfeld, Frenda, & Galynker (2008); Strassberg, Eastvold, Kenney, & Suchy (2012); Suchy, Whittaker, Strassberg, & Eastvold (2009a, b); Turner, Rettenberger, Lohmann, Eher, & Briken (2014)
Studies examining personality traits in sex offenders against children.	Franzen (2014); Giang (2018); R. Jordan (2012); Stoll (2008)
Those with pedophilia were more likely to be left-handed and have shorter height. However, the study by Jung, Klaver, and Pham (2014) did not find support the association between height and pedophilic interests. *Comment*: These retrospective and correlational studies are not definitive and do not refute the observation that sexual interests change.	Fazio, Dyshniku, Lykins, & Cantor (2017); Fazio, Lykins, & Cantor (2014); Garcia (2009); Jung et al. (2014); McPhail & Cantor (2015)
Studies comparing pedophilic disorder to substance (mainly opiate) addictions. One study (Hamdi & Knight, 2012) also examined the use of substances by child sex offenders. *Comment*: These are important studies highlighting the importance of considering concurrent or comorbid disorders in the differential diagnosis.	Cohen, Forman, et al. (2010); Cohen & Galynker (2012); Cohen, Grebchenko, Steinfeld, Frenda, & Galynker (2008); Cohen, Nesci, Steinfeld, Haeri, & Galynker (2010); Green (2018); Hamdi & Knight (2012)
Deterioration or trauma to the temporal and/or frontal lobes of the brain has been associated with new onset of pedophilia and increased risk of committing a sexual offense.	

Summary	Reference
Comment: These case reports support the premise that sexual interest can be altered, including by neurologic insults. Fortunately, neurologic trauma can be managed and treated.	Abdo (2013); Alnemari, Mansour, Buehler, & Gaudin (2016); Fumagalli, Pravettoni, & Priori (2015); Gilbert & Focquaert (2015); Mendez & Shapira (2011); Poeppl et al. (2015); Rainero et al. (2011); Rodriguez, Boyce, & Hodges (2017); Sartori, Scarpazza, Codognotto, & Pietrini (2016); Scarpazza, Pennati, & Sartori (2018)
Articles and studies examining the executive functioning of sex offenders with and without pedophilia as well as non-offender controls. Overall, it has been found that sex offenders against children (both pedophilic and non-pedophilic) have poorer executive skills compared to those of non-offending controls. *Comment*: These findings are consistent with the observation that the decision to commit a sex crime may be determined by other factors besides those that influence sexual interest and its stability.	Becerra-García & Egan (2014); Eastvold (2010); Eastvold, Suchy, & Strassberg (2011); K. Jordan, Fromberger, von Herder, et al. (2016); Rosburg et al. (2018); Suchy, Eastvold, Strassberg, & Franchow (2014); Suchy, Whittaker, Strassberg, & Eastvold (2009a,b); Thompson (2016)
Insight into Committing an Offense Against Children	
Studies examining the decision-making process involved in committing offenses toward children and the motives behind these offenses. Simply having a sexual interest in children is not the sole motivation for committing offenses against children.	Beauregard, Leclerc, & Lussier (2012); Konrad, Kuhle, Amelung, & Beier (2018); Kruger & Schiffer (2011); Sullivan & Sheehan (2016); Williams (2017); Winder, Gough, & Seymour-Smith (2015)
Studies examining the beliefs and attitudes of men with pedophilia concerning sexual acts with children.	Jahnke & Malón (2019); Spriggs, Cohen, Valencia, Zimri, & Galynker (2018)
Literature reviews and investigations into the cognitive distortions of sex offenders against children. Failure to identify and treat cognitive distortions can hinder treatment progress.	Carvalho & Nobre (2014); Drapeau, Beretta, de Roten, Koerner, & Despland (2008); Geradt, Jahnke, Heinz, & Hoyer (2018); Hamo & Idisis (2017); Knott, Impey, Fisher, Delpero, & Fedoroff (2016); Marshall,

Summary	Reference
	Marshall, & Kingston (2011); Navathe, Ward, & Gannon (2008); Nunes & Jung (2013); Paquette, Cortoni, Proulx, & Longpre (2014); Sigre-Leirós, Carvalho, & Nobre (2015, 2016); Szumski & Zielona-Jenek (2016)
Studies concerning victim gender. Results showed that "crossover" (male and female victims) was significantly more likely as victims' ages decreased. Offenders with victims who were aged 6 years or younger were more likely to have male and female victims and to self-identify as having a "bisexual orientation." *Comment*: Many risk assessment instruments assign higher risk to so-called homosexual offenders. However, these studies suggest that "orientation" is being confused with interest and age of victim by both the offenders and the researchers.	Bailey, Hsu, & Bernhard (2016); Carlstedt et al. (2009); Levenson, Becker, & Morin (2008); Mitchell, Bravo, & Galupo (2017); Sim & Proeve (2010)
Studies comparing intrafamilial and extrafamilial child sex offenders. *Comment*: It is important not to confuse intra- and extrafamilial child sex offenders with "incest" that can be independent of age.	Becerra-García & Egan (2014); Bogaerts, Buschman, Kunst, & Winkel (2010); Seto, Babchishin, Pullman, & McPhail (2015); Titcomb, Goodman-Delahunty, & De Puiseau (2012)
Studies concerning clerics who sexually offended against a child. *Comment*: Religion does not cause pedophilia, but religious orders may attract people with pedophilia who ironically were hoping to escape their pedophilic interests via celibacy. These studies provide evidence that treatment based on "management" of pedophilic interest(s) with no attempt to change them may be ineffective.	Cartor, Cimbolic, & Tallon (2008); Firestone, Moulden, & Wexler (2009); Plante (2015)

Summary	Reference
Studies including women who sexually offended against children. See also Fedoroff, Fishell, and Fedoroff (1999).	Almond, McManus, Giles, & Houston (2017); Bader, Welsh, & Scalora (2010); Gannon, Hoare, Rose, & Parrett (2012); Gannon & Rose (2009); Gannon, Rose, & Williams (2009); Gillespie et al. (2015); Mackelprang (2016); Shaffer (2018)
Online Child Sex Offenders	
Literature reviews concerning online sexual offenses against children and online child sex offenders.	Babchishin, Hanson, & Hermann (2011); Beech, Elliott, Birgden, & Findlater (2008); Henshaw, Ogloff, & Clough (2017); Houtepen, Sijtsema, & Bogaerts (2014); Jewkes & Wykes (2012); Kloess, Beech, & Harkins (2014); Leclerc, Proulx, & Beauregard (2009); Niveau (2010); Prat & Jonas (2013); Vlachopoulou & Missionier (2018)
Studies related to child pornography offenders.	Burgess, Mahoney, Visk, & Morgenbesser (2008); Merdian, Curtis, Thakker, Wilson, & Boer (2013); Prat & Jonas (2012a, 2012b); Ray, Kimonis, & Donoghue (2010); Sheldon & Howitt (2008); Teeter-Witt (2016); Wolak, Finkelhor, & Mitchell (2011)
Those who possess child pornography (with no known prior sexual offences) typically do not transition to contact sexual offenses.	Endrass et al. (2009); Temporini (2012)
However, child sexual aggression has been associated with pedophilic interests, cognitive distortions, antisocial personality disorder, and use of child pornography.	Huang (2017); Lee, Li, Lamade, Schuler, & Prentky (2012); Smid, Schepers, Kamphuis, van Linden, & Bartling (2015)
A "subculture" of online "pedophile forums" supports emotional and sexual relationships with children in both online and offline settings.	Holt, Blevins, & Burkert (2010); O'Halloran & Quayle (2011)
Studies examining offenders' strategies to induce victims to comply with their requests, and characteristics of "online solicitors."	Kloess et al. (2017); Schulz, Bergen, Schuhmann, & Hoyer (2017)

Summary	Reference
Studies comparing contact sex offenders with online child sex offenders.	Babchishin et al. (2011); Babchishin, Hanson, & VanZuylen (2015); Burgess, Carretta, & Burgess (2012); Faust, Bickart, Renaud, & Camp (2015); Long, Alison, & McManus (2013); Magaletta, Faust, Bickart, & McLearen (2014); McCarthy (2011); Neutze, Grundmann, Scherner, & Beier (2012); Neutze, Seto, Schaefer, Mundt, & Beier (2011)
Diagnosis	
DSM Criticisms	
Discusses pedophilic disorder and describes those who are highly aroused by children as having a "powerful biological craving."	Berlin (2014)
Articles that discuss the forensic and clinical consequences of having the diagnosis of pedophilic disorder.	Malón (2012); Seto (2009); Wakefield (2012)
Articles reviewing the reliability and validity of the DSM-5 diagnosis of pedophilic disorder.	Blanchard (2010); Krueger, Kaplan, & First (2009); Mokros, Habermeyer, & Küchenhoff (2017); Perillo, Spada, Calkins, & Jegic (2014); Seto et al. (2016)
Articles proposing changes to the diagnostic criteria in the DSM-5, some of which include the addition of Tanner stages, behavioral indicators of child sexual attractions, use of child pornography, and online solicitations.	Balon (2014); Berlin (2011); First (2011); Mongeau & Rouleau (2014); Seto (2010)
Notes that pedophilic disorder does not have the option of being categorized as "in remission" in the DSM-5.	Briken, Fedoroff, & Bradford (2014)
Possible Variations	
Tests whether individuals with pedophilia have more paraphilias compared to individuals with hebephilia.	Burke (2013)
Suggests obsessive–compulsive disorder (OCD) and/or obsessive-compulsive personality disorder (OCPD) can be misdiagnosed as pedophilia.	Bogaerts, Daalder, Vanheule, Desmet, & Leeuw (2008); Bruce, Ching, & Williams (2018); Carlson (2012); Glazier (2018); Glazier, Swing, & McGinn (2015)

Summary	Reference
Case study of a man with an intellectual disability, "koro-like symptoms," and pedophilia.	Faccini (2009)
Factitious disorder presenting as pedophilia. Malingered pedophilia has also been described (Fedoroff, Hanson, McGuire, Malin, & Berlin, 1992).	Porter & Feldman (2011)
Assessment	
Articles considering whether pedophilic disorder is dimensional or categorical. The majority of studies have found that pedophilic disorder falls best into a dimensional structure.	Blanchard (2013); Blanchard et al. (2009); Mackaronis, Strassberg, & Marcus (2011); Poeppl et al. (2013); Stephens, Leroux, Skilling, Cantor, & Seto (2017)
Articles examining the classification of child sex offenders.	Baltieri & Boer (2015); Feelgood & Hoyer (2008); King (2011); Mandeville-Norden & Beech (2009); Marshall, Smallbone, & Marshall (2015); McPhail, Olver, Brouillette-Alarie, & Looman (2018)
Studies comparing offenses motivated by pedophilia to offenses that are opportunistic.	Gerwinn et al. (2018); Pearson (2013)
Studies comparing sex offenders against children to sex offenders against adults.	Schmidt, Mokros, & Banse (2013); Spehr, Hill, Habermann, Briken, & Bernter (2010)
The use of artificial intelligence to detect those with pedophilia.	Kouros (2013)
The use of highly immersive virtual reality to differentiate individuals with pedophilia from others.	Renaud et al. (2010)
Examines the use of computer-generated images of males and females in various developmental stages to assess pedophilia.	Dombert et al. (2013)
Examines the use of computer-generated characters to accurately discriminate individuals with pedophilia from others.	Marschall-Lévesque, Rouleau, & Renaud (2018)
Studies of the Not-Real-People (NRP) phallometric stimuli.	Dombert et al. (2015); Mokros et al. (2011)

Summary	Reference
Comment: NRP stimuli consist primarily of ethically approved audiotapes of adult–child sexual encounters constructed by splicing the voices of child actors protected from the sexual aspects of the stimuli into sexual scenarios.	
Studies examining phallometric testing to assess child sexual interest.	Babchishin, Curry, Fedoroff, Bradford, & Seto (2017); Cantor & McPhail (2015); Lalumière (2015); Lykins et al. (2010a, 2010b); McPhail et al. (2019); Moulden, Firestone, Kingston, & Bradford (2009); Müller et al. (2014); Renaud et al. (2013); Stephens, Cantor, Goodwill, & Seto (2017)
Articles examining neuroimaging techniques (magnetic resonance imaging [MRI] or functional MRI) to identify or assess pedophilia. *Comment*: Although important, none of these studies definitively investigate whether sexual interest can be modified.	Cantor & Blanchard (2012); Cantor et al. (2008, 2015, 2016); Cazala et al. (2018); Fonteille, Cazala, Moulier, & Stoléru (2012); Gerwinn et al. (2015); Habermeyer, Esposito, Händel, Lemoine, Klarhöfer, et al. (2013); Habermeyer, Esposito, Händel, Lemoine, Kuhl, et al. (2013); Kärgel et al. (2015, 2017); Lett et al. (2018); Massau et al. (2017a,b); Poeppl et al. (2011, 2013); Polisois-Keating & Joyal (2013); Ponseti et al. (2012, 2014, 2016, 2018); Sartorius et al. (2008); Schiffer et al. (2008a, 2008b, 2017); Tenbergen et al. (2015); Wiebking & Northoff (2013)
Studies using eye movements and/or pupil dilation to assess pedophilic sexual interests.	Beech, Kalmus, et al. (2008); Ciardha, Attard-Johnson, & Bindemann (2018); Fromberger et al. (2012, 2013)
Studies investigating viewing time measures of child sex offenders.	Boardman (2010); Casey (2008); Crosby (2008); Gray et al. (2015); Mokros et al. (2013); Schmidt, Babchishin, & Lehmann (2017); Worsham (2011)

Summary	Reference
Studies examining the use of implicit association tasks to identify pedophilic interests.	Babchishin, Nunes, & Hermann (2013); Babchishin, Nunes, Hermann, & Malcom (2015); Babchishin, Nunes, & Kessous (2014); Brown, Gray, & Snowden (2009); Ciardha & Gormley (2012); Hempel, Buck, Goethals, & Van Marle (2013); Mokros, Dombert, Osterheider, Zappalà, & Santtila (2010); Schmidt, Gykiere, Vanhoeck, Mann, & Banse (2014); van Leeuwen et al. (2013); Weidacker et al. (2017); Zappalà, Antfolk, Dombert, Mokros, & Santtila (2016)
Dream analysis of males diagnosed with pedophilia. A common theme was ambivalence toward their mothers and to adult relationships with women.	Kaplan (2012)
Developed and validated a measure to assess level of self-efficacy in modifying pedophilic interests.	Tozdan, Jakob, Schuhmann, Budde, & Briken (2015)
Assessing Recidivism and Risk Levels	
Studies of sexual recidivism and risk. Overall, rates of recidivism are low for sex offenders against children.	Beggs & Grace (2008); Craig (2008); Kingston, Fedoroff, Firestone, Curry, & Bradford (2008); Kingston, Firestone, Wexler, & Bradford (2008); McLawsen (2010); McLawsen, Scalora, & Darrow (2012); Phenix & Sreenivasan (2009); Rettenberger, Briken, Turner, & Eher (2015); Tan & Grace (2008); Vess & Skelton (2010)
Researchers tested the use of virtual reality scenarios to track treatment progress of sex offenders against children.	Fromberger, Meyer, Jordan, & Müller (2018)
Some scales developed to assess risk of sexual recidivism:	
Correlates of Admission of Sexual Interest in Children (CASIC)	Seto & Eke (2017)

Summary	Reference
MOLEST scales RAPE scales Risk Matrix 2000 STATIC-99 Violence Risk Scale: Sexual Offender Version (VRS:SO) PCL-R Stable-2007 Screening Scale for Pedophilic Interests (SSPI) and version 2	Nunes, Pettersen, Hermann, Looman, & Spape (2016) Osborn, Elliott, Middleton, & Beech (2010) Beggs & Grace (2010); Eher, Olver, Heurix, Schilling, & Rettenberger (2015) Eher et al. (2015) Eher et al. (2015); Helmus, Ó Ciardha, & Seto (2015) Eher et al. (2015); Helmus et al. (2015); Seto, Sandler, & Freeman (2017); Seto, Stephens, Lalumière, & Cantor (2017)
Rapid Risk Assessment of Sex Offender Recidivism (RRASOR) A risk measure for child pornography reoffenses, Child Pornography Offender Risk Tool (CPORT). *Comment*: A checklist completed by the investigator that the authors correctly indicate has not been sufficiently validated for clinical use without significant caution.	Wilson, Abracen, Looman, Picheca, & Ferguson (2011) Seto & Eke (2015)
Treatment	
Discusses some treatments available to men with pedophilic interests.	Seto & Ahmed (2014); Stolpmann, Briken, & Müller (2017)
Articles examining the roles of health care professionals in treating individuals with pedophilic interests.	Bach & Demuth (2018); Bleistein (2012)
Asked 14 women convicted of sex offenses against children about treatment goals. Results showed women believed in changing themselves, developing better relationships with men, and learning to cope with the psychological effects of their convictions.	Lawson & Rowe (2010)
Discusses whether deep brain stimulation should be used to treat parkinsonian patients with known or suspected pedophilia.	Müller, Walter, & Christen (2014)

Summary	Reference
Pharmacological Treatment	
Investigated the prevalence of pharmacological treatment for paraphilic disorders in German outpatient treatment centers.	Turner, Hertz, Sauter, Briken, & Rettenberger (2018)
Tested the use of divalproex sodium and quetiapine to treat a person with pedophilia and bipolar disorder.	Wang, Kao, & Liu (2014)
Studies examining the use of luteinizing hormone-releasing hormone agonists to treat patients with pedophilia.	Briken & Berner (2012); Habermeyer et al. (2012); Moulier et al. (2012); Schiffer, Gizewski, & Kruger (2009); Turner & Briken (2018); Witztum, Daie, & Rosler (2012)
Articles and studies examining the use of anti-androgens to treat sex offenders.	Amelung, Kuhle, Konrad, Pauls, & Beier (2012); Jordan, Fromberger, Laubinger, Dechent, & Müller (2014); Jordan, Fromberger, Stolpmann, & Müller (2011); Kingston et al. (2012); Panesar, Allard, Pai, & Valachova (2011); Silvani, Mondaini, & Zucchi (2015)
Psychological and Behavioral Therapy	
Articles examining the influence of therapy on recidivism rates. Although sex offenders have low recidivism rates in general, it was found that treatment groups (compared to untreated groups) tended to have lower recidivism rates. One meta-analysis (Grønnerød, Grønnerød, & Grøndahl, 2015) found that the evidence for treatment effects was inconclusive.	Abracen, Looman, Ferguson, Harkins, & Mailloux (2011); Codispoti (2008); Grønnerød et al. (2015); Harkins & Beech (2008); Walton & Chou (2015)
Studies of "self-efficacy" in individuals who are attempting to change their pedophilic interests.	Farmer, Beech, & Ward (2012); Tozdan & Briken (2015a,b); Tozdan et al. (2018)
Articles examining the changeability and therefore treatability of pedophilic interests.	Blagden, Mann, Webster, Lee, & Williams (2017); Fedoroff (2018); Fedoroff, Curry, Ranger, & Bradford (2016); Mokros & Habermeyer (2016)

Summary	Reference
Case study of psychoanalysis to treat pedophilia.	Campbell (2014)
Description of a group of people with pedophilia who view sexual relations between children and adults as wrong. This group self-identify as "virtuous pedophiles." Some use religion to cope with their pedophilic interests. They were found to have fewer cognitive distortions and low levels of distress.	Cranney (2017)
Discusses the use of the restorative justice model and its application to sexual abuse by the clergy.	Noll & Harvey (2008)
Utilized "satiation" therapy with a 19-year-old male sex offender. His sexual interests changed from male children to adult male peers.	Hunter, Ram, & Ryback (2008)
Reintegration	
Found the good lives model was associated with positive community reintegration.	Willis & Ward (2011)
Child sex offenders who did not recidivate had higher quality reintegration planning. The following combination was associated with low recidivism: successful accommodation, employment, and social support.	Russell, Seymour, & Lambie (2013); Willis & Grace (2009)
Investigated the impact of the Sex Offender Registration and Notification Act (SORNA) on registered men with pedophilia. Results showed that SORNA had a negative impact on their psychosocial functioning and did not reduce sexual offending.	Moster (2015); Palermo (2012); Sandler, Freeman, & Socia (2008)
Prevention	
Discusses methods and approaches of preventing child sexual abuse and the limitations of those approaches.	Cohen-Almago (2013); Finkelhor (2009); Houtepen, Sijtsema, & Bogaerts (2016); Lasher & Stinson (2017)

Summary	Reference
Studies that are related to the Prevention Project Dunkelfeld, which launched in Germany with the goal of preventing child sexual abuse by treating people with pedophilic and hebephilic interests before they committed offenses.	Beier, Ahlers, et al. (2009); Beier, Neutze, et al. (2009); Beier et al. (2015, 2016); Schaefer et al. (2010)
Explored the barriers that prevented individuals with pedophilic interests from seeking professional help. Obstacles included shame, secrecy, and other personal, social, and legal consequences.	Levenson, Willis, & Vicencio (2017)
Interviewed staff who were working at an anonymous helpline for people with pedophilic interests and examined how staff can help prevent child sexual abuse by helping those with pedophilic interests get the interventions they need.	Goodier & Lievesley (2018)
Books and Book Chapters	
Baltieri, D. A., Anrade, A. G., & Boer, D. P. (2011). Ethical issues regarding the implementation of sex offender treatment in Brazil. In D. P. Boer, R. Eher, L. A. Craig, M. H. Miner, & F. Pfafflin (Eds.), *International perspectives on the assessment and treatment of sexual offenders: Theory, practice, and research* (pp. 575–585). Malden, MA: Wiley-Blackwell.	
Bradford, J. M. W., Fedoroff, P., & Firestone, P. (2008). Sexual violence and the clinician. In R. I. Simon & K. Tardiff (Eds.), *Textbook of violence assessment and management* (pp. 441–460). Arlington, VA: American Psychiatric Publishing.	
Cantor, J. M. (2014). "Gold star pedophiles" in general sex therapy practice. In Y. M. Binik & K. S. K. Hall (Eds.), *Principles and practice of sex therapy* (5th ed., pp. 219–234). New York, NY: Guilford.	
Duncan, K. A. (2010). *Female sexual predators: Understanding them to protect our children and youths.* Santa Barbara, CA: ABC-CLIO.	
Elliott, I. A., & Babchishin, K. M. (2012). Psychological profiles and processes in viewers of internet child pornography. In B. K. Schwartz (Ed.), *The sex offender: Current trends in policy and treatment practice* (Vol. 7, pp. 1–15). Kingston, NJ: Civic Research Institute.	
Fedoroff, J. P., & Marshall, W. L. (2010). Paraphilias. In D. McKay, J. S. Abramowitz, & S. Taylor (Eds.), Cognitive–behavioral therapy for refractory cases: Turning failure into success (pp. 369–384). Washington, DC: American Psychological Association.	

Flak, V. E., Beech, A. R., & Humphreys, G. W. (2009). The rapid serial visual presentation test of sexual interest in child molesters. In D. Thornton & D. R. Laws (Eds.), *Cognitive approaches to the assessment of sexual interest in sexual offenders* (pp. 145–158). Malden, MA: Wiley-Blackwell.

Gacono, C. B., Meloy, J. R., & Bridges, M. R. (2008). A Rorschach understanding of psychopaths, sexual homicide perpetrators, and nonviolent pedophiles. In C. B. Gacono & F. B. Evans (Eds.), *The handbook of forensic Rorschach assessment* (pp. 379–393). New York, NY: Taylor & Francis.

Graf, M., & Dittmann, V. (2011). Forensic-psychiatric treatment for internet sex offenders: Ten years of experience. In D. P. Boer, R. Eher, L. A. Craig, M. H. Miner, & F. Pfafflin (Eds.), *International perspectives on the assessment and treatment of sexual offenders: Theory, practice, and research* (pp. 575–585). Malden, MA: Wiley-Blackwell.

Hoffer, T. A., & Shelton, J. L. E. (2013). *Suicide among child sex offenders*. New York, NY: Springer.

Jordan, K., Fromberger, P., & Müller, J. L. (2016). Structural and functional magnetic resonance imaging in assessing sexual preference. In D. P. Boer (Ed.), *The Wiley handbook on the theories, assessment and treatment of sexual offending* (pp. 925–964). Malden, MA: Wiley.

Khoury, J. M., Roque, M. A. V., & Garcia, F. D. (2016). Pedophilic disorder. In R. Balon (Ed.), *Practical guide to paraphilia and paraphilic disorders* (pp. 141–154). Cham, Switzerland: Springer.

Kolod, S. (2016). Reluctance to finding myself in the other: Treating an alleged paedophile. In B. Willock, L. C. Bohm, & R. C. Curtis (Eds.), *Psychoanalytic perspectives on identity and difference* (pp. 81–87). New York, NY: Routledge.

Laws, D. R., & O'Donohue, W. T. (Eds.). (2008). *Sexual deviance: Theory, assessment, and treatment* (2nd ed.). New York, NY: Guilford.

MacDonell, L., & Bolton, C. (2018). Dual histories of abuse and perpetration. In R. B. Gartner (Ed.), *Healing sexually betrayed men and boys: Treatment for sexual abuse, assault, and trauma* (pp. 289–317). New York, NY: Routledge.

Malesky, A. L., Jr., Ennis, L., & Gress, C. L. Z. (2009). Child pornography and the internet. In F. M. Saleh, A. J. Grudzinskas, Jr., J. M. Bradford, & D. Brodsky (Eds.), Sex offenders: Identification, risk assessment, treatment, and legal issues (pp. 302–323). New York, NY: Oxford University Press.

Maram, W. B. (2016). Psychophysiological assessment of sexual offenders: A practitioner's perspective. In A. Phenix & H. M. Hoberman (Eds.), *Sexual offending* (pp. 331–352). New York, NY: Springer.

Marshall, W. L., O'Brien, M. D., & Marshall, L. E. (2009). Modifying sexual preferences. In A. R. Beech, L. A. Craig, & K. D. Browne (Eds.), *Assessment and treatment of sex offenders: A handbook* (pp. 311–327). New York, NY: Wiley.

McCartan, K. F. (2008). Current understandings of paedophilia and the resulting crisis in modern society. In J. M. Caroll & M. K. Alena (Eds.), *Psychological sexual dysfunctions* (pp. 51–84). Hauppauge, NY: Nova.

Nunes, K. L. (2009). Measuring child molesters' implicit cognitions about self and children. In D. Thornton & D. R. Laws (Eds.), *Cognitive approaches to the assessment of sexual interest in sexual offenders* (pp. 125–143). Malden, MA: Wiley-Blackwell.

Quayle, E. (2011). Pedophilia, child porn, and cyberpredators. In C. D. Bryant (Ed.), *The Routledge handbook of deviant behavior* (pp. 390–396). New York, NY: Routledge.

Renaud, P., Joyal, C., Stoleru, S., Goyette, M., Weiskopf, N., & Birbaumer, N. (2011). Real-time functional magnetic imaging—Brain–computer interface and virtual reality: Promising tools for the treatment of pedophilia. *Progress in Brain Research, 192,* 263–272.

Rowland, D. L., & Incrocci, L. (2008). *Handbook of sexual and gender identity disorders.* Hoboken, NJ: Wiley.

Seto, M. C. (2008). *Pedophilia and sexual offending against children: Theory, assessment, and intervention.* Washington, DC: American Psychological Association.

Seto, M. C. (2013). *Internet sex offenders* (pp. 169–192). Washington, DC: American Psychological Association.

Seto, M. C. (2018). *Pedophilia and sexual offending against children: Theory, assessment, and intervention* (2nd ed., pp. 251–252). Washington, DC: American Psychological Association.

Shetty, A., Nayak, A., Travers, R., Vaidya, H., & Wylie, K. (2014). Pedophilia. In G. Corona, E. A. Jannini, & M. Maggi (Eds.), Emotional, physical and sexual abuse: Impact in children and social minorities (pp. 1–17). Cham, Switzerland: Springer.

Steele, B. R., & Ryan, G. (2010). Deviancy: Development gone wrong. In G. Ryan, T. Leversee, & S. Lane (Eds.), *Juvenile sexual offending: Causes, consequences, and correction* (pp. 55–69). Hoboken, NJ: Wiley.

Stephens, S., & Seto, M. C. (2016). Hebephilic sexual offending. In A. Phenix & H. M. Hoberman (Eds.), *Sexual offending: Predisposing antecedents, assessments, and management* (pp. 29–43). New York, NY: Springer.

Wiebking, C., Sartorius, A., Dressing, H., & Northoff, G. (2012). Pedophilia. In J. R. Simpson (Ed.), *Neuroimaging in forensic psychiatry: From the clinic to the courtroom* (pp. 99–111). Malden, MA: Wiley-Blackwell.

Williams, S. E., Gannon, T. A., Ward, T., & Collie, R. M. (2008). Child molesters' cognitive distortions: A brief research review. In J. P. Tsai (Ed.), *Leading-edge cognitive disorders research* (pp. 155–167). Hauppauge, NY: Nova.

Wollert, R., Waggoner, J., & Smith, J. (2012). Federal internet child pornography offenders—Limited offense histories and low recidivism rates. In B. K. Schwartz (Ed.), *The sex offender: Current trends in policy and treatment practice* (Vol. 7, pp. 1–21). Kingston, NJ: Civic Research Institute.
Wood, H. (2010). Applied analytic work in forensic settings: The understanding and treatment of paedophilia. In A. Lemma & M. Patrick (Eds.), *Off the couch: Contemporary psychoanalytic applications* (pp. 143–159). New York, NY: Routledge.

References

Abdo, C. H. N. (2013). Sexuality and couple intimacy in dementia. *Current Opinion in Psychiatry, 26*(6), 593–598.

Abel, G. G., Jordan, A., Hand, C. G., Holland, L. A., & Phipps, A. (2001). Classification models of child molesters utilizing the Abel Assessment for Sexual Interest. *Child Abuse & Neglect, 25,* 703–718.

Abracen, J., Looman, J., Ferguson, M., Harkins, L., & Mailloux, D. (2011). Recidivism among treated sexual offenders and comparison subjects: Recent outcome data from the Regional Treatment Centre (Ontario) High-Intensity Sex Offender Treatment Programme. *Journal of Sexual Aggression, 17*(2), 142–152.

Aho, J. (2013). A comparison of levels of aggression between pedophilic and non-pedophilic child molesters. Doctoral dissertation, Alliant International University, California School of Forensic Studies, Irvine, CA.

Alanko, K., Gunst, A., Mokros, A., & Santtila, P. (2016). Genetic variants associated with male pedophilic sexual interest. *Journal of Sexual Medicine, 13*(5), 835–842.

Alanko, K., Salo, B., Mokros, A., & Santtila, P. (2013). Evidence for heritability of adult men's sexual interest in youth under age 16 from a population-based extended twin design. *Journal of Sexual Medicine, 10*(4), 1090–1099.

Almond, L., McManus, M. A., Giles, S., & Houston, E. (2017). Female sex offenders: An analysis of crime scene behaviors. *Journal of Interpersonal Violence, 32*(24), 3839–3860.

Alnemari, A. M., Mansour, T. R., Buehler, M., & Gaudin, D. (2016). Neural basis of pedophilia: Altered sexual preference following traumatic brain injury. *International Journal of Surgery Case Reports, 25,* 221–224.

Amelung, T., Kuhle, L. F., Konrad, A., Pauls, A., & Beier, K. M. (2012). Androgen deprivation therapy of self-identifying, help-seeking pedophiles in the Dunkelfeld. *International Journal of Law and Psychiatry, 35*(3), 176–184.

American Psychiatric Association. (1994). *Diagnostic and statistical manual of mental disorders* (4th ed.). Washington, DC: Author.

American Psychiatric Association. (2000). *Diagnostic and statistical manual of mental disorders* (4th ed., text revision). Washington, DC: Author.

American Psychiatric Association. (2013a). *Diagnostic and statistical manual of mental disorders* (5th ed.). Arlington, VA: American Psychiatric Publishing.

American Psychiatric Association (2013b, October 31). *APA statement on DSM-5 text error.* Press release.

Andrews, D. A., Bonta, J., & Wormith, J. S. (2011, June 1). The risk–need–responsivity (RNR) model: Does adding the Good Lives Model contribute to effective crime prevention? *Criminal Justice and Behavior,* **38**(7), 735–755. doi:10.1177/0093854811406356

Babchishin, K. M., Curry, S. D., Fedoroff, J. P., Bradford, J., & Seto, M. C. (2017). Inhibiting sexual arousal to children: Correlates and its influence on the validity of penile plethysmography. *Archives of Sexual Behavior, 46*(3), 671–684.

Babchishin, K. M., Hanson, R. K., & Hermann, C. A. (2011). The characteristics of online sex offenders: A meta-analysis. *Sexual Abuse, 23*(1), 92–123.

Babchishin, K. M., Hanson, R. K., & VanZuylen, H. (2015). Online child pornography offenders are different: A meta-analysis of the characteristics of online and offline sex offenders against children. *Archives of Sexual Behavior, 44*(1), 45–66.

Babchishin, K. M., Nunes, K. L., & Hermann, C. A. (2013). The validity of Implicit Association Test (IAT) measures of sexual attraction to children: A meta-analysis. *Archives of Sexual Behavior, 42*(3), 487–499.

Babchishin, K. M., Nunes, K. L., Hermann, C. A., & Malcom, J. R. (2015). Implicit sexual interest in children: Does separating gender influence discrimination when using the Implicit Association Test? *Journal of Sexual Aggression, 21*(2), 194–208.

Babchishin, K. M., Nunes, K. L., & Kessous, N. (2014). A multimodal examination of sexual interest in children: A comparison of sex offenders and non-sex offenders. *Sexual Abuse, 26*(4), 343–374.

Babchishin, K. M., Seto, M. C., Fazel, S., & Långström, N. (2019). Are there early risk markers for pedophilia? A nationwide case–control study of child sexual exploitation material offenders. *Journal of Sex Research, 56*(2), 203–212.

Bach, M. H., & Demuth, C. (2018). Therapists' experiences in their work with sex offenders and people with pedophilia: A literature review. *Europe's Journal of Psychology, 14*(2), 498–514.

Bader, S. M., Welsh, R., & Scalora, M. J. (2010). Recidivism among female child molesters. *Violence and Victims, 25*(3), 349–362.

Bailey, J. M., Bernhard, P. A., & Hsu, K. J. (2016). An internet study of men sexually attracted to children: Correlates of sexual offending against children. *Journal of Abnormal Psychology, 125*(7), 989–1000.

Bailey, J. M., Hsu, K. J., & Bernhard, P. A. (2016). An internet study of men sexually attracted to children: Sexual attraction patterns. *Journal of Abnormal Psychology, 125*(7), 976–988.

Balon, R. (2014). Politics of diagnostic criteria: Specifiers of pedophilic disorder in DSM-5. *Archives of Sexual Behavior, 43*(7), 1235.

Baltieri, D. A., Anrade, A. G., & Boer, D. P. (2011). Ethical issues regarding the implementation of sex offender treatment in Brazil. In D. P. Boer, R. Eher, L. A. Craig, M. H. Miner, & F. Pfafflin (Eds.), *International perspectives on the assessment and treatment of sexual offenders: Theory, practice, and research* (pp. 575–585). Malden, MA: Wiley-Blackwell.

Baltieri, D. A., & Boer, D. P. (2015). Two clusters of child molesters based on impulsiveness. *Revista Brasileira de Psiquiatria, 37*(2), 139–145.

Bao, A. M., & Swaab, D. F. (2010). Sex differences in the brain, behavior, and neuropsychiatric disorders. *The Neuroscientist, 16*(5), 550–565.

Beauregard, E., Leclerc, B., & Lussier, P. (2012). Decision making in the crime commission process: Comparing rapists, child molesters, and victim-crossover sex offenders. *Criminal Justice and Behavior, 39*(10), 1275–1295.

Becerra-García, J. A., & Egan, V. (2014). Neurocognitive functioning and subtypes of child molesters: Poorer working memory differentiates incestuous from non-incestuous offenders. *Psychiatry, Psychology and Law, 21*(4), 585–590.

Beech, A. R., Elliott, I. A., Birgden, A., & Findlater, D. (2008). The internet and child sexual offending: A criminological review. *Aggression and Violent Behavior, 13*(3), 216–228.

Beech, A. R., Kalmus, E., Tipper, S. P., Baudouin, J. Y., Flak, V., & Humphreys, G. W. (2008). Children induce an enhanced attentional blink in child molesters. *Psychological Assessment, 20*(4), 397–402.

Beggs, S. M., & Grace, R. C. (2008). Psychopathy, intelligence, and recidivism in child molesters: Evidence of an interaction effect. *Criminal Justice and Behavior, 35*(6), 683–695.

Beggs, S. M., & Grace, R. C. (2010). Assessment of dynamic risk factors: An independent validation study of the Violence Risk Scale: Sexual Offender Version. *Sexual Abuse, 22*(2), 234–251.

Beier, K. M., Ahlers, C. J., Goecker, D., Neutze, J., Mundt, I. A., Hupp, E., & Schaefer, G. A. (2009). Can pedophiles be reached for primary prevention of child sexual abuse? First results of the Berlin Prevention Project Dunkelfeld (PPD). *Journal of Forensic Psychiatry & Psychology, 20*(6), 851–867.

Beier, K. M., Grundmann, D., Kuhle, L. F., Scherner, G., Konrad, A., & Amelung, T. (2015). The German Dunkelfeld Project: A pilot study to prevent child sexual abuse and the use of child abusive images. *Journal of Sexual Medicine, 12*(2), 529–542.

Beier, K. M., Neutze, J., Mundt, I. A., Ahlers, C. J., Goecker, D., Konrad, A., & Schaefer, G. A. (2009). Encouraging self-identified pedophiles and hebephiles to seek professional help: First results of the Prevention Project Dunkelfeld (PPD). *Child Abuse and Neglect: The International Journal, 33*(8), 545–549.

Beier, K. M., Oezdemir, U. C., Schlinzig, E., Groll, A., Hupp, E., & Hellenschmidt, T. (2016). "Just dreaming of them": The Berlin Project for Primary Prevention of Child Sexual Abuse by Juveniles (PPJ). *Child Abuse & Neglect, 52*, 1–10.

Berlin, F. S. (2011). Commentary on pedophilia diagnostic criteria in DSM-5. *Journal of the American Academy of Psychiatry and the Law Online, 39*(2), 242–244.

Berlin, F. S. (2014). Pedophilia and DSM-5: The importance of clearly defining the nature of a pedophilic disorder [Editorial]. *Journal of the American Academy of Psychiatry and the Law, 42*, 404–407.

Berryessa, C. (2014). Potential implications of research on genetic or heritable contributions to pedophilia for the objectives of criminal law. *Recent Advances in DNA & Gene Sequences, 8*(2), 65–77.

Blagden, N. J., Mann, R., Webster, S., Lee, R., & Williams, F. (2017). "It's not something I chose you know": Making sense of pedophiles' sexual interest in children and the impact on their psychosexual identity. *Sexual Abuse, 30*(6), 728–754.

Blanchard, R. (2010). The DSM diagnostic criteria for pedophilia. *Archives of Sexual Behavior, 39*(2), 304–316. doi:10.1007/s10508-009-9536-0

Blanchard, R. (2013). A dissenting opinion on DSM-5 pedophilic disorder. *Archives of Sexual Behavior, 42*(5), 675–678.

Blanchard, R., Kuban, M. E., Blak, T., Cantor, J. M., Klassen, P. E., & Dickey, R. (2009). Absolute versus relative ascertainment of pedophilia in men. *Sexual Abuse, 21*(4), 431–441.

Bleistein, L. A. (2012). The reintegration process of male pedophiles. Doctoral dissertation, Alliant International University, California School of Forensic Studies, Irvine, CA (ProQuest Dissertations, Accession No. 3482838).

Boardman, R. D. (2010). Creating an expected profile for Affinity 2.5 from a sample of non-pedophilic, exclusively heterosexual, college-age males. Doctoral dissertation, Brigham Young University, Provo, UT (ProQuest Dissertations, Accession No. 3376127).

Bogaerts, S., Buschman, J., Kunst, M. J. J., & Winkel, F. W. (2010). Intra- and extra-familial child molestation as pathways building on parental and relational deficits and personality disorders. *International Journal of Offender Therapy and Comparative Criminology, 54*(4), 478–493.

Bogaerts, S., Daalder, A., Vanheule, S., Desmet, M., & Leeuw, F. (2008). Personality Disorders in a Sample of Paraphilic and Nonparaphilic Child Molesters: A Comparative Study. *International Journal of Offender Therapy and Comparative Criminology, 52*(1), 21–30. https://doi.org/10.1177/0306624X07308261

Bradford, J. M., Pawlak, A., & Curry, S. (1997). Evaluation of the Sexual Behaviors Clinic: Assessment of child molesters. Unpublished manuscript.

Bradford, J. M. W., Fedoroff, P., & Firestone, P. (2008). Sexual violence and the clinician. In R. I. Simon & K. Tardiff (Eds.), *Textbook of violence assessment and management* (pp. 441–460). Arlington, VA: American Psychiatric Publishing.

Briken, P., & Berner, W. (2012). Double-blind, controlled, clinical trial planned in Germany to investigate the efficacy of psychotherapy combined with triptorelin in adult male patients with severe pedophilic disorders: Presentation of the study protocol. *Israel Journal of Psychiatry and Related Sciences, 49*(4), 306–313.

Briken, P., Fedoroff, J. P., & Bradford, J. W. (2014). Why can't pedophilic disorder remit? *Archives of Sexual Behavior, 43*(7), 1237–1239.

Brown, A. S., Gray, N. S., & Snowden, R. J. (2009). Implicit measurement of sexual associations in child sex abusers: Role of victim type and denial. *Sexual Abuse, 21*(2), 166–180.

Bruce, S. L., Ching, T. H., & Williams, M. T. (2018). Pedophilia-themed obsessive–compulsive disorder: Assessment, differential diagnosis, and treatment with exposure and response prevention. *Archives of Sexual Behavior, 47*(2), 389–402.

Burgess, A. W., Carretta, C. M., & Burgess, A. G. (2012). Patterns of federal internet offenders: A pilot study. *Journal of Forensic Nursing, 8*(3), 112–121.

Burgess, A. W., Mahoney, M., Visk, J., & Morgenbesser, L. (2008). Cyber child sexual exploitation. *Journal of Psychosocial Nursing and Mental Health Services, 46*(9), 38–45.

Burke, S. (2013). Pedophilia and *hebephilia*: An *analysis* of *deviant sexual interest using* the Abel Assessment for Sexual Interest-2. Doctoral dissertation, Alliant International University, California School of Forensic Studies, Irvine, CA.

Camilleri, J., & Quinsey, V. (2008). Pedophilia: Assessment and treatment. In D. R. Laws & W. T. Donohue (Eds.), *Sexual deviance: Theory, assessment, and treatment* (2nd ed., pp. 183–212). New York, NY: Guilford.

Campbell, D. (2014). Doubt in the psychoanalysis of a paedophile. *International Journal of Psychoanalysis, 95*(3), 441–463.

Cantor, J. M. (2012). Is homosexuality a paraphilia? The evidence for and against. *Archives of Sexual Behavior, 41*, 237–247. https://doi.org/10.1007/s10508-012-9900-3

Cantor, J. M. (2014). "Gold star pedophiles" in general sex therapy practice. In Y. M. Binik & K. S. K. Hall, (Eds.), *Principles and practice of sex therapy* (5th ed., pp. 219–234). New York, NY: Guilford.

Cantor, J. M., & Blanchard, R. (2012). White matter volumes in pedophiles, hebephiles, and teleiophiles. *Archives of Sexual Behavior, 41*(4), 749–752.

Cantor, J. M., & Fedoroff, J. P. (2018). Can pedophiles change response to opening arguments and conclusions. *Current Sexual Health Reports, 10*(4), 213–220. https://doi.org/10.1007/s11930-018-0167-0

Cantor, J. M., Kabani, N., Christensen, B. K., Zipursky, R. B., Barbaree, H. E., Dickey, R., . . . Richards, B. A. (2008). Cerebral white matter deficiencies in pedophilic men. *Journal of Psychiatric Research, 42*(3), 167–183.

Cantor, J. M., Lafaille, S. J., Hannah, J., Kucyi, A., Soh, D. W., Girard, T. A., & Mikulis, D. J. (2016). Independent component analysis of resting-state functional magnetic resonance imaging in pedophiles. *Journal of Sexual Medicine, 13*(10), 1546–1554.

Cantor, J. M., Lafaille, S., Soh, D. W., Moayedi, M., Mikulis, D. J., & Girard, T. A. (2015). Diffusion tensor imaging of pedophilia. *Archives of Sexual Behavior, 44*(8), 2161–2172.

Cantor, J. M., & McPhail, I. V. (2015). Sensitivity and specificity of the phallometric test for hebephilia. *Journal of Sexual Medicine, 12*(9), 1940–1950.

Capra, G. A., Forresi, B., & Caffo, E. (2014). Current scientific research on paedophilia: A review. *Journal of Psychopathology, 20*, 17–26.

Carlson, S. (2012). Obsessive–compulsive disorder: Homosexual and pedophilic obsessions in a 25-year-old male. In P. Levounis, J. Drescher, & M. E. Barber (Eds.), *The LGBT casebook* (pp. 161–169). Arlington, VA: American Psychiatric Publishing.

Carlstedt, A., Nilsson, T., Hofvander, B., Brimse, A., Innala, S., & Anckarsäter, H. (2009). Does victim age differentiate between perpetrators of sexual child abuse? A study of mental health, psychosocial circumstances, and crimes. *Sexual Abuse, 21*(4), 442–454.

Cartor, P., Cimbolic, P., & Tallon, J. (2008). Differentiating pedophilia from ephebophilia in cleric offenders. *Sexual Addiction & Compulsivity, 15*(4), 311–319.

Carvalho, J., & Nobre, P. J. (2014). Early maladaptive schemas in convicted sexual offenders: Preliminary findings. *International Journal of Law and Psychiatry, 37*(2), 210–216.

Casey, K. A. (2008). The Abel Assessment for Sexual Interests: Impact of antisocial personality features and pedophilic tendencies on test performance. Doctoral dissertation (ProQuest Information & Learning, Accession No. 3299504).

Cazala, F., Fonteille, V., Moulier, V., Pélégrini-Issac, M., De Beaurepaire, C., Abondo, M., . . . Thevenon, C. (2018). Brain responses to pictures of children in men with pedophilic disorder: A functional magnetic resonance imaging study. *European Archives of Psychiatry and Clinical Neuroscience* [Epub ahead of print].

Ciardha, C. Ó., Attard-Johnson, J., & Bindemann, M. (2018). Latency-based and psychophysiological measures of sexual interest show convergent and concurrent validity. *Archives of Sexual Behavior, 47*(3), 637–649.

Ciardha, C. Ó., & Gormley, M. (2012). Using a pictorial-modified Stroop task to explore the sexual interests of sexual offenders against children. *Sexual Abuse, 24*(2), 175–197.

Codispoti, V. L. (2008). Pharmacology of sexually compulsive behavior. *Psychiatric Clinics of North America, 31*(4), 671–679.

Cohen, L. J., Forman, H., Steinfeld, M., Fradkin, Y., Frenda, S., & Galynker, I. (2010). Comparison of childhood sexual histories in subjects with pedophilia or opiate addiction and healthy controls: Is childhood sexual abuse a risk factor for addictions? *Journal of Psychiatric Practice, 16*(6), 394–404.

Cohen, L. J., & Galynker, I. (2012). Identifying psychological traits potentially subserving aberrant motivation or inhibitory failure in pedophilic behavior. *Israel Journal of Psychiatry and Related Sciences, 49*(4), 280–290.

Cohen, L. J., Grebchenko, Y. F., Steinfeld, M., Frenda, S. J., & Galynker, I. I. (2008). Comparison of personality traits in pedophiles, abstinent opiate addicts, and healthy controls: Considering pedophilia as an addictive behavior. *Journal of Nervous and Mental Disease, 196*(11), 829–837.

Cohen, L. J., Nesci, C., Steinfeld, M., Haeri, S., & Galynker, I. (2010). Investigating the relationship between sexual and chemical addictions by comparing executive function in pedophiles, opiate addicts and healthy controls. *Journal of Psychiatric Practice, 16*(6), 405–412.

Cohen-Almagor, R. (2013). Online child sex offenders: Challenges and counter-measures. *Howard Journal of Criminal Justice, 52*(2), 190–215.

Connolly, M., & Woollons, R. (2008). Childhood sexual experience and adult offending: An exploratory comparison of three criminal groups. *Child Abuse Review, 17*(2), 119–132.

Craig, L. A. (2008). How should we understand the effect of age on sexual recidivism? *Journal of Sexual Aggression, 14*(3), 185–198.

Cranney, S. (2017). Why did God make me this way? Religious coping and framing in the Virtuous Pedophile Community. *Journal for the Scientific Study of Religion, 56*(4), 852–868.

Crosby, D. (2008). *Non-pedophilic heterosexual male response to the Affinity 2.0.* Doctoral dissertation, Brigham Young University, Provo, UT (ScholarsArchive, Accession No. 1471).

Diamond, L. M. (2016). Sexual fluidity in males and females. *Current Sexual Health Reports, 8*, 249–256.

Diamond, L. M. (2018). Sexual fluidity. In J. Christer & C. Golden (Eds.), *Lectures on the psychology of women* (5th ed., pp. 49–62). Long Grove, IL: Waveland.

Diamond, M. (2009). Pornography, public acceptance and sex related crime: A review. *International Journal of Law and Psychiatry, 32*(5), 304–314.

Diamond, M., & Uchiyama, A. (1999). Pornography, rape, and sex crimes in Japan. *International Journal of Law and Psychiatry, 22*(1), 1–22.

Demidova, L., Murphy, L., Dwyer, G., Klapilova, K., & Fedoroff, J. (2019). Internatinal review of sexual behavior assessment labs. *Internatinal Review of Psychiatry, 31*(2), 114–125.

Dombert, B., Antfolk, J., Kallvik, L., Zappalà, A., Osterheider, M., Mokros, A., & Santtila, P. (2015). Identifying pedophilic interest in sex offenders against children with the indirect choice reaction time task. *European Journal of Psychological Assessment, 33*, 345–351.

Dombert, B., Mokros, A., Bruckner, E., Schlegl, V., Antfolk, J., . . . Santtila, P. (2013). The Virtual People Set: Developing computer-generated stimuli for the assessment of pedophilic sexual interest. *Sexual Abuse: Journal of Research and Treatment, 25*(6), 557–582.

Dombert, B., Schmidt, A. F., Banse, R., Briken, P., Hoyer, J., Neutze, J., & Osterheider, M. (2016). How common is men's self-reported sexual interest in prepubescent children? *Journal of Sex Research, 53*(2), 214–223.

Drapeau, M., Beretta, V., de Roten, Y., Koerner, A., & Despland, J. N. (2008). Defense styles of pedophilic offenders. *International Journal of Offender Therapy and Comparative Criminology, 52*(2), 185–195.

Duncan, K. A. (2010). *Female sexual predators: Understanding them to protect our children and youths*. Santa Barbara, CA: ABC-CLIO.

Dyshniku, F., Murray, M. E., Fazio, R. L., Lykins, A. D., & Cantor, J. M. (2015). Minor physical anomalies as a window into the prenatal origins of pedophilia. *Archives of Sexual Behavior, 44*(8), 2151–2159.

Eastvold, A. (2010). *Executive function and processing speed profiles of pedophilic and nonpedophilic child molesters.* Doctoral dissertation, University of Utah, Salt Lake City, UT (ProQuest Dissertations, Accession No. 3377898).

Eastvold, A., Suchy, Y., & Strassberg, D. (2011). Executive function profiles of pedophilic and nonpedophilic child molesters. *Journal of the International Neuropsychological Society, 17*(2), 295–307.

Eher, R., Olver, M. E., Heurix, I., Schilling, F., & Rettenberger, M. (2015). Predicting reoffense in pedophilic child molesters by clinical diagnoses and risk assessment. *Law and Human Behavior, 39*(6), 571–580.

Elliott, I. A., & Babchishin, K. M. (2012). Psychological profiles and processes in viewers of internet child pornography. In B. K. Schwartz (Ed.), *The sex offender: Current trends in policy and treatment practice* (Vol. 7, pp. 1–15). Kingston, NJ: Civic Research Institute.

Endrass, J., Urbaniok, F., Hammermeister, L. C., Benz, C., Elbert, T., Laubacher, A., & Rossegger, A. (2009). The consumption of internet child pornography and violent and sex offending. *BMC Psychiatry, 9*(1), 43.

Faccini, L. (2009). The incredible case of the shrinking penis: A Koro-like syndrome in an person with intellectually disability. *Sexuality and Disability, 27*(3), 173–178.

Farmer, M., Beech, A. R., & Ward, T. (2012). Assessing desistance in child molesters: A qualitative analysis. *Journal of Interpersonal Violence, 27*(5), 930–950.

Faust, E., Bickart, W., Renaud, C., & Camp, S. (2015). Child pornography possessors and child contact sex offenders: A multilevel comparison of demographic characteristics and rates of recidivism. *Sexual Abuse, 27*(5), 460–478.

Fazio, R. L. (2018). Toward a neurodevelopmental understanding of pedophilia [Invited commentary]. *Journal of Sexual Medicine, 15*(9), 1205–1207.

Fazio, R. L., Dyshniku, F., Lykins, A. D., & Cantor, J. M. (2017). Leg length versus torso length in pedophilia: Further evidence of atypical physical development early in life. *Sexual Abuse, 29*(5), 500–514.

Fazio, R. L., Lykins, A. D., & Cantor, J. M. (2014). Elevated rates of atypical handedness in paedophilia: Theory and implications. *Laterality: Asymmetries of Body, Brain and Cognition, 19*(6), 690–704.

Fedoroff, J. P. (2016). Managing versus successfully treating paraphilic disorders: The paradigm is changing. In S. B. Levine, C. B. Risen, & S. E. Althof (Eds.), *Handbook of Clinical Sexuality for Mental Health Professionals* (pp. 345–361). New York, NY: Taylor & Francis Group.

Fedoroff, J. P. (2018a). More puzzles: A response to Seto's (2017) "The puzzle of male chronophilias." *Archives of Sexual Behavior, 47*(8), 2171–2173. doi:10.1007/s10508-018-1242-3

Fedoroff, J. P. (2018b). Can people with pedophilia change? Yes they can! *Current Sexual Health Reports, 10*(4), 207–212. https://doi.org/10.1007/s11930-018-0166-1

Fedoroff, J. P., Curry, S., Müller, K., Ranger, R., Briken, P., & Bradford, J.B. (2015). Evidence that arousal to pedophilic stimuli can change: Response to Bailey, Cantor and Lalumiére. *Archives of Sexual Behavior, 44*(1), 259–263.

Fedoroff, J. P., Curry, S., Ranger, R., & Bradford, J. (2016). Regression to the mean or the Semmelweis reflex? *Archives of Sexual Behavior, 45*(7), 1869. doi.org/10.1007/s10508-016-0786-3

Fedoroff, J. P., Fishell, A., & Fedoroff, B. (1999). A case series of women evaluated for paraphilic sexual disorders. *Canadian Journal of Human Sexuality, 8*, 127–140.

Fedoroff, J. P., Hanson, A., McGuire, M., Malin, H. M., & Berlin, F. (1992). Simulated paraphilias—A preliminary study of patients who imitate or exaggerate paraphilic symptoms and behaviours. *Journal of Forensic Sciences, 37*, 902–911.

Fedoroff, J. P., Kuban, M., & Bradford, J. M. (2009). Laboratory measurement of penile response in the assessment of sexual interests. In F. Saleh, A. Grudzinskas, Jr., J. Bradford, & D. Brodsky (Eds.), *Sex offenders: Identification, risk assessment, treatment and legal issues* (pp. 89–100). New York, NY: Oxford University Press.

Fedoroff, J. P., & Marshall, W. L. (2010). Paraphilias. In D. McKay, J. S. Abramowitz, & S. Taylor (Eds.), *Cognitive-behavioral therapy for refractory cases: Turning failure into success* (pp. 369–384). Washington, DC: American Psychological Association.

Fedoroff, J. P., & Pinkus, S. (1996). The genesis of pedophilia: Testing the abuse to abuser hypothesis. *Journal of Offender Rehabilitation, 23,* 85–101.

Feelgood, S., & Hoyer, J. (2008). Child molester or paedophile? Sociolegal versus psychopathological classification of sexual offenders against children. *Journal of Sexual Aggression, 14*(1), 33–43.

Finkelhor, D. (2009). The prevention of childhood sexual abuse. *The Future of Children, 19*(2), 169–194.

Finkelhor, D., & Jones, L. (2004, January). *Explanations for the decline in child sexual abuse* (Juvenile Justice Bulletin No. NCJ199298, pp. 1–12). Washington, DC: US Government Printing Office.

Firestone, P., Moulden, H. M., & Wexler, A. F. (2009). Clerics who commit sexual offenses: Offender, offense, and victim characteristics. *Journal of Child Sexual Abuse, 18*(4), 442–454.

First, M. B. (2011). The inclusion of child pornography in the DSM-5 diagnostic criteria for pedophilia: Conceptual and practical problems. *Journal of the American Academy of Psychiatry and the Law Online, 39*(2), 250–254.

Flak, V. E., Beech, A. R., & Humphreys, G. W. (2009). The rapid serial visual presentation test of sexual interest in child molesters. In D. Thornton & D. R. Laws (Eds.), *Cognitive approaches to the assessment of sexual interest in sexual offenders* (pp. 145–158). Malden, MA: Wiley-Blackwell.

Fonteille, V., Cazala, F., Moulier, V., & Stoléru, S. (2012). Pedophilia: Contribution of neurology and neuroimaging techniques. *L'Encephale, 38*(6), 496–503.

Franzen, A. G. (2014). An evaluation of the utility of the MMPI-2 *Personality* Psychopathology *Five* (PSY-5) scales on a pedophile sample as compared to non-sex offending criminal sample. Doctoral dissertation, Alliant International University, California School of Forensic Studies, Irvine, CA.

Fromberger, P., Jordan, K., Steinkrauss, H., Von Herder, J., Stolpmann, G., Kröner-Herwig, B., & Müller, J. L. (2013). Eye movements in pedophiles: Automatic and controlled attentional processes while viewing prepubescent stimuli. *Journal of Abnormal Psychology, 122*(2), 587–599.

Fromberger, P., Jordan, K., Steinkrauss, H., von Herder, J., Witzel, J., Stolpmann, G., . . . Müller, J. L. (2012). Diagnostic accuracy of eye movements in assessing pedophilia. *Journal of Sexual Medicine, 9*(7), 1868–1882.

Fromberger, P., Meyer, S., Jordan, K., & Müller, J. L. (2018). Behavioral monitoring of sexual offenders against children in virtual risk situations: A feasibility study. *Frontiers in Psychology,* 9, 224. https://doi.org/10.3389/fpsyg.2018.00224

Fumagalli, M., Pravettoni, G., & Priori, A. (2015). Pedophilia 30 years after a traumatic brain injury. *Neurological Sciences, 36*(3), 481–482

Gacono, C. B., Meloy, J. R., & Bridges, M. R. (2008). A Rorschach understanding of psychopaths, sexual homicide perpetrators, and nonviolent pedophiles. In C. B. Gacono & F. B. Evans (Eds.), *The handbook of forensic Rorschach assessment* (pp. 379–393). New York, NY: Taylor & Francis.

Gannon, T. A., Hoare, J. A., Rose, M. R., & Parrett, N. (2012). A re-examination of female child molesters' implicit theories: Evidence of female specificity? *Psychology, Crime & Law, 18*(2), 209–224.

Gannon, T. A., & Rose, M. R. (2009). Offense-related interpretative bias in female child molesters: A preliminary study. *Sexual Abuse, 21*(2), 194–207.

Gannon, T. A., Rose, M. R., & Williams, S. E. (2009). Do female child molesters implicitly associate children and sex? A preliminary investigation. *Journal of Sexual Aggression, 15*(1), 55–61.

García, J. A. B. (2009). Etiology of pedophilia from a neurodevelopmental perspective: Markers and brain alterations. *Revista de Psiquiatría y Salud Mental (English Edition), 2*(4), 190–196.

Garrett, L. H. (2010). A phenomenological exploration of reflections on lived space by child sexual abusers. *Issues in Mental Health Nursing, 31*(12), 758–762.

Geradt, M., Jahnke, S., Heinz, J., et al. (2018). Is contact with children related to legitimizing beliefs toward sex with children among men with pedophilia? *Arch Sex Behav*, *47*, 375. https://doi.org/10.1007/s10508-017-1042-1

Gerwinn, H., Pohl, A., Granert, O., van Eimeren, T., Wolff, S., Jansen, O., . . . Ponseti, J. (2015). The (in) consistency of changes in brain macrostructure in male paedophiles: A combined T1-weighted and diffusion tensor imaging study. *Journal of Psychiatric Research*, *68*, 246–253.

Gerwinn, H., Weiß, S., Tenbergen, G., Amelung, T., Födisch, C., Pohl, A., . . . Wittfoth, M. (2018). Clinical characteristics associated with paedophilia and child sex offending—Differentiating sexual preference from offence status. *European Psychiatry*, *51*, 74–85.

Giang, H. (2018). A comparison of pedophilic and non-pedophilic males using the MMPI-2. Doctoral dissertation, Alliant International University, California School of Forensic Studies, Irvine, CA (ProQuest Dissertations, Accession No. 10276550).

Gilbert, F., & Focquaert, F. (2015). Rethinking responsibility in offenders with acquired paedophilia: Punishment or treatment? *International Journal of Law and Psychiatry*, *38*, 51–60.

Gillespie, S. M., Williams, R., Elliott, I. A., Eldridge, H. J., Ashfield, S., & Beech, A. R. (2015). Characteristics of females who sexually offend: A comparison of solo and co-offenders. *Sexual Abuse*, *27*(3), 284–301.

Glazier, K. (2018). Testing the efficacy of an education-based training tool to improve diagnostic accuracy of obsessive-compulsive disorder. Doctoral dissertation, Yeshiva University, New York, NY (ProQuest Dissertations, Accession No. 10596612).

Glazier, K., Swing, M., & McGinn, L. K. (2015). Half of obsessive–compulsive disorder cases misdiagnosed: Vignette-based survey of primary care physicians. *Journal of Clinical Psychiatry*, *76*(6), e761–e767.

Goldie, T. (2015). *The man who invented gender: Engaging the ideas of John Money*. Vancouver, British Columbia, Canada: University of British Columbia Press.

Goodier, S., & Lievesley, R. (2018). Understanding the needs of individuals at risk of perpetrating child sexual abuse: A practitioner perspective. *Journal of Forensic Psychology Research and Practice*, *18*(1), 77–98.

Graf, M., & Dittmann, V. (2011). Forensic–psychiatric treatment for internet sex offenders: Ten years of experience. In D. P. Boer, R. Eher, L. A. Craig, M. H. Miner, & F. Pfafflin (Eds.), *International perspectives on the assessment and treatment of sexual offenders: Theory, practice, and research* (pp. 575–585). Malden, MA: Wiley-Blackwell.

Gray, S. R., Abel, G. G., Jordan, A., Garby, T., Wiegel, M., & Harlow, N. (2015). Visual Reaction Time as a predictor of sexual offense recidivism. *Sexual Abuse*, *27*(2), 173–188.

Green, C. R. (2018). A comparison of MMPI-2 profiles of individuals with pedophilic disorder and chemically dependent substance abusers. Doctoral dissertation, Alliant International University, California School of Forensic Studies, Irvine, CA (Accession No. 10620339).

Grønnerød, C., Grønnerød, J. S., & Grøndahl, P. (2015). Psychological treatment of sexual offenders against children: A meta-analytic review of treatment outcome studies. *Trauma, Violence, & Abuse*, *16*(3), 280–290.

Grundmann, D., Krupp, J., Scherner, G., Amelung, T., & Beier, K. M. (2016). Stability of self-reported arousal to sexual fantasies involving children in a clinical sample of pedophiles and hebephiles. *Archives of Sexual Behavior*, *45*(5), 1153–1162.

Grundmann, D., Krupp, J., Scherner, G., Amelung, T., & Beier, K. M. (2017). Response to Tozdan and Briken's (2016) "Accepting sexual interest in children as unchangeable: One claim fits for all?" *Archives of Sexual Behavior*, *46*(2), 335.

Habermeyer, B., Esposito, F., Händel, N., Lemoine, P., Klarhöfer, M., Mager, R., . . . Graf, M. (2013). Immediate processing of erotic stimuli in paedophilia and controls: A case control study. *BMC Psychiatry*, *13*(1), 88.

Habermeyer, B., Esposito, F., Händel, N., Lemoine, P., Kuhl, H. C., Klarhöfer, M., . . . Graf, M. (2013). Response inhibition in pedophilia: An fMRI pilot study. *Neuropsychobiology*, *68*(4), 228–237.

Habermeyer, B., Händel, N., Lemoine, P., Klarhöfer, M., Seifritz, E., Dittmann, V., & Graf, M. (2012). LH-RH agonists modulate amygdala response to visual sexual stimulation: A single case fMRI study in pedophilia. *Neurocase*, *18*(6), 489–495.

Hamdi, N. R., & Knight, R. A. (2012). The relationships of perpetrator and victim substance use to the sexual aggression of rapists and child molesters. *Sexual Abuse, 24*(4), 307–327.

Hamo, G., & Idisis, Y. (2017). Pedophiles in the Ultra-Orthodox Haredi Sector in Israel: Thought processes regarding their actions. *Journal of Child Sexual Abuse*, 26(4), 407–427.

Hanson, R. K., Harris, A. J. R., Letourneau, E., Helmus, L. M., & Thornton, D. (2018). Reductions in risk based on time offense-free in the community: Once a sexual offender, not always a sexual offender. *Psychology, Public Policy, and Law, 24*(1), 48–63. http://dx.doi.org/10.1037/law0000135

Harkins, L., & Beech, A. R. (2008). Examining the impact of mixing child molesters and rapists in group-based cognitive–behavioral treatment for sexual offenders. *International Journal of Offender Therapy and Comparative Criminology, 52*(1), 31–45.

Heitzman, J., Lew-Starowicz, M., Pacholski, M., & Lew-Starowicz, Z. (2014). Children sexual abuse in Poland—Study of 257 sexual offenders against minors. *Psychiatria Polska, 48*(1), 105–120.

Helmus, L., Ó Ciardha, C., & Seto, M. C. (2015). The Screening Scale for Pedophilic Interests (SSPI): Construct, predictive, and incremental validity. *Law and Human Behavior, 39*(1), 35–43.

Hempel, I. S., Buck, N. M. L., Goethals, K. R., & Van Marle, H. J. C. (2013). Unraveling sexual associations in contact and noncontact child sex offenders using the single category—Implicit association test. *Sexual Abuse, 25*(5), 444–460.

Henshaw, M., Ogloff, J. R., & Clough, J. A. (2017). Looking beyond the screen: A critical review of the literature on the online child pornography offender. *Sexual Abuse, 29*(5), 416–445.

Hoffer, T. A., & Shelton, J. L. E. (2013). *Suicide among child sex offenders*. New York, NY: Springer.

Holt, T. J., Blevins, K. R., & Burkert, N. (2010). Considering the pedophile subculture online. *Sexual Abuse, 22*(1), 3–24.

Houssier, F., Duchet, C., Chagnon, J. Y., Robert, P., & Marty, F. (2011). A skin on fire: The link between thermal metaphors and early trauma in a case of pedophilia. *Bulletin of the Menninger Clinic, 75*(1), 46–63.

Houtepen, J. A., Sijtsema, J. J., & Bogaerts, S. (2014). From child pornography offending to child sexual abuse: A review of child pornography offender characteristics and risks for cross-over. *Aggression and Violent Behavior, 19*(5), 466–473.

Houtepen, J. A., Sijtsema, J. J., & Bogaerts, S. (2016). Being sexually attracted to minors: Sexual development, coping with forbidden feelings, and relieving sexual arousal in self- identified pedophiles. *Journal of Sex & Marital Therapy, 42*(1), 48–69.

Hsu, K. J., & Bailey, J. M. (2017). Autopedophilia: Erotic-target identity inversions in men sexually attracted to children. *Psychological Science, 28*(1), 115–123.

Huang, J. (2017). Relationship between child sexual aggression intention and practice and its impact factors. *Bulletin of Educational Psychology, 49*(2), 193–214.

Hunter, J. A., Ram, N., & Ryback, R. (2008). Use of satiation therapy in the treatment of adolescent-manifest sexual interest in male children: A single-case, repeated measures design. *Clinical Case Studies, 7*(1), 54–74.

Ibiloglu, A. O., Atli, A., Oto, R., & Ozkan, M. (2018). Multifaceted glance on childhood sexual abuse and incest. *Psikiyatride Guncel Yaklasimlar, 10*(1), 84–98.

Jahnke, S. (2018). The stigma of pedophilia: Clinical and forensic implications. *European Psychologist, 23*(2), 144–153.

Jahnke, S., & Malón, A. (2019). How pedophilic men think about adult–child sex: Effects of child gender and physical maturity. *Psychology, Crime & Law, 25*, 90–107.

Jahnke, S., Philipp, K., & Hoyer, J. (2015). Stigmatizing attitudes towards people with pedophilia and their malleability among psychotherapists in training. *Child Abuse & Neglect, 40*, 93–102.

Jahnke, S., Schmidt, A. F., Geradt, M., & Hoyer, J. (2015). Stigma-related stress and its correlates among men with pedophilic sexual interests. *Archives of Sexual Behavior, 44*(8), 2173–2187.

Jakubczyk, A., Krasowska, A., Bugaj, M., Kopera, M., Klimkiewicz, A., Łoczewska, A., . . . Sołowiej, M. (2017). Paraphilic sexual offenders do not differ from control subjects with respect to dopamine- and serotonin-related genetic polymorphisms. *Journal of Sexual Medicine, 14*(1), 125–133.

Janssen, D. F. (2015). "Chronophilia": Entries of erotic age preference into descriptive psychopathology. *Medical History, 59*(4), 575–598.

Jewkes, Y., & Wykes, M. (2012). Reconstructing the sexual abuse of children: "Cyber-paeds," panic and power. *Sexualities, 15*(8), 934–952.

Jordan, K., Fromberger, P., Laubinger, H., Dechent, P., & Müller, J. L. (2014). Changed processing of visual sexual stimuli under GnRH-therapy—A single case study in pedophilia using eye tracking and fMRI. *BMC Psychiatry, 14*(1), 142.

Jordan, K., Fromberger, P., & Müller, J. L. (2016). Structural and functional magnetic resonance imaging in assessing sexual preference. In D. P. Boer (Ed.), *The Wiley handbook on the theories, assessment and treatment of sexual offending* (pp. 925–964). Malden, MA: Wiley.

Jordan, K., Fromberger, P., Müller, I., Wernicke, M., Stolpmann, G., & Müller, J. L. (2018). Sexual interest and sexual self-control in men with self-reported sexual interest in children—A first eye tracking study. *Journal of Psychiatric Research, 96*, 138–144.

Jordan, K., Fromberger, P., Stolpmann, G., & Müller, J. L. (2011). The role of testosterone in sexuality and paraphilia—A neurobiological approach. Part II: Testosterone and paraphilia. *Journal of Sexual Medicine, 8*(11), 3008–3029.

Jordan, K., Fromberger, P., von Herder, J., Steinkrauss, H., Nemetschek, R., Witzel, J., & Müller, J. L. (2016). Impaired attentional control in pedophiles in a sexual distractor task. *Frontiers in Psychiatry, 7*, 193.

Jordan, R. J. (2012). *Use of the Rorschach and MMPI-2 in distinguishing pedophilic and teleiophilic sexual offenders.* Doctoral dissertation, Alliant International University, California School of Professional Psychology, Irvine, CA.

Jumper, S., Babula, M., & Casbon, T. (2012). Diagnostic profiles of civilly committed sexual offenders in Illinois and other reporting jurisdictions: What we know so far. *International Journal of Offender Therapy and Comparative Criminology, 56*(6), 838–855.

Jung, S., Klaver, E., & Pham, A. (2014). Pedophilia and its (non-)association with physical height among sex offenders. *Deviant Behavior, 35*(4), 323–331.

Kaplan, H. G. (2012). Dreams as windows into the lived experience of males with pedophilia: A depth psychologically oriented, phenomenological study. Doctoral dissertation, Pacifica Graduate Institute, Santa Barbara, CA (ProQuest Dissertations, Accession No. 3475567).

Kärgel, C., Massau, C., Weiß, S., Walter, M., Borchardt, V., Krueger, T. H., . . . Gerwinn, H. (2017). Evidence for superior neurobiological and behavioral inhibitory control abilities in non-offending as compared to offending pedophiles. *Human Brain Mapping, 38*(2), 1092–1104.

Kärgel, C., Massau, C., Weiß, S., Walter, M., Kruger, T. H., & Schiffer, B. (2015). Diminished functional connectivity on the road to child sexual abuse in pedophilia. *Journal of Sexual Medicine, 12*(3), 783–795.

Khoury, J. M., Roque, M. A. V., & Garcia, F. D. (2016). Pedophilic disorder. In R. Balon (Ed.), *Practical guide to paraphilia and paraphilic disorders* (pp. 141–154). Cham, Switzerland: Springer.

King, M. W. (2011). Neurodevelopmental vulnerability for pedophilia: A taxometric investigation of its latent structure. Doctoral dissertation, University of Maine, Orono, ME (ProQuest Dissertations, Accession No. 3415477).

Kingston, D. A., Fedoroff, P., Firestone, P., Curry, S., & Bradford, J. M. (2008). Pornography use and sexual aggression: The impact of frequency and type of pornography use on recidivism among sexual offenders. *Aggressive Behavior, 34*(4), 341–351.

Kingston, D. A., Firestone, P., Wexler, A., & Bradford, J. M. (2008). Factors associated with recidivism among intrafamilial child molesters. *Journal of Sexual Aggression, 14*(1), 3–18.

Kingston, D. A., Seto, M. C., Ahmed, A. G., Fedoroff, P., Firestone, P., & Bradford, J. M. (2012). The role of central and peripheral hormones in sexual and violent recidivism in sex offenders. *Journal of the American Academy of Psychiatry and the Law Online, 40*(4), 476–485.

Kloess, J. A., Beech, A. R., & Harkins, L. (2014). Online child sexual exploitation: Prevalence, process, and offender characteristics. *Trauma, Violence, & Abuse, 15*(2), 126–139.

Kloess, J. A., Seymour-Smith, S., Hamilton-Giachritsis, C. E., Long, M. L., Shipley, D., & Beech, A. R. (2017). A qualitative analysis of offenders' modus operandi in sexually exploitative interactions with children online. *Sexual Abuse, 29*(6), 563–591.

Knack, N., Winder, B., Murphy, L., & Fedoroff, J. (2019). Primary and secondary prevention of child abuse. *Internatinal Review of Psychiatry, 31*(2), 181–194.

Knott, V., Impey, D., Fisher, D., Delpero, E., & Fedoroff, P. (2016). Pedophilic brain potential responses to adult erotic stimuli. *Brain Research, 1632*, 127–140.

Kolod, S. (2016). Reluctance to finding myself in the other: Treating an alleged paedophile. In B. Willock, L. C. Bohm, & R. C. Curtis (Eds.), *Psychoanalytic perspectives on identity and difference* (pp. 81–87). New York, NY: Routledge.

Konrad, A., Haag, S., Scherner, G., Amelung, T., & Beier, K. M. (2017). Previous judicial detection and paedophilic sexual interest partially predict psychological distress in a non-forensic sample of help-seeking men feeling inclined to sexually offend against children. *Journal of Sexual Aggression, 23*(3), 266–277.

Konrad, A., Kuhle, L. F., Amelung, T., & Beier, K. M. (2018). Is emotional congruence with children associated with sexual offending in pedophiles and hebephiles from the community? *Sexual Abuse: Journal of Research and Treatment, 30*(1), 3–22. http://dx.doi.org/10.1177/1079063215620397

Kouros, N. (2013). AI to pose as young girl to detect paedophiles. *Monash Bioethics Review, 31*(2), 28–29.

Krueger, R. B., Kaplan, M. S., & First, M. B. (2009). Sexual and other axis I diagnoses of 60 males arrested for crimes against children involving the internet. *CNS Spectrums, 14*(11), 623–631.

Kruger, T. H., & Schiffer, B. (2011). Neurocognitive and personality factors in homo-and heterosexual pedophiles and controls. *Journal of Sexual Medicine, 8*(6), 1650–1659.

Kutchinsky, B. (1971). *Towards an explanation of the decrease in registered sex crimes in Copenhagen: Technical report of the Commission on Obscenity and Pornography* (Vol. 7, pp. 263–310). Washington, DC: US Government Printing Office.

Lalumière, M. L. (2015). The lability of pedophilic interests as measured by phallometry. *Archives of Sexual Behavior, 44*(1), 255–258.

Lamy, S., Delavenne, H., & Thibaut, F. (2016). A case of female hypersexuality and child abuse and a review. *Archives of Women's Mental Health, 19*(4), 701–703.

Lasher, M. P., & Stinson, J. D. (2017). Adults with pedophilic interests in the United States: Current practices and suggestions for future policy and research. *Archives of Sexual Behavior, 46*(3), 659–670.

Laws, D. R., & O'Donohue, W. T. (Eds.). (2008). *Sexual deviance: Theory, assessment, and treatment* (2nd ed.). New York, NY: Guilford.

Lawson, L., & Rowe, S. (2010). Treatment of females convicted of molesting children. *Journal of Forensic Nursing, 6*(4), 180–187.

Leclerc, B., Proulx, J., & Beauregard, E. (2009). Examining the modus operandi of sexual offenders against children and its practical implications. *Aggression and Violent Behavior, 14*(1), 5–12.

Lee, A. F., Li, N. C., Lamade, R., Schuler, A., & Prentky, R. A. (2012). Predicting hands-on child sexual offenses among possessors of internet child pornography. *Psychology, Public Policy, and Law, 18*(4), 644–672.

Lett, T. A., Mohnke, S., Amelung, T., Brandl, E. J., Schiltz, K., Pohl, A., . . . Wittfoth, M. (2018). Multimodal neuroimaging measures and intelligence influence pedophile child sexual offense behavior. *European Neuropsychopharmacology, 28*(7), 818–827.

Levenson, J. S., Becker, J., & Morin, J. W. (2008). The relationship between victim age and gender crossover among sex offenders. *Sexual Abuse, 20*(1), 43–60.

Levenson, J. S., Willis, G. M., & Vicencio, C. P. (2017). Obstacles to help-seeking for sexual offenders: Implications for prevention of sexual abuse. *Journal of Child Sexual Abuse, 26*(2), 99–120.

Long, M. L., Alison, L. A., & McManus, M. A. (2013). Child pornography and likelihood of contact abuse: A comparison between contact child sexual offenders and noncontact offenders. *Sexual Abuse, 25*(4), 370–395.

Łucka, I., & Dziemian, A. (2014). Pedophilia—A review of literature, casuistic, doubts. *Psychiatria Polska, 48*(1), 121–134.

Ly, T., Murphy, L. & Fedoroff, J. P. (2016). Understanding online child sexual exploitation. *Current Psychiatry Reports, 18*, 74.

Lykins, A. D., Cantor, J. M., Kuban, M. E., Blak, T., Dickey, R., Klassen, P. E., & Blanchard, R. (2010a). The relation between peak response magnitudes and agreement in diagnoses obtained from two different phallometric tests for pedophilia. *Sexual Abuse, 22*(1), 42–57.

Lykins, A. D., Cantor, J. M., Kuban, M. E., Blak, T., Dickey, R., Klassen, P. E., & Blanchard, R. (2010b). Sexual arousal to female children in gynephilic men. *Sexual Abuse, 22*(3), 279–289.

MacDonell, L., & Bolton, C. (2018). Dual histories of abuse and perpetration. In R. B. Gartner (Ed.), *Healing sexually betrayed men and boys: Treatment for sexual abuse, assault, and trauma* (pp. 289–317). New York, NY: Routledge.

Mackaronis, J. E., Strassberg, D. S., & Marcus, D. K. (2011). The latent structure of Multiphasic Sex Inventory–Assessed Pedophilic Interest. *Psychological Assessment, 23*(4), 1017.

Mackelprang, E. (2016). What's the difference? A comparison of the MSI II protocols of male and female sexual offenders. Doctoral dissertation.

Magaletta, P. R., Faust, E., Bickart, W., & McLearen, A. M. (2014). Exploring clinical and personality characteristics of adult male internet-only child pornography offenders. *International Journal of Offender Therapy and Comparative Criminology, 58*(2), 137–153.

Malesky, A. L., Jr., Ennis, L., & Gress, C. L. Z. (2009). Child pornography and the internet. In F. M. Saleh, A. J. Grudzinskas, Jr., J. M. Bradford, & D. Brodsky (Eds.), *Sex offenders: Identification, risk assessment, treatment, and legal issues* (pp. 302–323). New York, NY: Oxford University Press.

Malón, A. (2012). Pedophilia: A diagnosis in search of a disorder. *Archives of Sexual Behavior, 41*(5), 1083–1097.

Mandeville-Norden, R., & Beech, A. R. (2009). Development of a psychometric typology of child molesters: Implications for treatment. *Journal of Interpersonal Violence, 24*(2), 307–325.

Maram, W. B. (2016). Psychophysiological assessment of sexual offenders: A practitioner's perspective. In A. Phenix & H. M. Hoberman (Eds.), *Sexual offending* (pp. 331–352). New York, NY: Springer.

Marschall-Lévesque, S., Rouleau, J. L., & Renaud, P. (2018). Increasing valid profiles in phallometric assessment of sex offenders with child victims: Combining the strengths of audio stimuli and synthetic characters. *Archives of Sexual Behavior, 47*(2), 417–428.

Marshall, W. L., Marshall, L. E., & Kingston, D. A. (2011). Are the cognitive distortions of child molesters in need of treatment? *Journal of Sexual Aggression, 17*(2), 118–129.

Marshall, W. L., O'Brien, M. D., & Marshall, L. E. (2009). Modifying sexual preferences. In A. R. Beech, L. A. Craig, & K. D. Browne (Eds.), *Assessment and treatment of sex offenders: A handbook* (pp. 311–327). New York, NY: Wiley.

Marshall, W. L., Smallbone, S., & Marshall, L. E. (2015). A critique of current child molester subcategories: A proposal for an alternative approach. *Psychology, Crime & Law, 21*(3), 205–218.

Massau, C., Kärgel, C., Weiß, S., Walter, M., Ponseti, J., Krueger, T., . . . Schiffer, B. (2017). Neural correlates of moral judgment in pedophilia. *Social Cognitive and Affective Neuroscience, 12*(9), 1490–1499.

Massau, C., Tenbergen, G., Kärgel, C., Weiß, S., Gerwinn, H., Pohl, A., . . . Ristow, I. (2017). Executive functioning in pedophilia and child sexual offending. *Journal of the International Neuropsychological Society, 23*(6), 460–470.

McCartan, K. F. (2008). Current understandings of paedophilia and the resulting crisis in modern society. In J. M. Caroll & M. K. Alena (Eds.), *Psychological sexual dysfunctions* (pp. 51–84). Hauppauge, NY: Nova.

McCarthy, J. A. (2011). The relationship between possessing child pornography and child molestation. Doctoral dissertation, City University of New York, New York, NY (ProQuest Dissertations, Accession No. 3412742).

McLawsen, J. E. (2010). Factors associated with the civil commitment of sex offenders: A comparison between four states. Doctoral dissertation, University of Nebraska–Lincoln, Lincoln, NE (ProQuest Dissertations, Accession No. 3404022).

McLawsen, J. E., Scalora, M. J., & Darrow, C. (2012). Civilly committed sex offenders: A description and interstate comparison of populations. *Psychology, Public Policy, and Law, 18*(3), 453–476.

McPhail, I. V., & Cantor, J. M. (2015). Pedophilia, height, and the magnitude of the association: A research note. *Deviant Behavior, 36*(4), 288–292.

McPhail, I. V., Hermann, C. A., Fernane, S., Fernandez, Y. M., Nunes, K. L., & Cantor, J. M. (2019). Validity in phallometric testing for sexual interests in children: A meta-analytic review. *Assessment, 26*(3), 535–551. doi:10.1177/1073191117706139

McPhail, I. V., Olver, M. E., Brouillette-Alarie, S., & Looman, J. (2018). Taxometric analysis of the latent structure of pedophilic interest. *Archives of Sexual Behavior, 47*(8), 2223–2240.

Mendez, M., & Shapira, J. S. (2011). Pedophilic behavior from brain disease. *Journal of Sexual Medicine, 8*(4), 1092–1100.

Merdian, H. L., Curtis, C., Thakker, J., Wilson, N., & Boer, D. P. (2013). The three dimensions of online child pornography offending. *Journal of Sexual Aggression, 19*(1), 121–132.

Mitchell, R. C., Bravo, A. P., & Galupo, M. P. (2017). Sexual desire among an online sample of men sexually attracted to children. *Journal of Child Sexual Abuse, 26*(6), 643–656.

Mitchell, R. C., & Galupo, M. P. (2016). Interest in child molestation among a community sample of men sexually attracted to children. *Journal of Sexual Aggression, 22*(2), 224–232.

Mitchell, R. C., & Galupo, M. P. (2018). The perceived role of general self-regulation and prosocial support on the decision not to act among men sexually attracted to children. *International Journal of Offender Therapy and Comparative Criminology, 62*(10), 2897–2916.

Mokros, A., Butz, M., Dombert, B., Santtila, P., Bäuml, K. H., & Osterheider, M. (2011). Judgment of age and attractiveness in a paired comparison task: Testing a picture set developed for diagnosing paedophilia. *Legal and Criminological Psychology, 16*(2), 323–334.

Mokros, A., Dombert, B., Osterheider, M., Zappalà, A., & Santtila, P. (2010). Assessment of pedophilic sexual interest with an attentional choice reaction time task. *Archives of Sexual Behavior, 39*(5), 1081–1090.

Mokros, A., Gebhard, M., Heinz, V., Marschall, R. W., Nitschke, J., Glasgow, D. V., . . . Laws, D. R. (2013). Computerized assessment of pedophilic sexual interest through self-report and viewing time: Reliability, validity, and classification accuracy of the affinity program. *Sexual Abuse, 25*(3), 230–258.

Mokros, A., & Habermeyer, E. (2016). Regression to the mean mimicking changes in sexual arousal to child stimuli in pedophiles. *Archives of Sexual Behavior, 45*(7), 1863–1867.

Mokros, A., Habermeyer, E., & Küchenhoff, H. (2017). The uncertainty of psychological and psychiatric diagnoses. *Psychological Assessment, 30*(4), 556–560.

Money, J. (1986). *Lovemaps: Clinical concepts of sexual/erotic health and pathology, paraphilia, and gender transposition in childhood, adolescence, and maturity*. New York, NY: Prometheus.

Mongeau, V., & Rouleau, J. L. (2014). DSM-5 pedophilic disorder: Are the age and number of victims significant variables? *Archives of Sexual Behavior, 43*(7), 1247–1252.

Moster, A. N. (2015). Registered pedophiles' thoughts on the efficacy, justification, and psychosocial impact of SORNA (Sex Offender Registration and Notification Act) and their sensitivity to sexual and non-sexual violence. Doctoral dissertation, University of Rhode Island, Kingston, RI.

Moulden, H. M., Firestone, P., Kingston, D., & Bradford, J. (2009). Recidivism in pedophiles: An investigation using different diagnostic methods. *Journal of Forensic Psychiatry & Psychology, 20*(5), 680–701.

Moulier, V., Fonteille, V., Pélégrini-Issac, M., Cordier, B., Baron-Laforêt, S., Boriasse, E., . . . Stoléru, S. (2012). A pilot study of the effects of gonadotropin-releasing hormone agonist therapy on brain activation pattern in a man with pedophilia. *International Journal of Offender Therapy and Comparative Criminology, 56*(1), 50–60.

Müller, K., Curry, S., Ranger, R., Briken, P., Bradford, J., & Fedoroff, J. P. (2014). Changes in sexual arousal as measured by penile plethysmography in men with pedophilic sexual interest. *Journal of Sexual Medicine, 11*(5), 1221–1229.

Müller, S., Walter, H., & Christen, M. (2014). When benefitting a patient increases the risk for harm for third persons—The case of treating pedophilic parkinsonian patients with deep brain stimulation. *International Journal of Law and Psychiatry, 37*(3), 295–303.

Murphy, L., Curry, S., Klapilova, K., Dwyer, G., Zikanova, T., & Fedoroff, J. (2019). Stimuli used in the meaqsurement of problematic sexual interests. *Internatinal Review of Psychiatry, 31*(2), 126–140.

Murphy, L., Ranger, R., & Fedoroff, J. P. (2014). Legal and clinical issues in interpreting child pornography on the internet. In F. Saleh, A. Grudzinskas, & A. Judge (Eds.), *Adolescent sexual behavior in the digital world* (pp. 213–243). New York, NY: Oxford University Press.

Murphy, L., Ranger, R., Stewart, H., Dwyer, G., & Fedoroff, J. P. (2015). Assessment of problematic sexual interests with the penile plethysmograph: An overview of assessment laboratories. *Current Psychiatry Reports, 17*(5), 1–5.

Nabokov, V. (1955). *Lolita*. Paris, Feance: Olympia Press.

Navathe, S., Ward, T., & Gannon, T. (2008). Cognitive distortions in child sex offenders: An overview of theory, research & practice. *Journal of Forensic Nursing, 4*(3), 111–122.

Neutze, J., Grundmann, D., Scherner, G., & Beier, K. M. (2012). Undetected and detected child sexual abuse and child pornography offenders. *International Journal of Law and Psychiatry, 35*(3), 168–175.

Neutze, J., Seto, M. C., Schaefer, G. A., Mundt, I. A., & Beier, K. M. (2011). Predictors of child pornography offenses and child sexual abuse in a community sample of pedophiles and hebephiles. *Sexual Abuse, 23*(2), 212–242.

Niveau, G. (2010). Cyber-pedocriminality: Characteristics of a sample of internet child pornography offenders. *Child Abuse & Neglect: The International Journal, 34*(8), 570–575.

Noll, D. E., & Harvey, L. (2008). Restorative mediation: The application of restorative justice practice and philosophy to clergy sexual abuse cases. *Journal of Child Sexual Abuse, 17*(3–4), 377–396.

Nunes, K. L. (2009). Measuring child molesters' implicit cognitions about self and children. In D. Thornton & D. R. Laws (Eds.), *Cognitive approaches to the assessment of sexual interest in sexual offenders* (pp. 125–143). Malden, MA: Wiley-Blackwell.

Nunes, K. L., Hermann, C. A., Malcom, J. R., & Lavoie, K. (2013). Childhood sexual victimization, pedophilic interest, and sexual recidivism. *Child Abuse & Neglect, 37*(9), 703–711.

Nunes, K. L., & Jung, S. (2013). Are cognitive distortions associated with denial and minimization among sex offenders? *Sexual Abuse, 25*(2), 166–188.

Nunes, K. L., Pettersen, C., Hermann, C. A., Looman, J., & Spape, J. (2016). Does change on the MOLEST and RAPE scales predict sexual recidivism? *Sexual Abuse, 28*(5), 427–447.

O'Halloran, E., & Quayle, E. (2010). A content analysis of a "boy love" support forum: Revisiting Durkin and Bryant. *Journal of Sexual Aggression, 16*(1), 71–85.

Osborn, J., Elliott, I., Middleton, D., & Beech, A. (2010). The use of actuarial risk assessment measures with UK internet child pornography offenders. *Journal of Aggression, Conflict and Peace Research, 2*(3), 16–24.

Palermo, G. B. (2012). An old problem seeking a new solution: Sex offenders. *International Journal of Offender Therapy and Comparative Criminology, 56*(1), 3–5.

Panesar, N., Allard, B., Pai, N., & Valachova, I. (2011). Cyproterone acetate in paraphilia. *Australian and New Zealand Journal of Psychiatry, 45*(5), 428.

Paquette, S., Cortoni, F., Proulx, J., & Longpre, N. (2014). An examination of implicit theories among francophone child molesters. *Journal of Sexual Aggression, 20*(2), 182–196.

Pearson, H. E. (2013). Correlates of the MMPI-2 and the AASI-2 with child molester typology. Doctoral dissertation, Alliant International University, California School of Forensic Studies, Irvine, CA.

Perillo, A. D., Spada, A. H., Calkins, C., & Jeglic, E. L. (2014). Examining the scope of questionable diagnostic reliability in Sexually Violent Predator (SVP) evaluations. *International Journal of Law and Psychiatry, 37*(2), 190–197.

Phenix, A., & Sreenivasan, S. (2009). A practical guide for the evaluation of sexual recidivism risk in mentally retarded sex offenders. *Journal of the American Academy of Psychiatry and the Law Online, 37*(4), 509–524.

Plante, T. G. (2015). Four lessons learned from treating Catholic priest sex offenders. *Pastoral Psychology, 64*(3), 407–412.

Poeppl, T. B., Eickhoff, S. B., Fox, P. T., Laird, A. R., Rupprecht, R., Langguth, B., & Bzdok, D. (2015). Connectivity and functional profiling of abnormal brain structures in pedophilia. *Human Brain Mapping, 36*(6), 2374–2386.

Poeppl, T. B., Nitschke, J., Dombert, B., Santtila, P., Greenlee, M. W., Osterheider, M., & Mokros, A. (2011). Functional cortical and subcortical abnormalities in pedophilia: A combined study using a choice reaction time task and fMRI. *Journal of Sexual Medicine, 8*(6), 1660–1674.

Poeppl, T. B., Nitschke, J., Santtila, P., Schecklmann, M., Langguth, B., Greenlee, M. W., . . . Mokros, A. (2013). Association between brain structure and phenotypic characteristics in pedophilia. *Journal of Psychiatric Research, 47*(5), 678–685.

Polisois-Keating, A., & Joyal, C. C. (2013). Functional neuroimaging of sexual arousal: A preliminary meta-analysis comparing pedophilic to non-pedophilic men. *Archives of Sexual Behavior, 42*(7), 1111–1113.

Ponseti, J., Bruhn, D., Nolting, J., Gerwinn, H., Pohl, A., Stirn, A., . . . Jansen, O. (2018). Decoding pedophilia: Increased anterior insula response to infant animal pictures. *Frontiers in Human Neuroscience, 11*, 645.

Ponseti, J., Granert, O., Jansen, O., Wolff, S., Beier, K., Neutze, J., . . . Bosinski, H. (2012). Assessment of pedophilia using hemodynamic brain response to sexual stimuli. *Archives of General Psychiatry, 69*(2), 187–194.

Ponseti, J., Granert, O., Van Eimeren, T., Jansen, O., Wolff, S., Beier, K., . . . Siebner, H. (2014). Human face processing is tuned to sexual age preferences. *Biology Letters, 10*(5), 20140200. doi:10.1098/rsbl.2014.0200

Ponseti, J., Granert, O., Van Eimeren, T., Jansen, O., Wolff, S., Beier, K., . . . Siebner, H. R. (2016). Assessing paedophilia based on the haemodynamic brain response to face images. *World Journal of Biological Psychiatry, 17*(1), 39–46.

Porter, T. M., & Feldman, M. D. (2011). A case of factitious pedophilia. *Journal of Forensic Sciences, 56*(5), 1380–1382.

Prat, S., & Jonas, C. (2012a). Characteristics of French users of child pornography: Description of a cohort subjected to forensic evaluation. *Medico-Legal Journal, 80*(4), 162–166.

Prat, S., & Jonas, C. (2012b). How to catch child pornographers in France? *The Entrapment. Legal Medicine, 14*(5), 276–277.

Prat, S., & Jonas, C. (2013). Psychopathological characteristics of child pornographers and their victims: A literature review. *Medicine, Science and the Law, 53*(1), 6–11.

Quayle, E. (2011). Pedophilia, child porn, and cyberpredators. In C. D. Bryant (Ed.), *The Routledge handbook of deviant behavior* (pp. 390–396). New York, NY: Routledge.

Rainero, I., Rubino, E., Negro, E., Gallone, S., Galimberti, D., Gentile, S., . . . Pinessi, L. (2011). Heterosexual pedophilia in a frontotemporal dementia patient with a mutation in the progranulin gene. *Biological Psychiatry, 70*(9), e43–e44.

Ray, J. V., Kimonis, E. R., & Donoghue, C. (2010). Legal, ethical, and methodological considerations in the internet-based study of child pornography offenders. *Behavioral Sciences & the Law, 28*(1), 84–105.

Renaud, P., Chartier, S., Rouleau, J., Proulx, J., Goyette, M., . . . Bouchard, S. (2013). Using immersive virtual reality and ecological psychology to probe into child molesters' phenomenology. *Journal of Sexual Aggression, 19*(1), 102–120.

Renaud, P., Goyette, M., Chartier, S., Zhornitski, S., Trottier, D., Rouleau, J. L., . . . Bouchard, S. (2010). Sexual affordances, perceptual-motor invariance extraction and intentional nonlinear dynamics: Sexually deviant and non-deviant patterns in male subjects. *Nonlinear Dynamics, Psychology, and Life Sciences, 14*(4), 463–489.

Renaud, P., Joyal, C., Stoleru, S., Goyette, M., Weiskopf, N., & Birbaumer, N. (2011). Real-time functional magnetic imaging—brain–computer interface and virtual reality: Promising tools for the treatment of pedophilia. *Progress in Brain Research, 192*, 263–272.

Rettenberger, M., Briken, P., Turner, D., & Eher, R. (2015). Sexual offender recidivism among a population-based prison sample. *International Journal of Offender Therapy and Comparative Criminology, 59*(4), 424–444.

Rice, M. E., Harris, G. T., Lang, C., & Chaplin, T. C. (2008). Sexual preferences and recidivism of sex offenders with mental retardation. *Sexual Abuse, 20*(4), 409–425.

Ristow, I., Li, M., Colic, L., Marr, V., Födisch, C., von Düring, F., . . . Beier, K. (2018). Pedophilic sex offenders are characterised by reduced GABA concentration in dorsal anterior cingulate cortex. *NeuroImage: Clinical, 18*, 335–341.

Rodriguez, M., Boyce, P., & Hodges, J. (2017). A neuropsychological study of older adult first-time sex offenders. *Neurocase, 23*(2), 154–161.

Rosburg, T., Deuring, G., Boillat, C., Lemoine, P., Falkenstein, M., Graf, M., & Mager, R. (2018). Inhibition and attentional control in pedophilic child sexual offenders: An event-related potential study. *Clinical Neurophysiology, 129*(9), 1990–1998.

Rowland, D. L., & Incrocci, L. (2008). *Handbook of sexual and gender identity disorders.* Hoboken, NJ: Wiley.

Russell, G., Seymour, F., & Lambie, I. (2013). Community reintegration of sex offenders of children in New Zealand. *International Journal of Offender Therapy and Comparative Criminology, 57*(1), 55–70.

Sandler, J. C., Freeman, N. J., & Socia, K. M. (2008). Does a watched pot boil? A time-series analysis of New York State's sex offender registration and notification law. *Psychology, Public Policy, and Law, 14*(4), 284.

Santtila, P., Antfolk, J., Räfså, A., Hartwig, M., Sariola, H., Sandnabba, N. K., & Mokros, A. (2015). Men's sexual interest in children: One-year incidence and correlates in a population-based sample of Finnish male twins. *Journal of Child Sexual Abuse, 24*(2), 115–134.

Sartori, G., Scarpazza, C., Codognotto, S., & Pietrini, P. (2016). An unusual case of acquired pedophilic behavior following compression of orbitofrontal cortex and hypothalamus by a Clivus chordoma. *Journal of Neurology, 263*, 1454–1455.

Sartorius, A., Ruf, M., Kief, C., Demirakca, T., Bailer, J., Ende, G., . . . Dressing, H. (2008). Abnormal amygdala activation profile in pedophilia. *European Archives of Psychiatry and Clinical Neuroscience, 258*(5), 271–277.

Scarpazza, C., Pennati, A., & Sartori, G. (2018). Mental insanity assessment of pedophilia—The importance of the trans-disciplinary approach: Reflections on two cases. *Frontiers in Neuroscience, 12*, 335.

Schaefer, G. A., Mundt, I. A., Feelgood, S., Hupp, E., Neutze, J., Ahlers, C. J., . . . Beier, K. M. (2010). Potential and Dunkelfeld offenders: Two neglected target groups for prevention of child sexual abuse. *International Journal of Law and Psychiatry, 33*(3), 154–163.

Schiffer, B., Amelung, T., Pohl, A., Kaergel, C., Tenbergen, G., Gerwinn, H., . . . Marr, V. (2017). Gray matter anomalies in pedophiles with and without a history of child sexual offending. *Translational Psychiatry, 7*(5), e1129.

Schiffer, B., Gizewski, E., & Kruger, T. (2009). Reduced neuronal responsiveness to visual sexual stimuli in a pedophile treated with a long-acting LH-RH agonist. *Journal of Sexual Medicine, 6*(3), 892–894.

Schiffer, B., Krueger, T., Paul, T., de Greiff, A., Forsting, M., Leygraf, N., . . . Gizewski, E. (2008). Brain response to visual sexual stimuli in homosexual pedophiles. *Journal of Psychiatry & Neuroscience, 33*(1), 23–33.

Schiffer, B., Paul, T., Gizewski, E., Forsting, M., Leygraf, N., Schedlowski, M., & Kruger, T. H. (2008). Functional brain correlates of heterosexual paedophilia. *Neuroimage, 41*(1), 80–91.

Schiffer, B., & Vonlaufen, C. (2011). Executive dysfunctions in pedophilic and nonpedophilic child molesters. *Journal of Sexual Medicine, 8*(7), 1975–1984.

Schmidt, A. F., Babchishin, K. M., & Lehmann, R. J. (2017). A meta-analysis of viewing time measures of sexual interest in children. *Archives of Sexual Behavior, 46*(1), 287–300.

Schmidt, A. F., Gykiere, K., Vanhoeck, K., Mann, R. E., & Banse, R. (2014). Direct and indirect measures of sexual maturity preferences differentiate subtypes of child sexual abusers. *Sexual Abuse, 26*(2), 107–128.

Schmidt, A. F., Mokros, A., & Banse, R. (2013). Is pedophilic sexual preference continuous? A taxometric analysis based on direct and indirect measures. *Psychological Assessment, 25*(4), 1146–1153.

Schulz, A., Bergen, E., Schuhmann, P., & Hoyer, J. (2017). Social anxiety and loneliness in adults who solicit minors online. *Sexual Abuse, 29*(6), 519–540.

Seto, M. C. (2008a). *Pedophilia and sexual offending against children: Theory, assessment, and intervention.* Washington, DC: American Psychological Association.

Seto, M. C. (2008b). Pedophilia: Psychopathology and theory. In D. R. Laws & W. T. Donohue (Eds.), *Sexual deviance: Theory, assessment, and treatment* (2nd ed., pp. 164–182). New York, NY: Guilford.

Seto, M. C. (2009). Pedophilia. *Annual Review of Clinical Psychology, 5*, 391–407.

Seto, M. C. (2010). Child pornography use and internet solicitation in the diagnosis of pedophilia. *Archives of Sexual Behavior, 39*(3), 591–593.

Seto, M. C. (2012). Is pedophilia a sexual orientation? *Archives of Sexual Behavior, 41*(1), 231–236.

Seto, M. C. (2013). *Internet sex offenders* (pp. 169–192). Washington, DC: American Psychological Association.

Seto, M. C. (2017). The puzzle of male chronophilias. *Archives of Sexual Behavior, 46*(1), 3–22.

Seto, M. C. (2018a). *Pedophilia and sexual offending against children: Theory, assessment, and intervention* (2nd ed., pp. 251–252). Washington, DC: American Psychological Association.

Seto, M. C. (2018b). Reply to "More puzzles: A response to Seto's (2017) "The puzzle of male chronophilias" (Fedoroff, 2018). *Archives of Sexual Behavior, 47*(8), 2175–2176. https://doi.org/10.1007/s10508-018-1298-0

Seto, M. C., & Ahmed, A. G. (2014). Treatment and management of child pornography use. *Psychiatric Clinics, 37*(2), 207–214.

Seto, M. C., Babchishin, K. M., Pullman, L. E., & McPhail, I. V. (2015). The puzzle of intrafamilial child sexual abuse: A meta-analysis comparing intrafamilial and extrafamilial offenders with child victims. *Clinical Psychology Review, 39*, 42–57.

Seto, M. C., & Eke, A. W. (2015). Predicting recidivism among adult male child pornography offenders: Development of the Child Pornography Offender Risk Tool (CPORT). *Law and Human Behavior, 39*(4), 416.

Seto, M. C., & Eke, A. W. (2017). Correlates of admitted sexual interest in children among individuals convicted of child pornography offenses. *Law and Human Behavior, 41*(3), 305–313.

Seto, M. C., Fedoroff, J. P., Bradford, J. M., Knack, N., Rodrigues, N. C., Curry, S., . . . Messina, S. (2016). Reliability and validity of the DSM-IV-TR and proposed DSM-5 criteria for pedophilia: Implications for the ICD-11 and the next DSM. *International Journal of Law and Psychiatry, 49*, 98–106.

Seto, M. C., Hermann, C. A., Kjellgren, C., Priebe, G., Svedin, C. G., & Långström, N. (2015). Viewing child pornography: Prevalence and correlates in a representative community sample of young Swedish men. *Archives of Sexual Behavior, 44*(1), 67–79.

Seto, M. C., Sandler, J. C., & Freeman, N. J. (2017). The revised screening scale for pedophilic interests: Predictive and concurrent validity. *Sexual Abuse, 29*(7), 636–657.

Seto, M. C., Stephens, S., Lalumière, M. L., & Cantor, J. M. (2017). The revised Screening Scale for Pedophilic Interests (SSPI–2): Development and criterion-related validation. *Sexual Abuse, 29*(7), 619–635.

Shaffer, B. M. (2018). Society's view of female child molesters compared to male child molesters. Doctoral dissertation, Alliant International University, California School of Forensic Studies, Irvine, CA (ProQuest Dissertations, Accession No. 10619915).

Sheilds, M., Tonmy, L., & Hovdestad, W. (2016). Is child sexual abuse declining in Canada? Results from nationally representative retrospective surveys. *Health Promotion and Chronic Disease Prevention in Canada, 36*(11), 252–260.

Sheldon, K., & Howitt, D. (2008). Sexual fantasy in paedophile offenders: Can any model explain satisfactorily new findings from a study of internet and contact sexual offenders? *Legal and Criminological Psychology, 13*(1), 137–158.

Shetty, A., Nayak, A., Travers, R., Vaidya, H., & Wylie, K. (2014). Pedophilia. In G. Corona, E. A. Jannini, & M. Maggi (Eds.), *Emotional, physical and sexual abuse: Impact in children and social minorities* (pp. 1–17). Cham, Switzerland: Springer.

Sigre-Leirós, V., Carvalho, J., & Nobre, P. (2015). Cognitive schemas and sexual offending: Differences between rapists, pedophilic and nonpedophilic child molesters, and nonsexual offenders. *Child Abuse & Neglect, 40*, 81–92.

Sigre-Leirós, V., Carvalho, J., & Nobre, P. (2016). Preliminary findings on men's sexual self-schema and sexual offending: Differences between subtypes of offenders. *Journal of Sex Research, 53*(2), 204–213.

Silvani, M., Mondaini, N., & Zucchi, A. (2015). Androgen deprivation therapy (castration therapy) and pedophilia: What's new. *Archivio Italiano di Urologia e Andrologia, 87*(3), 222–226.

Sim, D. J., & Proeve, M. (2010). Crossover and stability of victim type in child molesters. *Legal and Criminological Psychology, 15*(2), 401–413.
Smid, W., Schepers, K., Kamphuis, J. H., van Linden, S., & Bartling, S. (2015). Prioritizing child pornography notifications: Predicting direct victimization. *Sexual Abuse, 27*(4), 398–413.
Spehr, A., Hill, A., Habermann, N., Briken, P., & Berner, W. (2010). Sexual murderers with adult or child victims: Are they different? *Sexual Abuse, 22*(3), 290–314.
Spriggs, S. A., Cohen, L. J., Valencia, A., Zimri, Y., & Galynker, I. I. (2018). Qualitative analysis of attitudes toward adult–child sexual activity among minor-attracted persons. *Journal of Sex & Marital Therapy, 44*(8), 787–799.
Steele, B. R., & Ryan, G. (2010). Deviancy: Development gone wrong. In G. Ryan, T. Leversee, & S. Lane (Eds.), *Juvenile sexual offending: Causes, consequences, and correction* (pp. 55–69). Hoboken, NJ: Wiley.
Stephens, S., Cantor, J. M., Goodwill, A. M., & Seto, M. C. (2017). Multiple indicators of sexual interest in prepubescent or pubescent children as predictors of sexual recidivism. *Journal of Consulting and Clinical Psychology, 85*(6), 585–595.
Stephens, S., Leroux, E., Skilling, T., Cantor, J. M., & Seto, M. C. (2017). Taxometric analyses of pedophilia utilizing self-report, behavioral, and sexual arousal indicators. *Journal of Abnormal Psychology, 126*(8), 1114–1119.
Stephens, S., & Seto, M. C. (2016). Hebephilic sexual offending. In A. Phenix & H. M. Hoberman (Eds.), *Sexual offending: Predisposing antecedents, assessments, and management* (pp. 29–43). New York, NY: Springer.
Stoll, G. E. (2008). The Native American child molester: An exploration of psychopathology as measured by the Minnesota Multiphasic Personality Inventory and the Millon Clinical Multiaxial Inventory. Doctoral dissertation, Alliant International University, California School of Forensic Studies, Irvine, CA (ProQuest Dissertations, Accession No. 3276570).
Stolpmann, G., Briken, P., & Müller, J. L. (2017). Treatment structures for men with pedosexual problems [in German]. *Bundesgesundheisblatt Gesundheitsforschung Gesundheitsschutz, 60*(9), 1055–1062. doi:10.1007/s00103-017-2604-z
Strassberg, D. S., Eastvold, A., Kenney, J. W., & Suchy, Y. (2012). Psychopathy among pedophilic and nonpedophilic child molesters. *Child Abuse & Neglect, 36*(4), 379–382.
Suchy, Y., Eastvold, A. D., Strassberg, D. S., & Franchow, E. I. (2014). Understanding processing speed weaknesses among pedophilic child molesters: Response style vs. neuropathology. *Journal of Abnormal Psychology, 123*(1), 273–285.
Suchy, Y., Whittaker, W. J., Strassberg, D. S., & Eastvold, A. (2009a). Facial and prosodic affect recognition among pedophilic and nonpedophilic criminal child molesters. *Sexual Abuse, 21*(1), 93–110.
Suchy, Y., Whittaker, J. W., Strassberg, D. S., & Eastvold, A. (2009b). Neurocognitive differences between pedophilic and nonpedophilic child molesters. *Journal of the International Neuropsychological Society, 15*(2), 248–257.
Sullivan, J., & Sheehan, V. (2016). What motivates sexual abusers of children? A qualitative examination of the spiral of sexual abuse. *Aggression and Violent Behavior, 30*, 76–87.
Szumski, F., & Zielona-Jenek, M. (2016). Child molesters' cognitive distortions: Conceptualizations of the term. *Psychiatria Polska, 50*(5), 1053–1063.
Tan, L., & Grace, R. C. (2008). Social desirability and sexual offenders: A review. *Sexual Abuse, 20*(1), 61–87.
Teeter-Witt, A. (2016). The psychological experience of Internet child pornography offenders [Abstract]. Doctoral dissertation, Alliant International University, California School of Forensic Studies, Irvine, CA.
Temporini, H. (2012). Child pornography and the internet. *Psychiatric Clinics, 35*(4), 821–835.
Tenbergen, G., Wittfoth, M., Frieling, H., Ponseti, J., Walter, M., Walter, H., . . . Kruger, T. H. (2015). The neurobiology and psychology of pedophilia: Recent advances and challenges. *Frontiers in Human Neuroscience, 9*, 344.
Thibaut, F., de la Barra, F., Gordon, H., Cosyns, P., & Bradford, J. (2010). The World Federation of Societies of Biological Psychiatry (WFSBP) guidelines for the biological treatment of paraphilias. *The World Journal of Biological Psychiatry, 11*, 604–655. doi:10.3109/15622971003671628

Thompson, D. K. (2016). *IQ and neuropsychological profiles of sexual offenders against children and adolescents: A meta-analysis.* Doctoral dissertation, University of the Rockies, Denver, CO (ProQuest Dissertations, Accession No. 3719616).

Titcomb, C., Goodman-Delahunty, J., & De Puiseau, B. W. (2012). Pretrial diversion for intrafamilial child sexual offending: Does biological paternity matter? *Criminal Justice and Behavior, 39*(4), 552–570.

Tousseul, S. (2018). Are prohibited sexualities pathological? [in French]. *Cliniques Mediterraneennes: Psychanalyse et Psychopathologie Freudiennes, 97*(1), 243–255.

Tozdan, S., & Briken, P. (2015a). "I believed I could, so I did"—A theoretical approach on self-efficacy beliefs to positively influence men with a risk to sexually abuse children. *Aggression and Violent Behavior, 25*, 104–112.

Tozdan, S., & Briken, P. (2015b). The earlier, the worse? Age of onset of sexual interest in children. *Journal of Sexual Medicine, 12*(7), 1602–1608.

Tozdan, S., & Briken, P. (2017). Accepting sexual interest in children as unchangeable: One claim fits for all? Comments on Grundmann, Krupp, Scherner, Amelung, and Beier's (2016) "Stability of self-reported arousal to sexual fantasies involving children in a clinical sample of pedophiles and hebephiles." *Archives of Sexual Behavior, 46*(2), 331–333.

Tozdan, S., Jakob, C., Schuhmann, P., Budde, M., & Briken, P. (2015). Specific self-efficacy for modifying sexual interest in children (SSIC): Construction and validation of a measuring instrument. *Psychotherapie, Psychosomatik, Medizinische Psychologie, 65*(9–10), 345–352.

Tozdan, S., Kalt, A., Dekker, A., Keller, L. B., Thiel, S., Müller, J. L., & Briken, P. (2018). Why information matters: Examining the consequences of suggesting that pedophilia is immutable. *International Journal of Offender Therapy and Comparative Criminology, 62*(5), 1241–1261.

Turner, D., & Briken, P. (2018). Treatment of paraphilic disorders in sexual offenders or men with a risk of sexual offending with luteinizing hormone-releasing hormone agonists: An updated systematic review. *Journal of Sexual Medicine, 15*(1), 77–93.

Turner, D., Hertz, P. G., Sauter, J., Briken, P., & Rettenberger, M. (2018). Pharmacological treatment of sexual offenders in German outpatient treatment centers. *International Clinical Psychopharmacology, 33*(6), 349–335. doi:10.1097/YIC.0000000000000222

Turner, D., Rettenberger, M., Lohmann, L., Eher, R., & Briken, P. (2014). Pedophilic sexual interests and psychopathy in child sexual abusers working with children. *Child Abuse & Neglect, 38*(2), 326–335.

van Leeuwen, M. L., van Baaren, R. B., Chakhssi, F., Loonen, M. G., Lippman, M., & Dijksterhuis, A. (2013). Assessment of implicit sexual associations in non-incarcerated pedophiles. *Archives of Sexual Behavior, 42*(8), 1501–1507.

Vess, J., & Skelton, A. (2010). Sexual and violent recidivism by offender type and actuarial risk: Reoffending rates for rapists, child molesters and mixed-victim offenders. *Psychology, Crime & Law, 16*(7), 541–554.

Vlachopoulou, X., & Missionier, S. (2018). The pedophile act and the psychopathological issues of downloading: A virtual protector? [in French]. *Annales Medico-Psychologiques, 176*(3), 301–304.

Wakefield, J. C. (2012). The DSM-5's proposed new categories of sexual disorder: The problem of false positives in sexual diagnosis. *Clinical Social Work Journal, 40*(2), 213–223.

Walter, G., & Pridmore, S. (2012). Suicide and the publicly exposed pedophile. *Malaysian Journal of Medical Sciences, 19*(4), 50–56.

Walton, J. S., & Chou, S. (2015). The effectiveness of psychological treatment for reducing recidivism in child molesters: A systematic review of randomized and nonrandomized studies. *Trauma, Violence, & Abuse, 16*(4), 401–417.

Walton, J. S., & Duff, S. (2017). "I'm not homosexual or heterosexual, I'm paedosexual": Exploring sexual preference for children using interpretive phenomenology. *Journal of Forensic Practice, 19*(2), 151–161.

Wang, S. C., Kao, Y. C., & Liu, Y. P. (2014). Divalproex sodium and quetiapine treatment of a pedophile with bipolar spectrum disorder. *Journal of Neuropsychiatry and Clinical Neurosciences, 26*(3), E47–E48.

Weidacker, K., Kärgel, C., Massau, C., Weiß, S., Kneer, J., Krueger, T. H. C., & Schiffer, B. (2017). Approach and avoidance tendencies toward picture stimuli of (pre-)pubescent children and adults: An investigation in pedophilic and nonpedophilic samples. *Sexual Abuse, 30*(7), 781–802. doi:10.1177/1079063217697134

Wiebking, C., & Northoff, G. (2013). Neuroimaging in pedophilia. *Current Psychiatry Reports, 15*(4), 351. doi:10.1007/s11920-013-0351-x

Wiebking, C., Sartorius, A., Dressing, H., & Northoff, G. (2012). Pedophilia. In J. R. Simpson (Ed.), *Neuroimaging in forensic psychiatry: From the clinic to the courtroom* (pp. 99–111). Malden, MA: Wiley-Blackwell.

Williams, L. H. (2017). Talk of pedophilia: The reflexive management of desire. *Deviant Behavior, 38*(12), 1406–1418.

Williams, S. E., Gannon, T. A., Ward, T., & Collie, R. M. (2008). Child molesters' cognitive distortions: A brief research review. In J. P. Tsai (Ed.), *Leading-edge cognitive disorders research* (pp. 155–167). Hauppauge, NY: Nova.

Willis, G. M., & Grace, R. C. (2009). Assessment of community reintegration planning for sex offenders: Poor planning predicts recidivism. *Criminal Justice and Behavior, 36*(5), 494–512.

Willis, G. M., & Ward, T. (2011). Striving for a good life: The good lives model applied to released child molesters. *Journal of Sexual Aggression, 17*(3), 290–303.

Wilson, R. J., Abracen, J., Looman, J., Picheca, J. E., & Ferguson, M. (2011). Pedophilia: An evaluation of diagnostic and risk prediction methods. *Sexual Abuse, 23*(2), 260–274.

Winder, B., Gough, B., & Seymour-Smith, S. (2015). Stumbling into sexual crime: The passive perpetrator in accounts by male internet sex offenders. *Archives of Sexual Behavior, 44*(1), 167–180.

Witztum, E., Daie, N., & Rosler, A. (2012). History of abuse and organic difficulties in a convenience sample of 46 ultra-Orthodox males with pedophilia. *Israel Journal of Psychiatry and Related Sciences, 49*(4), 262–269.

Wolak, J., Finkelhor, D., & Mitchell, K. (2011). Child pornography possessors: Trends in offender and case characteristics. *Sexual Abuse, 23*(1), 22–42.

Wollert, R., Waggoner, J., & Smith, J. (2012). Federal internet child pornography offenders—Limited offense histories and low recidivism rates. In B. K. Schwartz (Ed.), *The sex offender: Current trends in policy and treatment practice* (Vol. 7, pp. 1–21). Kingston, NJ: Civic Research Institute.

Wood, H. (2010). Applied analytic work in forensic settings: The understanding and treatment of paedophilia. In A. Lemma & M. Patrick (Eds.), *Off the couch: Contemporary psychoanalytic applications* (pp. 143–159). New York, NY: Routledge.

Wood, H. (2013). Internet pornography and paedophilia. *Psychoanalytic Psychotherapy, 27*(4), 319–338.

World Health Organization. (2004). *International statistical classification of diseases and related health problems* (10th rev.). Geneva, Switzerland: Author.

Worsham, M. (2011). Creating an expected profile for Affinity 2.5 from a sample of non-pedophilic, exclusively heterosexual, college-age females. Doctoral dissertation, Brigham Young University, Provo, UT (ProQuest Dissertations, Accession No. 3427215).

Wurtele, S. K., Simons, D. A., & Moreno, T. (2014). Sexual interest in children among an online sample of men and women: Prevalence and correlates. *Sexual Abuse, 26*(6), 546–568.

Wurtele, S. K., Simons, D. A., & Parker, L. J. (2018). Understanding men's self-reported sexual interest in children. *Archives of Sexual Behavior, 47*(8), 2255–2264.

Zappalà, A., Antfolk, J., Dombert, B., Mokros, A., & Santtila, P. (2016). Identifying deviant sexual interest in a sex offender sample using dual-target rapid serial visual presentation task. *Journal of Forensic Psychiatry & Psychology, 27*(2), 281–307.

7

Sexual Masochism and Sexual Sadism Disorder

Sadism is all right in its place, but it should be directed to proper ends.
—Sigmund Freud (1935; as cited in Wortis, 1954, p. 153)

Introduction

If this is the first chapter you flipped to while browsing this book, do not be alarmed. Sexual masochism and sexual sadism seem to be universally interesting. In part, this is because sexual sadism and masochism encompass a very wide range of sexual interest(s). The words "sadism" and "masochism" are also used to describe nonsexual situations in the English language (e.g., "My new boss is a sadist" or "I am a masochist when it comes to taking on new projects at work"). This chapter may be confusing because the concepts of "sadism" and "masochism" are discussed as they relate both to "sexual sadism disorder" and "sexual masochism disorder" as defined in the Fifth edition of the *Diagnostic and Statistical Manual of Mental Disorders* (DSM-5; American Psychiatric Association, 2013) and to bondage and discipline, dominance and submission, sadism and masochism (BDSM). The concepts are further compounded by issues of degree of consent. It is important to distinguish between act and intent. The same act—for example, disrobing a sexual partner—may be part of conventional "vanilla" sexual behavior, part of a negotiated and consensual BDSM "scene," or a criminal offense committed by a person with sexual sadistic disorder if the act is non-consensual.

The terms sadism and masochism were eponymously coined by Richard von Krafft-Ebbing (1886/1999) after two contemporary writers who were sociopolitical commentators: Donatien Alphonse Francois, the Marquis de Sade (1740—1814), and Leopold von Sacher-Masoch (1836–1895). In retrospect, both of these writers had lives and views that were as apparently paradoxical as the concept of sadomasochism. Much of de Sade's writing parodied the social hierarchies of the French aristocracy to which he belonged and from which he benefited, and also the Roman Catholic Church, which included a convent in which he grew up. He championed personal freedom but spent 27 years of his life imprisoned for blasphemy and sex crimes under the regimes of both Louis XV and, after the French Revolution, the first Emperor of France, Napoleon Bonaparte. Although de Sade is linked to sadism, he personally lived much of his life in chains deprived of interpersonal sexual interactions of any type. He wrote about whipping women but was himself the victim of flagellation by nuns.

Von Sacher-Masoch (1836–1895) was a writer who espoused humanitarianism and who is best known for his novel, *Venus in Furs* (1932), which describes the life of a man who arranges to sign a contract with a woman to treat him as her slave and for her to humiliate and torture him. It parallels Von Sacher-Masoch's personal life, in which he attempted to convince two women in two separate relationships to treat him as a slave. The first woman was his wife, Aurora Rumelin, who in her own fictionalized account of their marriage described her husband's unwanted and uninvited attempts to force her to satisfy his masochistic interests (W. Sacher-Masoch, 1906). The second woman was Fanny Pistor, for whom Sacher-Masoch left his wife. It is of interest that in *Venus in Furs*, Von Sacher-Masoch's autobiographical, masochistic protagonist, Severin, loses his interest in masochism when his sadistic mistress falls in love with another man, arranges for her lover to whip him, and then leaves him. The memoir ends with his comment,

> I had to smile, and as I fell to musing the beautiful woman suddenly stood before me in her velvet jacket trimmed with ermine, with the whip in her hand. And I continued to smile at the woman I had once loved so insanely, at the fur-jacket that had once so entranced me, at the whip, and ended by smiling at myself and saying: The cure was cruel, but radical; but the main point is, I have been cured. (p. 144)

Although Sachor-Masoch's name has been linked to masochism, he is reported to have been displeased when Von Krafft-Ebing coined his name for the condition. It is also notable that by his wife's account, Sachor-Masoch was perceived as manipulative and coercive. His pattern of imposing his sexual interests on others is opposite to the stereotypic view of people with masochism as being submissive and unassertive.

A third literary contribution to the world of sadomasochism is equally paradoxic. The first "support group" for people with self-defined masochism, The Eulenspiegel Society (TES), was named after Eulenspiegel, who was described as a Germanic "folklore prankster." Aschenbrenner, J. (1994). The TES began as a group for people with masochism, but soon people who identified a sadists were included as their welcome guests. The TES derives its name from a tale in which Eulenspiegel is joyful as he ascends a mountain. A passerby asks why he is so happy while doing such an onerous task as climbing a mountain, and Eulenspiegel says he is happy because he knows that soon he will be going downhill. He adds that he is always upset when he reaches the bottom of a hill because he knows this means he inevitably will have to walk uphill, which is much less pleasant. The founders of TES believed the identification of pleasure due to adversity reflected the way they derived sexual pleasure from seemingly aversive situations. Of course, many people with masochism would object to that characterization, insisting the pleasure is due to adversity itself and not to its anticipated ending.

Readers will note that the concepts of sadism, masochism, and sadomasochism are named after individuals whose interests and motivations may seem confusing, overlapping, and paradoxical. The issues are further complicated by the concept of consent. People who identify as belonging to the group of communities known as BDSM identify mutual revocable consent as crucial to their interests (sometimes referred to as RACK, which is an acronym for "risk-aware consensual kink"). Members of BDSM communities frequently refer to the expectation and requirement that all acts be "safe, sane and consensual" (Jacques, 1993; Stein, 2002). Many of the major themes seen in sadomasochistic literature are reflected in children's fairy stories and "vanilla" (conventional) culture, such as the ideas of "falling in love," "love at first sight," "being taken," and "to honor and obey."

The DSM-5 makes an attempt to distinguish between consensual sexual interests and non-consensual ones in its definitions of sadistic disorders and masochist disorders. The DSM-5 defines *masochism disorder* as a condition lasting at least 6 months, consisting of "recurrent and intense sexual arousal from the act of being humiliated, beaten, bound, or otherwise made to suffer as manifested by fantasies, urge or behaviors" (APA, 2013, p. 694). The B criteria state the condition causes clinically significant distress or impairment in social, occupational, or other important areas of functioning" (p. 694). There are no specified age limits. There are three specifiers: "with asphyxiophilia"(achieving sexual arousal by restriction breathing), "in a controlled environment," and "in full remission" (5 or more years with no category B criteria) (p. 694).

The DSM-5 states the prevalence of masochistic behaviors is 2.2% of males and 1.3% of females in the past 12 months (APA, 2013, p. 694). The text states that "very little" is known about the persistence of masochistic disorders, which the text states have a mean age of onset of 19.3 years.

The DSM-5 defines *sexual sadism disorder* as a condition lasting at least 6 months, consisting of "recurrent and intense sexual arousal from the physical or psychological suffering of another person as manifested by fantasies, urges or behaviors" (APA, 2013, p. 695). The B criteria state the "individual has acted on these sexual interests with a nonconsenting person, or the sexual urges or fantasies cause clinically significant distress or impairment in social, occupational or other important areas of functioning" (p. 685). There are two specifiers: "in a controlled environment" and "in full remission" (no non-consensual acts and no distress for at least 5 years) (p. 695).

The DSM-5 claims the prevalence of sexual sadism disorder varies between 2% to 30% and that only 10% of civilly committed sex offenders have sexual sadism, but it adds that 37–75% of sexually motivated homicides are committed by people with sexual sadism disorder (APA, 2013, p. 696). Like sexual masochism disorder, sexual sadism disorder is reported to begin at the mean age of 19.4 years and "may fluctuate" (p. 697).

In contrast, the 10th revision of the *International Classification of Diseases* (ICD-10; World Health Organization, 2004) combines sexual masochism and sexual sadism into a single condition grouped under the category of disorders of adult personality and behavior. *Sadomasochism* is defined as

> a preference for sexual activity which involves the infliction of pain or humiliation, or bondage. If the subject prefers to be the recipient of such stimulation this is called masochism, if the provider, sadism. Often an individual obtains sexual excitement from both sadistic and masochistic activities. (F.65.5)

In the ICD-11 definition, mutual consent is implied by the word "preference." The ICD-11 will therefore likely eliminate sadomasochism from its list of paraphilic disorders based on the notion that people with sadomasochism do not necessarily have distress or non-consenting victims (Reiersøl & Skeid, 2006). The diagnosis will likely be replaced by two new ones: "coercive sexual sadism disorder" and "other paraphilic disorder involving non-consenting individuals."

In the Sexual Behaviours Clinic (SBC), the old view of sadism and masochism as illustrated in Figure 7.1, is challenged. Many patients present with the belief that they are either extremely sadistic or masochistic with little regard to the orthogonal aspect of how consenting they or their partner(s) is to activities in which they may engage. Instead, SBC patients are invited to consider the paradigm as illustrated in Figure 7.2, in which extreme sadism and masochism look more alike compared to sexual interests that do not explicitly focus on sadistic or masochistic interests and acts—so-called vanilla sex.

Note again that degree of dominance and submission is orthogonal to the degree of consent (they can vary independently). Dividing these factors into separate characteristics often makes it easier for patients who want to change their interests or behaviors to focus on what exactly it is that they and their partner(s) wish to change.

Variations

The concept of sadomasochism (SM) from a forensic perspective was reviewed several years ago (Fedoroff, 2008). The concept of consensual bondage, domination, submission, sadism, and masochism (BDSM; in a subsample of men who have sex with men) has been reviewed more recently (Holmes, Murray, Knack, Mecier, & Fedoroff, 2017a, 2017b).

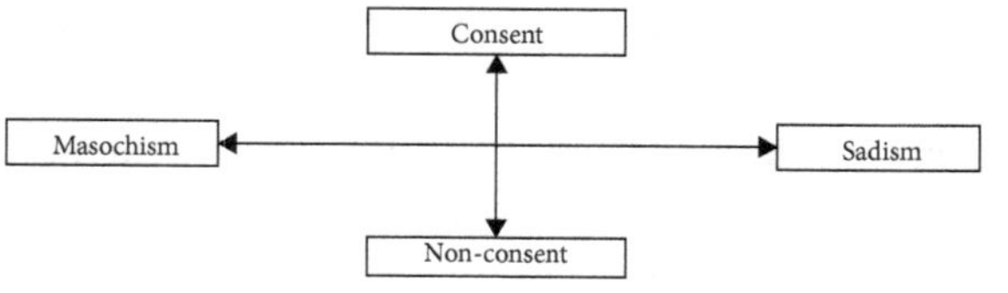

Figure 7.1 The old view of masochism and sadism.

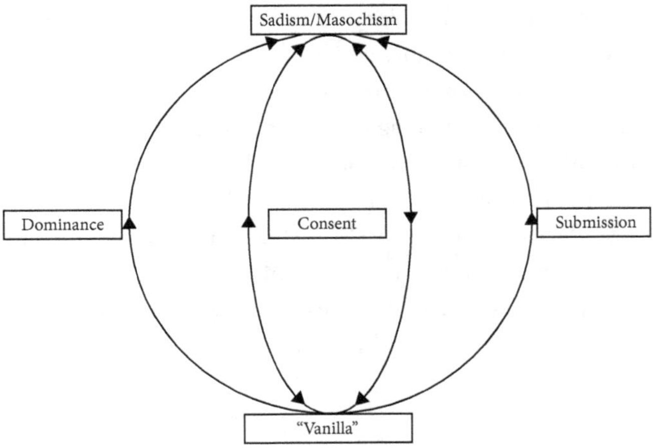

Figure 7.2 The SBC view of sadism and masochism.

It is important in any discussion of S/M and BDSM to distinguish between motivations, behaviors, and intentions. Diagnosis of S/M and/or identification of non-pathologic BDSM interests on the basis of behavior alone is treacherous. Consider, for example, Case Report 7.1, which presents the classic dilemma posed to medical students.

In this section, the terms *sadism* and *masochism* refer to sexual arousal from dominating or humiliating or of being dominated or humiliated, respectively. They are used generically without consideration of whether or not consent is obtained.

Case Report 7.1

You are a doctor in the busy emergency room of a teaching hospital. A young semiconscious man arrives by ambulance. He has sustained a brain concussion and has a broken arm. After he is stabilized and wakes up, he tells you he was playing football.

Do you refer him to psychiatry? What if instead of playing football, he tells you that he was involved in a consenting BDSM scene in which there was an accident. Would you refer him then? What if he tells you he was in a BDSM scene and intentionally asked to have his arm broken? What if he has done this more than once? What if instead of a young man, it was a young woman?

In Case Report 7.1, the medical problems (concussion and broken arm) are the same. The possibility of reoccurrence or worsening of the identified problems (especially concussion) is the same if the man returns to playing football or another sexual "scene" with the same elements. In North American society, behaviors motivated by sports are typically tolerated and encouraged. Behaviors motivated by sexual arousal are viewed with more concern.

In sports and sex, *intent* is a defining concept. An act intended to cause harm by inflicting lasting physical injury is against the rules in both arenas. This is especially true in BDSM, which, as noted previously, traditionally values consent as fundamental to sexual interactions.

Details of popular activities in the BDSM community are constantly changing due to cultural changes. However, a mainstay of BDSM iconography is the imagined fashions prevalent in the worlds of de Sade and von Sachor-Masoch, such as corsets, capes, and riding boots (Lewandowski, 2011).

Case Report 7.2

A middle-aged man self-referred to the SBC. He arrived a half-hour early. He was wearing a suit and tie. He was thin and appeared anxious. He admitted he was anxious but not about his sexual interest that he proudly declared was masochistic. He was successful in his profession and had been fortunate to find a woman who identified as sadistic and they were married.

He explained that he had always known he was intensely and persistently sexually aroused by the idea of being abducted, controlled, and forced to do things (sexual or otherwise) against his will. He described elaborate fantasies involving being left bound and naked in the basement by his wife while she went shopping. The idea of not knowing when or if she would return was extremely arousing, especially the idea that he might starve or lose his job.

So, what was the problem? He explained that his wife objected to him "pushing" her to do sadistic things to him. She called him a "smart ass masochist" because he constantly pushed her to do more than she desired. If she tied him up in the basement and left him for an hour, he would ask for 2 hours. If she left him for 2 hours, he would ask to be abandoned for 4 hours. Recently, he had been telling her that he wanted her to take him to a BDSM club and humiliate him in front of other club members. In a recent argument, she told him she would leave him permanently if he did not stop making demands on her.

On the second visit, he was accompanied by his wife, who was neatly groomed and had a self-confident demeanor. She weighed more than her husband. She confirmed that she identified as sadistic. Unlike her husband, she had not realized she was a sadist until her husband introduced her to the "scene." She was aroused by the effect her sadistic actions had on her husband. The problem, she explained, was that for her sadism was sexual:

> I do not want to go to a BDSM club where people dress up in leather and pretend to be sadists or masochists but they are just vanillas who want to role-play. To me sadomasochism is too sexual to want to take it public.

She confirmed her husband's impression that she was annoyed when her husband asked to be abused: "If he is asking for it, who is in charge?" She also believed that her husband's insistence that she starve him was a veiled criticism of her weight and "failure" to control her own eating.

Case Report 7.2 illustrates several important aspects of sadism and masochism. The first is that sadism and masochism, rather than being polar opposites, are better understood as a continuum. Extreme sadism is indistinguishable from extreme masochism. The husband in Case Report 7.2 identified as masochistic but in fact was aroused by controlling his wife's behaviors. His wife identified as sadistic but was aroused by her husband's arousal. Suppose they went to a restaurant and he gave her the menu and told her to order as much or as little as she wanted him to have for supper that evening. Would an observer know who was the person with sadism and who was the person with masochism?

A second important aspect to note is that sadism and masochism are not necessarily criminal. In Case Report 7.2, the man and woman were a law-abiding, religious couple with conservative political beliefs. Both valued consent and respected it. In fact, the husband justified the demands he made on his wife by the fact that he was the one who suffered for her enjoyment: "I am not one of those guys who tells women they have to have sex. I tell my wife she does not have to have sex with me." It is notable that he never commented on his wife's weight, but his wife mistakenly interpreted his actions as critical, which he indignantly denied.

A third aspect of sadism and masochism illustrated by the couple discussed in Case Report 7.2 is the fact that analysis is complicated by the level of their sexual interests. The wife correctly noted that many people in the BDSM scene have little or no interest in sexual sadomasochism and simply enjoy dressing up and role playing the way people may enjoy attending cocktail parties or masquerade balls. Alternatively, some people take BDSM far beyond the bedroom, assuming BDSM as a self-identity. The DSM-5 describes people who may engage in the same activities as people in BDSM communities but, because their arousal is due to nonconsent, have little in common phenomenologically with BDSM.

As a final comment, much of sadism and masochism is contextual. A "vanilla" couple is having drinks with a BDSM "lifestyle" couple in which the wife identifies as the husband's slave and obediently obeys his orders. The vanilla wife notices the attention the sadistic husband pays to his masochistic wife, perhaps with some envy. But she comments to the BDSM couple,

> You know you two are really not as BDSM as my husband and I are. Your husband has to order you to do something. I already know what my husband wants and do it for him before he realizes it. He doesn't need to order me. Isn't that what love is?

Sexual Masochism

Although it is possible to understand why sexual sadism that involves non-consent is worthy of diagnosis, many wonder why sexual masochism should be pathologized.

Case Report 7.3

An energetic woman arrived at the SBC. She wasted no time in describing her problem. "Doctor I am getting scared." She explained she was scared for two reasons. The first involved concern about a series of devices that she referred to as "contraptions." They consisted of cords and pulleys that she had arranged to put herself into forms of bondage from which she had been having increasing difficulty escaping. Of particular concern were the contraptions that involved strangulation. She admitted masturbating while strangling herself. She said being anoxic not only increased her ability to reach orgasm but also heightened the intensity of the orgasms.

Her second concern involved her pattern of dressing provocatively and intentionally going to dangerous places such as back alleys in the hope of being raped. She realized this was a dangerous activity, but she found the excitement she experienced difficult to resist. On questioning, she admitted that her fantasies involved being not only raped but also strangled and killed.

Treatment began with her agreeing to dismantle her contraptions. She was told to buy a "magic wand" vibrator to use when she masturbated. These are external vibrators that are powered by an electrical cord instead of batteries. They are very effective in assisting women to reach orgasm. She also agreed to stop endangering herself when she went for walks. Instead, she was encouraged to challenge her "Madonna–whore" self-concept and accept the idea that she could have fulfilling sex without compromising her identity as a feminist. She responded extremely well to therapy that she described as empowering because it did not challenge her masochistic fantasies but instead permitted her to experience sex in a continuous rather than dichotomous paradigm.

Sexual Homicide

A recurring theme in the literature on sexual sadism is the way in which it relates to sex crimes. The relationship between sexual sadism and sexual homicide is reviewed by Briken, Bourget, and Dufour (2014). Surprisingly, the literature is confused by the lack of a definition of sexual homicide that is sufficiently specific.

Ressler, Burgess, and Douglas (1988) provided nine criteria, but those criteria consist mainly of observations that may be made at the crime scene, such as "semen on or near the victim's body."

This is problematic because spousal homicide is very different from sadistic homicide committed by offenders such as Jack the Ripper. A second problem in the literature is the fact that sex offenders who kill their victims are often retrospectively labeled as sadistic due to the brutality of the crime. It is important not to equate the apparent "brutality" of a crime with the motivation for the crime. A third issue is the fact that people with sadism who commit crimes are only studied after they have been convicted and spent time in custody. People who commit sex crimes have a higher frequency of sustaining head injury while in custody. Therefore, brain imaging studies showing right-sided temporal lobe abnormalities need to be reviewed with caution (Harenski, Thornton, Harenski, Decety, & Kiehl, 2012; Hucker et al., 1988; Langevin, Ben-Aron, Wright, Marchese, & Handy, 1988).

Assessment and Treatment Recommendations

As with all paraphilias that involve sexual interests that would be criminal if acted upon, it is important to establish that sexual fantasies per se are never criminal. Individuals with sadistic interests can be assured that the reason they were arrested is not because of their sadistic thoughts but, rather, because they acted on their interests in a non-consenting manner. The aim of therapy therefore starts with the insistence that the person assume responsibility for any current or future sexual behaviors. Again, they should be reminded that sexual behaviors are voluntary and therefore under their control. If they report their sex drive is too high, and they are unwilling or unable to manage their sex drive by conventional means such as masturbation to orgasm, high sex drive can be reliably treated with anti-androgens and gonadotropin-releasing hormone medications (see Chapter 2, this book). Treatment with these medications is more likely to be accepted if they are presented as voluntary, temporary, and reversible interventions. Sadistic interests do not need to be changed unless they are dependent on or conducive to engaging in non-consensual activities. Helping people with sadistic interests understand that sexual relations with a consenting partner are more likely to result in fulfilling sexual relations is key to effective treatment.

Madonna–Whore Syndrome

A common finding in people with sadistic interests is some variant of the Madonna–whore syndrome (MWS).

Case Report 7.4

A married man scheduled an urgent appointment for "sexual addiction." When seen, he was wearing business attire. He explained that although he was self-employed and his business was going well, he was in financial difficulty. He was spending thousands of dollars on a woman who danced at a strip bar.

He described a lively sexual history when he was single. He was very sexually interested in his wife when he first met her, but she was religious and they agreed to wait until they were married before they had sex. Once married, they decided to have children. There were some fertility problems, and sex with his wife, timed to her ovulations, became a chore for him. When she became pregnant, their sexual relations declined and then stopped when she had their daughter. At the same time that he stopped having sex with his wife, he started to leave his work in the early afternoon to secretly go to a strip bar where he met the dancer. Their relationship became sexual, but he justified it by reminding himself that it was "purely business" and had no effect on the love he felt for his wife.

Case Report 7.4 is an example of a person with the MWS, which has numerous variants. The cardinal feature is a pattern of dichotomizing women into those who are maternal ("good girls" or mothers) and those who are sexual ("bad girls" or whores). Men with this syndrome typically have no problems before they marry. However, either at the time of marriage or at the time of the birth of the first child, their partner changes from someone who is sexual to someone who is "mother." Women can also have the syndrome, but usually it involves a change in how they view themselves rather than their partner.

Returning to people with sexual sadism, many who present with problems do so because they have a variant of MWS. Treatment in these cases usually focuses on improving the relationship.

Case Report 7.5

A man was referred by a member of the BDSM group to which he belonged. He was a student. He self-identified as a sadist. He had never had sexual intercourse. He explained that he found it disgusting to think of having sex with a woman who wanted to have sex. He was especially mortified by the idea of sex with a woman who specifically wanted to have sex with him. He said he wanted to find a virgin who he would fall in love with at the same time that she fell in love with him, "at first sight."

In the meantime, he engaged in "scenes" in which he attempted to force women to literally stigmatize themselves by branding, piercing, or tattooing. The BDSM community had become concerned by his fits of rage not only when women refused to do his bidding but also when they complied. In treatment, it became clear that he dichotomized women into "good girls" and "bad girls." The fact that the women were doing something they did not want to do allowed him to think of them as potential sexual partners.

Sadistic fantasies are one way for people with MWS to overcome the problem of excluding everyone who wants to have sex from being a potential sexual partner. Specifically, if a man believes that only "bad girls" want to have sex, forcing a woman to have sex may allow him to continue to think of her as a "good girl" because she did not consent. The same can be said for masochistic fantasies and interests. For example, a woman with the syndrome can permit herself to be sexual by adopting a masochistic persona in which she is being "taken against her will."

People with MWS often present with self-diagnosed "sex addiction" in which they label their sexual interests as pathologic. Treatment in these cases begins with helping the person reinterpret their sexual feelings as normal and their "addiction" as more akin to sexual frustration. In the SBC, sexual addiction is treated most effectively by permitting the patient to lawfully reduce their sexual frustrations.

Prognosis

This chapter began with the statement that sadism and masochism are paradoxical. This is also true concerning treatment. As with most of the paraphilias, what is known about treatment is based on experience derived from treating convicts. Unfortunately, crime is not a psychiatric disorder and therefore crime itself is not the subject of treatment. People who commit sex crimes are often labeled sadistic, but this does a disservice to sadism. People who commit sex crimes are criminals and not necessarily sadomasochistic.

Sexual sadism is best treated in conjunction with sexual masochism because the two are closely related. The first step in treatment is to identify why the sadistic or masochistic interests are causing problems. If crimes are being committed, they should be stopped immediately, and any identifiable victims should be helped without delay. This is not only ethical but also therapeutic.

Once criminal activity has stopped, the pressure is lessened. Next, it is important to diagnose and treat any major psychiatric illnesses, including schizophrenia and mood disorders. People with clinical depression often experience a change in self-attitude such that they not only feel depressed but also become convinced that they deserve to be depressed. This state combined with a sense of hopelessness can lead to suicidal or homicidal behavior. As described in Chapter 2, change in self-attitude can lead to fixed false beliefs of being a bad person. This can include the idea of being a sadistic sex offender because "that is the worst thing anyone could be." It is very important for therapists to consider altered self-attitude secondary to major depression as a possible explanation for problematic sadistic or masochistic interests, especially in a person with no previous history of sadomasochistic interests. Once criminal activity and altered self-attitude have been addressed, therapists should turn their attention to improving the sexual well-being of their patients. What aspect of the sadomasochistic interest(s) is interfering with the establishment of fulfilling and healthy relationships? The sooner attention can be paid to this goal, the sooner the person will recover. Paradoxically, sadomasochistic interests tend to change from "harmful interests" to a way of viewing relationships and feeling connected that is more similar to "vanilla" than expected. Ultimately, all consensual sexual interests are analogously still varieties of ice cream. For people who present with concerns about sadomasochistic interests, the prognosis is excellent.

Review of the Literature

The following table summarizes the literature that has been published on sadomasochism from 2008 to 2018 based on PsycINFO and PubMed searches. The following key terms were used: "sadism disorder," "sexual sadism," "masochism disorder," "sexual masochism," and "sadomasochism."

Summary	Reference
Prevalence	
Telephone interviews were conducted with 19,307 participants between ages 16 and 59 years in Australia. It was found that 1.8% of sexually active people were involved in BDSM. It was also found that BDSM is not the result of past abuse or difficulty with "normal" sex.	Richters, de Visser, Rissel, Grulich, & Smith (2008)
In a sample of 1,027 Belgians, 46.8% had performed at least one BDSM-related activity, 12.5% regularly engaged in BDSM activity, and 7.6% identified as BDSM practitioners.	Holvoet et al. (2017)
Literature Reviews	
Literature review on theories of sadism and its etiology.	Fedoroff (2008)
Discusses sexual sadism and its history in relation to "being evil" and other so-called domains of sexual sadism.	Stone (2010)

Summary	Reference
Discusses BDSM and other deviant practices as a "leisure activity."	Williams (2009)
Practices and Culture	
Examined how non-sex offending sexual sadomasochists differ from convicted sex offenders in an outpatient treatment program. It was found that they significantly differed in anxiety, alcohol-related problems, and had "marginal differences" in anti-sociality.	Chapman-Haddock (2012)
In 902 BDSM and 434 control participants, it was found that BDSM practitioners were less neurotic, more extraverted, more open to new experiences, more conscientious, less sensitive to rejection, and had higher subjective well-being, but they were less "agreeable."	Wismeijer & van Assen (2013)
Discusses possible evolutionary roots for BDSM practices.	Jozifkova (2013)
A cross-sectional study examining women (58 bisexuals and 289 lesbians) who engage in BDSM.	Tomassilli, Golub, Bimbi, & Parsons (2009)
Study of 95 "swingers" and the prevalence of various sex acts including BDSM in this sample.	Houngbedji & Guillem (2016)
In a sample of 14,306 participants, it was found that the effect of power on arousal by sadistic thoughts was stronger for women, whereas the effect of power on arousal by masochistic thoughts was stronger in men.	Lammers & Imhoff (2016)
BDSM members describe BDSM communities as a place of acceptance, sexual expression, friendship, safety, and sharing educational knowledge.	Graham, Butler, McGraw, Cannes, & Smith (2016)
Observational study of a BDSM community in Berlin, Germany, investigating power dynamics and societal egalitarianism.	Martin (2012)
Qualitative study of 73 individuals in the BDSM community and whether they conceal their identities as BDSM community members.	Stiles & Clark (2011)
Use of the Sexual Fantasy Questionnaire to investigate BDSM fantasies.	G. Wilson (2010)
Society	
A case involving a consensual sadomasochistic act that took place in public in Toronto, Canada.	Olson (2017)

Summary	Reference
Study of 29 interviews of BDSM practitioners in a Swedish BDSM community concerning gender and equality.	Carlström (2017)
BDSM members face discrimination, violence, and harassment, so they are often stigmatized.	Iannotti (2015)
Examined whether BDSM activities can be understood as a recreational leisure activity.	Williams, Prior, Alvarado, Thomas, & Christensen (2016)
Compared consent that comes with legal (i.e., mixed martial arts) and potentially illegal BDSM practices.	Weinberg, J. (2016)
Found no significant change in attitudes of graduate psychology students toward consensual sadomasochism after taking a course on sadomasochism.	Domue (2015)
Examines visual representations of sadomasochism and the impact of UK legislation on viewing "extreme" pornography.	Wilkinson (2009)
Discusses managing BDSM stigma by creating an opportunity to talk about it through sex education.	Bezreh, Weinberg, & Edgar (2012)
Roles	
In this study, 14 BDSM practitioners were assigned to either the "top role" or the "bottom role." BDSM was associated with reductions in stress, negative affect, and increased sexual arousal.	Ambler et al. (2017)
Semistructured interviews with 9 dominants and 12 submissives on the roles they play in a BDSM relationship and how these roles fit with their personality.	Hébert & Weaver (2015)
Using semistructured interviews and public discussion board threads, Simula (2012) examined the role of gender in BDSM bisexuality and whether this gender role can change. It was found that participants usually differentiated "sex" from "sexual." Three types of BDSM bisexuality were identified.	Simula (2012)
Explanation of BDSM and the roles that partners play during sexual activity.	Airaksinen (2017)

Summary	Reference
Article illustrates how BDSM can be a phenomenological experience.	Turley (2016)
Discusses how abusive relationships can be disguised as consensual BDSM relationships.	Pitagora (2016a)
Using recorded event-related potentials and subjective ratings, this study found that females in the submissive role in BDSM practices tend to lessen their empathic responses to others' suffering.	Luo & Zhang (2017)
Mixed methods study examined 202 online participants and 25 semistructured interviews on switching BDSM roles and its relation to sexual orientation. It was found that men usually identified with dominant roles, whereas women usually identified with submissive roles. However, women and pansexual persons could switch identities.	Martinez (2018)
Consent	
Literature review on the associations between "kink" and "poly-oriented" relationships.	Pitagora (2016b)
Semistructured interviews about how BDSM members negotiate and maintain boundaries with their partner(s).	Holt (2016a)
Examines how BDSM members discuss and maintain boundaries for BDSM activities. It found that when boundary violations occur, they are handled by appointed community members.	Holt (2016b)
Sexual Sadism	
Describes acts of non-consensual sadism.	Palermo (2013)
Examines 5 female offenders diagnosed with sexual sadism.	Pflugradt & Allen (2012)
This study investigated personality differences between sadistic and non-sadistic sexual offenders using the Minnesota Multiphasic Personality Inventory (second edition). It was found that the sadistic offenders were more likely to be morally self-righteous, suspicious, delusional, have low morale, be hostile, have poor interpersonal skills, have severe emotional disturbances, and be lower on social introversion.	Battle (2014)

Summary	Reference
Compares 12 "sexual sadists" with 23 non-sadistic offenders on levels of empathy. After controlling for psychopathy, no differences in empathy were found between the two groups. The results suggest that sexual sadism is not related to impaired empathy.	Nitschke, Istrefi, Osterheider, & Mokros (2012)
In 100 male forensic patients, it was found that sexual sadism and psychopathy are separate latent variables. The findings support the pathway model that argues psychopathic affective deficits and behavioral disinhibition can be precursors to sadism.	Mokros, Osterheider, Hucker, & Nitschke (2011)
This study followed 22 homicidal juvenile sex offenders who had sexual sadism and psychopathic traits. It was found that those who had recidivated tended to have higher psychopathy levels.	Myers, Chan, Vo, & Lazarou (2010)
A dissertation that investigated the relations between psychopathy and "sexual sadism." Through the use of saliva samples and a social stress test, it was found that psychopathy and "sexual sadism" are two unique constructs that produce different physiological and biochemical results.	Robertson (2018)
Through two studies of male sex offenders, exploratory and confirmatory factor analyses show that "sadism" and "psychopathy" covary but remain separate constructs.	Robertson & Knight (2014)
Found that the Psychopathic Deviate Scale on the Minnesota Multiphasic Personality Inventory-2 (MMPI-2) was not significantly correlated with the Male and Female Sadomasochistic scales on the Abel Assessment for Sexual Interest-2 (AASI-2).	Dehnavifar (2013)
Compared single-victim and serial sexual homicide offenders. Serial sexual homicide offenders were more likely to have "deviant" sexual fantasies; victims who were strangers; verbally humiliated their victims; and had narcissistic, schizoid, and obsessive–compulsive traits and other paraphilias.	Chan, Beauregard, & Myers (2015)

Summary	Reference
Systematic review of 1,836 sexual murderers from 45 studies between 1985 and 2013. Serial sexual murderers tended to commit crimes reflecting their sadistic sexual fantasies and tended to plan their murders, whereas non-serial sexual murderers committed their crimes due to "impulsive anger."	James & Proulx (2016)
Article describes how dysfunctional anger may be related to sexual fantasies and sexual crimes.	Ahmed (2014)
Compared nonhomicidal and homicidal sexual offenders. Homicidal sexual offenders usually reported deviant sexual fantasies; admitted to the offense during apprehension; and were paranoid, schizotypal, borderline, histrionic, narcissistic, obsessive–compulsive, impulsive, and eccentric.	Chan & Beauregard (2016)
Investigated the relationship between psychopathy and sexual sadism in 10 serial sexual violent predators. It was found that 8 out of 10 participants had high levels of both psychopathy and sexual sadism.	E. Fischer (2008)
In a sample of 229 violent sexual offenders, it was found that they had persistently low self-esteem and persistent "deviant" sexual interests.	Healey & Beauregard (2015)
Examined the relationships between psychopathy, sadism, and sexual homicide and proposed a "psychopathic–sexually sadistic sexual homicide" offender profile. Case series explored the associations between crime scene behaviors and paraphilic interests in sexual homicide offenders.	Jones, Chan, Myers, & Heide (2013) Myers et al. (2008)
Case study of a child killer who had sexual sadism.	D. Wilson & Brookes (2011)
Sexual Masochism	
Examined the sexual arousal responses of 22 men and 15 women with conventional interests and 16 men and 17 women with masochistic sexual interests. Results showed that individuals usually responded more to their stated preferred sexual interests. However, those with masochistic interests responded equally to the conventional and masochistic sexual interest stimuli.	Chivers, Roy, Grimbos, Cantor, & Seto (2014)

Summary	Reference
Phenomenological study involving 4 females and 5 males, focusing on masochism as a form of addictive process.	Kurt & Ronel (2017)
Explored relationship between two masochists, compared to relationships that involve one partner being masochistic and the other being sadistic.	Hall (2014)
Etiology	
Suggests that the parasite *Toxoplasma* may increase sexual masochism in humans.	Flegr (2017)
Study explored women's BDSM behaviors. A positive association was found between erotica, BDSM behaviors, and physical satisfaction.	Kimberly, Williams, & Creel (2018)
Study of 120 male college students who were randomly assigned to a control group (viewed nonsexual and nonviolent material) or to one of the three pornography-viewing conditions: nonviolent, sadomasochistic, or violent pornography. All three groups that viewed pornography behaved more aggressively (determined by dart-throwing task).	Yang & Youn (2012)
Examined consensual sadomasochists and their attitudes toward their own body satisfaction and sexual objectification.	Martinez (2012)
Discusses sadomasochism as a defense for the superego and its relations to transference and countertransference.	Basseches & Sinkman (2010)
Author uses object relations and drive theory to explain how aggression mixes with sexual activity and becomes sexual sadism.	Juni (2009)
In a study of 5,990 Finnish participants, it was found that sadism and masochism were independent of genetic and environmental confounds.	Baur et al. (2016)
Suicide Ideation and Pain	
Study of BDSM and associations with suicide attempts in 576 BDSM practitioners recruited from online BDSM-related groups. Significant positive associations were found for males but none for females. BDSM-related acts in males were positively associated with specific components of suicide attempts.	Brown, Roush, Mitchell, & Cukrowicz (2017)

Summary	Reference
In 321 adults from the BDSM community, only 37% of the sample reported no suicide ideation. It was found that thwarted belongingness and perceived burdensomeness were positively associated with suicidal ideation.	Roush, Brown, Mitchell, & Cukrowicz (2017)
Dissertation that explored the phenomenon of erotic pain and how erotic pain was pathologized.	Hicks (2016)
Compared 17 masochistic participants and 17 controls to study if possible differences in pain perception and attitudes toward pain are context-related. Masochistic individuals had higher pain tolerance.	Defrin, Arad, Ben-Sasson, & Ginzburg (2015)
Analyzed four main explanations of pain in SM experiences. Pain was framed as a desirable, social, carnal, and emotional experience.	Newmahr (2010)
Recorded event-related potentials of female submissives who viewed various stimuli (including sexually sadistic stimuli) while being gagged or not gagged by a ball. It was found that the ball gag was related to late responses to others' suffering.	Luo & Zhang (2018)
Two studies involving 58 SM practitioners with physiological measures showed that after engaging in BDSM activity, it could enhance relationship closeness if SM activities went well but decrease relationship closeness if they went poorly.	Sagarin et al. (2009)
Diagnosis	
Diagnostic Concerns and DSM Criticisms	
An analysis of 1,020 Austrian male sexual offenders. It was found that sexual sadism was more in accordance with a dimensional interpretation rather than a categorical one.	Mokros, Schilling, Weiss, Nitschke, & Eher (2014)
Dimensional structure for sexual sadism may be more effective than a classificatory method of sadism.	Longpré, Guay, Knight, & Benbouriche (2018)
Discusses the concern of retaining paraphilias as mental disorders and suggests that the diagnosis should only be supported if there is empirical evidence.	Shindel & Moser (2011)

Summary	Reference
A literature review on the psychological well-being of members in the BDSM community and whether BDSM should be considered pathological.	Powls & Davies (2012)
Argues that consensual BDSM practices and fetishisms should not be pathologized.	Wright (2010)
Dissertation on the interdisciplinary overview of consensual BDSM practices and how BDSM is not a pathological sexual activity.	Rodemaker (2008)
Reviews the literature for sexual masochism from 1900 to 2008 and concludes that sexual masochism should be retained as a diagnosis.	Krueger (2010a)
Reviews the empirical literature for sexual sadism from 1900 to 2008 and concludes that sexual sadism should be retained as a diagnosis.	Krueger (2010b)
Discusses the DSM-5 criteria for sexual sadism and pedophilia.	Merrick (2016)
Low reliability for paraphilic diagnoses, especially sexual sadism.	Doren & Elwood (2009)
Severe sexual sadism is underdiagnosed. The authors found that two-thirds of sex offenders who were inpatients at high-security forensic institutions were not "identified" as sexual sadists.	Nitschke, Blendl, Ottermann, Osterheider, & Mokros (2009)
Argument that sexual sadism may be overdiagnosed in a proportion of those who are evaluated as sexual violent predators.	Frances & Wollert (2012)
Review of plethysmography studies shows that paraphilic coercive disorder can be discriminated from sadism, and it questions whether the DSM-5 should have coercive disorder as separate diagnosis.	Knight, Sims-Knight, & Guay (2013)
Discusses the difference between sexual sadism and paraphilia not otherwise specified, -non-consent. Sadistic acts are characterized by use of power and control to humiliate the victim.	Richards & Jackson (2011)
Diagnostic Variations	
Case study of a patient with autism and an amygdalohippocampal lesion who committed murder involving sadomasochistic behaviors.	Müller (2011)

Summary	Reference
Case of sadomasochism with borderline personality disorder.	Dulz (2009)
"Feederism" seen as a form of sexual masochism.	Terry & Vasey (2011)
Report on hypoxyphilia and its manifestation as an effect of sexual masochism.	Hucker (2011)
Sexual masochism was found to be more prevalent in 60 women with borderline personality disorder compared to 60 women with other personality disorders.	Frías, González, Palma, & Farriols (2017)
Phenomenological study involving 4 females and 5 males, focusing on masochism as an addictive process.	Kurt & Ronel (2017)
A review of sexual masochism disorder and asphyxiophilia.	Coluccia et al. (2016)
Case reports of 5 serial sexual murderers who engaged in autoerotic asphyxiation.	Myers et al. (2008)
The prevalence of personality disorders diagnosed in sexual murderers.	Koch, Berner, Hill, & Briken (2011)
Factitious disorder presenting as sexual sadism.	C. Fischer, Beckson, & Dietz (2017)
Assessment	
Scales	
Authors developed a 24-item checklist to assess sadomasochistic practices.	Weierstall & Giebel (2017)
Developed and validated the Attitudes about Sadomasochism Scale (ASMS). It was found that the ASMS was a reliable and valid measure for attitudes toward BDSM practices using 213 participants for exploratory analyses and 471 participants for validation analyses.	Yost (2010)
The Severe Sexual Sadism Scale is an observer rating of crime scene actions that is based on file information. The authors believe that its use can help diagnose sexual sadism if the patient is not willing to disclose violent sexual fantasies.	Nitschke, Mokros, Osterheider, & Marshall (2013)
Created an 11-item scale that identifies male forensic patients with sexual sadism.	Nitschke, Osterheider, & Mokros (2009)
Replication study on the one-dimensional scale structure of the Severe Sexual Sadism Scale using 105 Austrian sexual offenders.	Mokros, Schilling, Eher, & Nitschke (2012)

Summary	Reference
Phallometric	
Using phallometric testing on 128 sex offenders, it was found that sadistic offenders responded to the Oakridge and Barbaree stimulus set, whereas opportunistic offenders did not respond to either stimuli sets.	Looman, Dickie, & Maillet (2008)
Using phallometric testing, it was found that sexual sadists responded significantly to violence and injury compared to those who were non-sadists and those with sadistic interests.	Seto, Lalumière, Harris, & Chivers (2012)
A longitudinal study of 586 male sex offenders assessed between 1982 and 1992 found that sexual arousal to violence (via phallometric testing) was significantly associated with sexually violent recidivism.	Kingston, Seto, Firestone, & Bradford (2010)
Functional Magnetic Resonance Imaging	
Using functional magnetic resonance imaging, it was found that sadists ($n = 8$) showed more amygdala activation when viewing pain stimuli and rated pain pictures as higher on pain severity compared to non-sadists ($n = 7$). Sadists also showed activity in the anterior insula that was positively correlated with pain severity ratings.	Harenski, Thornton, Harenski, Decety, & Kiehl (2012)
Implicit Association Tests	
Three indirect measures (Implicit Association Test, Semantic Misattribution Procedure, and Viewing Time) were combined on an online platform to create an assessment battery for violent sexual interests. It was found that men responded to non-consensual sadistic sexual interest, whereas women responded to masochistic sexual interest.	Larue et al. (2014)
In 81 sex offenders and 48 male college students, it was found that sadistic offenders ($n = 19$) did not show any significant differences from non-sadists ($n = 62$) on the Sex and Aggression version of the Implicit Association Test, but sex offenders did score higher on this test compared to the students.	Reed (2015)
Behavioral and Crime Scene Indicators	
Found that professionals are able to reliably rate behaviors as sadistic or non-sadistic.	McLawsen, Jackson, Vannoy, Gagliardi, & Scalora (2008)

Summary	Reference
Using crime scene behaviors and criminal profiling, it was found that murders with a sexual motivation had elements that differed from murders that did not have sexual motives but which happened to occur in a sexual context.	Stefanska, Higgs, Carter, & Beech (2017)
In a meta-analysis and outcome study, it was found that a behavioral measure of sadism, rather than a clinical diagnosis, was associated with violent reoffending. However, the authors noted that at an individual level, it would be better to use a custom risk assessment instrument for violent sadists.	Eher et al. (2016)
Found four typologies of sexual homicide offenders using 342 males who were convicted for a violent sexual offense.	Healey, Beauregard, Beech, & Vettor (2016)
Based on a sample of 268 Canadian adult male offenders, crime scene indicators of sexual sadism could be differentiated from sexual homicide.	Healey, Lussier, & Beauregard (2013)
Associations	
Explored the use of the MMPI-2 and its associations with sadomasochistic behaviors. High-risk S&M behaviors in men were associated with antisocial behavior, psychoticism, and fearfulness. For women, high-risk S&M behaviors were associated with self-deprecation, discontent, competitiveness, anger, antisocial behaviors, and aberrant experiences.	Hopkins et al. (2016)
In 80 self-identified "dominants" and 190 self-identified "submissives," it was found that dominants scored significantly higher on desire for control, extraversion, self-esteem, and life satisfaction. "Submissives" scored higher for emotionality.	Hébert & Weaver (2014)
In 225 federal sex offenders from the Midwestern United States, it was found that sexual sadism was strongly associated with criminal behaviors (nonsexual) and was associated with sexual deviance and sexual violence. The authors noted that sexual sadism could be used as a risk factor when assessing recidivism.	DeLisi et al. (2017)

Summary	Reference
Using the Structured Risk Assessment: Forensic Version Light on 44 adult male sex offenders, it was found that those who responded to the sadomasochism scales on the AASI-2 were likely to have poor anger management, lack emotional intimacy, and have sexual preoccupation.	Trapold (2013)
Treatment	
Couples	
Case study of a couple in "kink-focused" and consensual nonmonogamy-focused therapy.	Sprott, Randall, Davison, Cannon, & Witherspoon (2017)
Suggests that couples could be misdiagnosed as sadomasochistic when they actually have a paranoid–masochistic dynamic. The author concludes that this misdiagnosis could be why some couples may be more difficult to treat.	Mendelsohn (2014)
Therapists' Experiences	
Examined the way in which dominatrices speak about BDSM and how dominatrices view themselves as "therapists" for their clients.	Lindemann (2011)
Semistructured interviews with 14 therapists who worked with BDSM clients. It was found that therapists who also engaged in BDSM usually had boundary issues with clients.	Lawrence & Love-Crowell (2008)
Dissertation on how a therapist's values may affect therapy with clients who practice consensual BDSM.	Garrott (2009)
Sadomasochism Case Study	
Case study on using self-psychology to treat individuals with narcissism, hypochondria, sex addiction, and sadomasochism.	Giugliano (2011)
Sadism	
Discusses a clinical view of sexual sadism and its relation to sexual homicide.	Briken, Bourget, Dufour (2014)
Masochism Case Studies	
Case study for treating a person with masochism, where self-regulation beliefs are targeted.	Novick & Novick (2012)

Summary	Reference
Use of cognitive–behavioral and dialectical–behavioral techniques to reduce self-mutilation in a case of a non-psychotic person with chronic depression, hypersexuality, and sexual masochism.	King (2014)
Case study of a 35-year-old Iranian man who had sexual masochism and comorbid disorders treated with cognitive–behavioral therapy (CBT) and education about "self-regulation" skills.	Khodayarifard, Pritz, Alavi, & Abedini (2013)
Case review of 3 women with sexual masochism who were sexually abused by a parent and who were treated with rational–emotive therapy and CBT.	Abrams & Stefan (2012)
Books and Book Chapters	
Apostolides, M. (2008). The pleasure of pain. In E. Goode & D. A. Vail (Eds.), *Extreme deviance* (pp. 207–212). Thousand Oaks, CA: Pine Forge Press.	
Barker, M., Iantaffi, A., & Gupta, C. (2008). Kinky clients, kinky counselling? The challenges and potentials of BDSM. In L. Moon (Ed.), *Feeling queer or queer feelings? Radical approaches to counselling sex, sexualities and genders* (pp. 106–124). New York, NY: Routledge.	
Berlin, M., & Monroe, D. (2010). Ruminations of a domiatrix: An interview with Mz. Berlin. In D. Monroe (Ed.), *Porn: How to think with kink* (pp. 247–256). Malden, MA: Wiley-Blackwell.	
Bradford, J. M. W., Fedoroff, P., & Firestone, P. (2008). Sexual violence and the clinician. In R. I. Simon & K. Tardiff (Eds.), *Textbook of violence assessment and management* (pp. 441–460). Arlington, VA: American Psychiatric Publishing.	
Hamilton, D. V., & Rosen, J. (2016). Sexual sadism disorder. In R. Balon (Ed.), *Practical guide to paraphilia and paraphilic disorders* (pp. 123–139). Cham, Switzerland: Springer.	
Hinman, M. (2013). Understanding clients with alternative expressions of sexuality using music. In S. Loue (Ed.), *Expressive therapies for sexual issues: A social work perspective* (pp. 137–155). New York, NY: Springer.	
Hucker, S. J. (2008). Sexual masochism: Assessment and treatment. In D. R. Laws & W. T. O'Donohue (Eds.), *Sexual deviance: Theory, assessment, and treatment* (2nd ed., pp. 264–271). New York, NY: Guilford.	
Hucker, S. J. (2008). Sexual masochism: Psychopathology and theory. In D. R. Laws & W. T. O'Donohue (Eds.), *Sexual deviance: Theory, assessment, and treatment* (2nd ed., pp. 250–263). New York, NY: Guilford.	

Hucker, S. J. (2008). Sexual sadism: Assessment and treatment. In D. R. Laws & W. T. O'Donohue (Eds.), *Sexual deviance: Theory, assessment, and treatment* (2nd ed., pp. 231–249). New York, NY: Guilford.

Hucker, S. J. (2009). Manifestations of sexual sadism: Sexual homicide, sadistic rape, and necrophilia. In F. M. Saleh, A. J. Grudzinskas, Jr., J. M. Bradford, & D. J. Brodsky (Eds.), *Sex offenders: Identification, risk assessment, treatment, and legal issues* (pp. 340–352). New York, NY: Oxford University Press.

"Jackie." (2008). The S&M experience. In E. Goode & D. A. Vail (Eds.), *Extreme deviance* (pp. 220–225). Thousand Oaks, CA: Pine Forge Press.

Leiser, R. (2018). Surprisingly straight: The pervasiveness of heteronormativity within BDSM and kink communities. In C. Stewart (Ed.), *Lesbian, gay, bisexual, and transgender Americans at risk: Problems and solutions—Adults, Generation X, and Generation Y* (Vol. 2, pp. 135–144). Santa Barbara, CA: Praeger/ABC-CLIO.

Lykins, A., & Hucker, S. J. (2014). Treatment of sexual masochism. In W. T. O'Donohue (Ed.), *Case studies in sexual deviance: Toward evidence-based practice* (pp. 102–116). New York, NY: Routledge.

Marshall, W. L., Hucker, S. J., Nitschke, J., & Mokros, A. (2017). Assessment of sexual sadism. In D. P. Boer, A. R. Beech, T. Ward, L. A. Craig, M. Rettenberger, L. E. Marshall, & W. L. Marshall (Eds.), *The Wiley handbook on the theories, assessment, and treatment of sexual offending* (Vols. 1–3, pp. 849–862). Malden, MA: Wiley-Blackwell.

McGrath, M., & Turvey, B. E. (2008). Sexual asphyxia. In B. E. Turvey (Ed.), *Criminal profiling: An introduction to behavioral evidence analysis* (3rd ed., pp. 605–628). San Diego, CA: Elsevier.

McLawsen, J., Jackson, R. L., & Vannoy, S. D. (2012). Perspectives on sexual sadism—The role of diagnostic experience. In J. McLawsen, R. L. Jackson, & S. D. Vannoy (Eds.), *The sex offender: Current trends in policy and treatment practice* (Vol. 7, pp. 1–20). Kingston, NJ: Civic Research Institute.

Myers, W. C., Bukhanovskiy, A., Justen, E., Morton, R. J., Tilley, J., Adams, K., . . . Hazelwood, R. R. (2008). The relationship between serial sexual murder and autoerotic asphyxiation. *Forensic Science International, 176*(2–3), 187–195.

Shipley, S. L., & Arrigo, B. A. (2015). Sexual homicide: A clinical and investigative analysis. In S. L. Shipley & B. A. Arrigo (Eds.), *The Routledge international handbook of biosocial criminology* (pp. 530–543). New York, NY: Routledge.

Wurmser, L. (2013). Trauma, archaic superego, and sadomasochism: Discussion of the case of Mariah. In H. I. Basseches, P. L. Ellman, & N. R. Goodman (Eds.), *Battling the life and death forces of sadomasochism: Clinical perspectives* (pp. 213–226). London, UK: Karnac Books.

Wylie, R. A., & Wylie, K. R. (2016). Sexual masochism disorder. In R. Balon (Ed.), *Practical guide to paraphilia and paraphilic disorders* (pp. 107–122). Cham, Switzerland: Springer.
Yates, P. M., Hucker, S .J., & Kingston, D. A. (2008). Sexual sadism: Psychopathology and theory. In R. D. Laws & W. T. O'Donohue (Eds.), *Sexual deviance: Theory, assessment, and treatment* (2nd ed., pp. 213–230). New York, NY: Guilford.

References

Abrams, M., & Stefan, S. (2012). Sexual abuse and masochism in women: Etiology and treatment. *Journal of Evidence-Based Psychotherapies, 12*(2), 231–239.

Ahmed, A. G. (2014). Dysfunctional anger and sexual violence. *Psychiatric Clinics of North America, 37*(2), 231–238.

Airaksinen, T. (2017). A philosophical and rhetorical theory of BDSM. *Journal of Mind and Behavior, 38*(1), 53–74.

Ambler, J. K., Lee, M. K., Klement, K. R., Loewald, T., Comber, E. M., Hanson, S. A., . . . Sagarin, B. J. (2017). Consensual BDSM facilitates role-specific altered states of consciousness: A preliminary study. *Psychology of Consciousness: Theory, Research, and Practice, 4*(1), 75–91.

American Psychiatric Association. (2013). *Diagnostic and statistical manual of mental disorders* (5th ed.). Arlington, VA: American Psychiatric Publishing.

Apostolides, M. (2008). The pleasure of pain. In E. Goode & D. A. Vail (Eds.), *Extreme deviance* (pp. 207–212). Thousand Oaks, CA: Pine Forge Press.

Aschenbrenner, J. (1994). Till Eulenspiegel The Medieval Jester, The Lighter and Darker Side of Humor: Mettlach Stein Number 2582, and Mettlach Steins Number 2035 and 2057.

Barker, M., Iantaffi, A., & Gupta, C. (2008). Kinky clients, kinky counselling? The challenges and potentials of BDSM. In L. Moon (Ed.), *Feeling queer or queer feelings? Radical approaches to counselling sex, sexualities and genders* (pp. 106–124). New York, NY: Routledge.

Basseches, H., & Sinkman, E. (Reporter). (2010). Battling the life and death forces of sadomasochism. *The International Journal of Psychoanalysis, 91*(4), 969–972. doi:10.1111/j.1745-8315.2010.00313.x

Battle, A. S. (2014). *Identifying personality differences between sadistic and non-sadistic sex offenders.* Doctoral dissertation, Alliant International University, California School of Forensic Studies, Irvine, CA (ProQuest Dissertations, Accession No. 3555198).

Baur, E., Forsman, M., Santtila, P., Johansson, A., Sandnabba, K., & Långström, N. (2016). Paraphilic sexual interests and sexually coercive behavior: A population-based twin study. *Archives of Sexual Behavior, 45*(5), 1163–1172.

Berlin, M., & Monroe, D. (2010). Ruminations of a domiatrix: An interview with Mz. Berlin. In D. Monroe (Ed.), *Porn: How to think with kink* (pp. 247–256). Malden, MA: Wiley-Blackwell.

Bezreh, T., Weinberg, T. S., & Edgar, T. (2012). BDSM disclosure and stigma management: Identifying opportunities for sex education. *American Journal of Sexuality Education, 7*(1), 37–61.

Bradford, J. M. W., Fedoroff, P., & Firestone, P. (2008). Sexual violence and the clinician. In R. I. Simon & K. Tardiff (Eds.), *Textbook of violence assessment and management* (pp. 441–460). Arlington, VA: American Psychiatric Publishing.

Briken, P., Bourget, D., & Dufour, M. (2014). Sexual sadism in sexual offenders and sexually motivated homicide. *Psychiatric Clinics, 37*(2), 215–230.

Brown, S. L., Roush, J. F., Mitchell, S. M., & Cukrowicz, K. C. (2017). Suicide risk among BDSM practitioners: The role of acquired capability for suicide. *Journal of Clinical Psychology, 73*(12), 1642–1654.

Carlström, C. (2017). Gender equal BDSM practice—A Swedish paradox? *Psychology & Sexuality, 8*(4), 268–279.

Chan, H. C., & Beauregard, E. (2016). Non-homicidal and homicidal sexual offenders: Prevalence of maladaptive personality traits and paraphilic behaviors. *Journal of Interpersonal Violence, 31*(13), 2259–2290.

Chan, H. C., Beauregard, E., & Myers, W. C. (2015). Single-victim and serial sexual homicide offenders: Differences in crime, paraphilias and personality traits. *Criminal Behaviour and Mental Health, 25*(1), 66–78.

Chapman-Haddock, C. (2012). *Consensual sexual sadomasochists and sexual offenders: An analysis of influential characteristics*. Doctoral dissertation, Alliant International University, California School of Forensic Studies, Irvine, CA (ProQuest Dissertations, Accession No. 3519208).

Chivers, M. L., Roy, C., Grimbos, T., Cantor, J. M., & Seto, M. C. (2014). Specificity of sexual arousal for sexual activities in men and women with conventional and masochistic sexual interests. *Archives of Sexual Behavior, 43*(5), 931–940.

Coluccia, A., Gabbrielli, M., Gualtieri, G., Ferretti, F., Pozza, A., & Fagiolini, A. (2016). Sexual masochism disorder with asphyxiophilia: A deadly yet underrecognized disease. *Case Reports in Psychiatry, 2016*, 5474862.

Defrin, R., Arad, M., Ben-Sasson, M. P., & Ginzburg, K. (2015). Attitudes and emotions towards pain and sensitivity to painful stimuli among people routinely engaging in masochistic behaviour. *European Journal of Pain, 19*(9), 1321–1330.

Dehnavifar, F. (2013). *A correlational study of sadomasochistic tendencies found on the Abel Assessment for Sexual Interest-2 (AASI-2) and scores on the Minnesota Multiphasic Personality Inventory-2 (MMPI-2)*. Doctoral dissertation, Alliant International University, California School of Forensic Studies, Irvine, CA (ProQuest Dissertations, Accession No. 3507227).

DeLisi, M., Drury, A., Elbert, M., Tahja, K., Caropreso, D., & Heinrichs, T. (2017). Sexual sadism and criminal versatility: Does sexual sadism spillover into nonsexual crimes? *Journal of Aggression, Conflict and Peace Research, 9*(1), 2–12.

Domue, N. (2015). *Attitudes of graduate psychology students towards consensual sadomasochism*. Doctoral dissertation, Chicago School of Professional Psychology, Chicago, IL (ProQuest Dissertations, Accession No. 3645225).

Doren, D., & Elwood, R. (2009). The diagnostic reliability of sexual sadism. *Sexual Abuse, 21*(3), 251–261.

Dulz, B. (2009). Extreme sadomasochistic sexuality [in German]. *PTT: Personlichkeitsstroungen Theorie und Therapie, 13*(4), 258–268.

Eher, R., Schilling, F., Hansmann, B., Pumberger, T., Nitschke, J., Habermeyer, E., & Mokros, A. (2016). Sadism and violent reoffending in sexual offenders. *Sexual Abuse, 28*(1), 46–72.

Fedoroff, J. P. (2008). Sadism, sadomasochism, sex, and violence. *Canadian Journal of Psychiatry, 53*(10), 637–646.

Fischer, C. A., Beckson, M., & Dietz, P. (2017). Factitious disorder in a patient claiming to be a sexually sadistic serial killer. *Journal of Forensic Sciences, 62*(3), 822–826.

Fischer, E. G. J. (2008). *Profiling sexually violent predators: A study to identify psychopathy and sexual sadism as baseline psychopathologies in predatory sexual serial offenders*. Doctoral dissertation, Capella University, Minneapolis, MN (ProQuest Dissertations, Accession No. 3296784).

Flegr, J. (2017). Does *Toxoplasma* infection increase sexual masochism and submissiveness? Yes and no. *Communicative & Integrative Biology, 10*(5–6), e1303590.

Frances, A., & Wollert, R. (2012). Sexual sadism: Avoiding its misuse in sexually violent predator evaluations. *Journal of the American Academy of Psychiatry and the Law Online, 40*(3), 409–416.

Frías, Á., González, L., Palma, C., & Farriols, N. (2017). Is there a relationship between borderline personality disorder and sexual masochism in Women? *Archives of Sexual Behavior, 46*(3), 747–754.

Garrott, R. (2009). *The effects of psychotherapists' values on their work with clients who practice consensual sexual sadomasochism*. (Accession No. 3322250).

Giugliano, J. R. (2011). Self-psychological treatment of a sex addict with sadomasochistic behaviours: A case report. *British Journal of Psychotherapy, 27*(4), 352–367.

Graham, B. C., Butler, S. E., McGraw, R., Cannes, S. M., & Smith, J. (2016). Member perspectives on the role of BDSM communities. *Journal of Sex Research, 53*(8), 895–909.

Hall, D. A. (2014). The fate of aggression in maso-masochistic relationships. *Psychoanalytic Quarterly, 83*(2), 345–373.

Hamilton, D. V., & Rosen, J. (2016). Sexual sadism disorder. In R. Balon (Ed.), *Practical guide to paraphilia and paraphilic disorders* (pp. 123–139). Cham, Switzerland: Springer.

Harenski, C. L., Thornton, D. M., Harenski, K. A., Decety, J., & Kiehl, K. A. (2012). Increased frontotemporal activation during pain observation in sexual sadism: Preliminary findings. *Archives of General Psychiatry, 69*(3), 283–292.

Healey, J., & Beauregard, E. (2015). The impact of persistent deviant sexual interests and persistent low self-esteem on sexual homicide. *Criminal Justice and Behavior, 42*(12), 1225–1242.

Healey, J., Beauregard, E., Beech, A., & Vettor, S. (2016). Is the sexual murderer a unique type of offender? A typology of violent sexual offenders using crime scene behaviors. *Sexual Abuse, 28*(6), 512–533.

Healey, J., Lussier, P., & Beauregard, E. (2013). Sexual sadism in the context of rape and sexual homicide: An examination of crime scene indicators. *International Journal of Offender Therapy and Comparative Criminology, 57*(4), 402–424.

Hébert, A., & Weaver, A. (2014). An examination of personality characteristics associated with BDSM orientations. *Canadian Journal of Human Sexuality, 23*(2), 106–115.

Hébert, A., & Weaver, A. (2015). Perks, problems, and the people who play: A qualitative exploration of dominant and submissive BDSM roles. *Canadian Journal of Human Sexuality, 24*(1), 49–62.

Hicks, V. (2016). *The eroticization of pain: A critical metabletic*. Doctoral dissertation, Chicago School of Professional Psychology, Chicago, IL (ProQuest Dissertations, Accession No. 3739928).

Hinman, M. (2013). Understanding clients with alternative expressions of sexuality using music. In S. Loue (Ed.), *Expressive therapies for sexual issues: A social work perspective* (pp. 137–155). New York, NY: Springer.

Holmes, D., Murray, S. J., Knack, N., Mecier, M., & Fedoroff, P. (2017a). BDSM, sexual subcultures, and the ethics of public health discourse. In D. Holmes, S. Murray, & T. Foth (Eds.), *Radical sex between men* (pp. 93–116). London, UK: Routledge.

Holmes, D., Murray, S. J., Knack, N., Mecier, M., & Fedoroff, P. (2017b). Degenitalizing the sexual: BDSM practices and the deteritorialization of bodies and pleasures. In D. Holmes, S. Murray, & T. Foth (Eds.), *Radical sex between men* (pp. 117–141). London, UK: Routledge.

Holt, K. (2016a). *Negotiating limits: Boundary management in the bondage/discipline/sadomasochism (BDSM) community*. Doctoral dissertation, City University of New York, New York, NY (ProQuest Dissertations, Accession No. 3703396).

Holt, K. (2016b). Blacklisted: Boundaries, violations, and retaliatory behavior in the BDSM community. *Deviant Behavior, 37*(8), 917–930.

Holvoet, L., Huys, W., Coppens, V., Seeuws, J., Goethals, K., & Morrens, M. (2017). Fifty shades of Belgian gray: The prevalence of BDSM-related fantasies and activities in the general population. *Journal of Sexual Medicine, 14*(9), 1152–1159.

Hopkins, T. A., Brawner, C. A., Meyer, M., Zawilinski, L., Carnes, P. J., & Green, B. A. (2016). MMPI-2 correlates of sadomasochism in a sexual addiction sample: Contrasting men and women. *Sexual Addiction & Compulsivity, 23*(1), 114–140.

Houngbedji, A., & Guillem, E. (2016). Profiles and sexual practices of current and past swingers interviewed on French websites. *Sexologies, 25*(1), e1–e4.

Hucker, S., Langevin, R., Dickey, R., Handy, L., Chambers, J., Wright, S., . . . Wortzman, G. (1988). Cerebral damage and dysfunction in sexually aggressive men. *Sex Abuse*, 1, 33–47.

Hucker, S. J. (2008a). Sexual sadism: Assessment and treatment. In D. R. Laws & W. T. O'Donohue (Eds.), *Sexual deviance: Theory, assessment, and treatment* (2nd ed., pp. 231–249). New York, NY: Guilford.

Hucker, S. J. (2008b). Sexual masochism: Psychopathology and theory. In D. R. Laws & W. T. O'Donohue (Eds.), *Sexual deviance: Theory, assessment, and treatment* (2nd ed., pp. 250–263). New York, NY: Guilford.

Hucker, S. J. (2008c). Sexual masochism: Assessment and treatment. In D. R. Laws & W. T. O'Donohue (Eds.), *Sexual deviance: Theory, assessment, and treatment* (2nd ed., pp. 264–271). New York, NY: Guilford.

Hucker, S. J. (2009). Manifestations of sexual sadism: Sexual homicide, sadistic rape, and necrophilia. In F. M. Saleh, A. J. Grudzinskas, Jr., J. M. Bradford, & D. J. Brodsky (Eds.), *Sex offenders: Identification, risk assessment, treatment, and legal issues* (pp. 340–352). New York, NY: Oxford University Press.

Hucker, S. J. (2011). Hypoxyphilia. *Archives of Sexual Behavior, 40*(6), 1323–1326.

Iannotti, L. (2015). *I didn't consent to that: A secondary analysis of discrimination against BDSM-identified individuals.* Doctoral dissertation, City University of New York, New York, NY (ProQuest Dissertations, Accession No. 3623553).

"Jackie." (2008). The S&M experience. In E. Goode & D. A. Vail (Eds.), *Extreme deviance* (pp. 220–225). Thousand Oaks, CA: Pine Forge Press.

Jacques, T. (1993). *On the safe edge: A manual for SM play*. Toronto, Ontario, Canada: WholeSM Publishing.

James, J., & Proulx, J. (2016). The modus operandi of serial and nonserial sexual murderers: A systematic review. *Aggression and Violent Behavior, 31*, 200–218.

Jones, S., Chan, H. C. O., Myers, W. C., & Heide, K. M. (2013). A proposed sexual homicide category: The psychopathic–sexually sadistic offender. *Criminal Psychology, 2*, 403–422.

Jozifkova, E. (2013). Consensual sadomasochistic sex (BDSM): The roots, the risks, and the distinctions between BDSM and violence. *Current Psychiatry Reports, 15*(9), 392.

Juni, S. (2009). The role of sexuality in sadism: Object relations and drive theory perspectives. *American Journal of Psychoanalysis, 69*(4), 314–329.

Khodayarifard, M., Pritz, A., Alavi, S. M., & Abedini, Y. (2013). A case study of cognitive–behavior therapy in Iran: Treatment of sexual masochism along with co-morbid disorders in a collectivist society. *International Journal of Psychotherapy, 17*(1), 53–63.

Kimberly, C., Williams, A. L., & Creel, S. (2018). Women's introduction to alternative sexual behaviors through erotica and its association with sexual and relationship satisfaction. *Sex Roles, 78*(1–2), 119–129.

King, P. R. (2014). Cognitive–behavioral intervention in a case of self-mutilation. *Clinical Case Studies, 13*(2), 181–189.

Kingston, D. A., Seto, M. C., Firestone, P., & Bradford, J. M. (2010). Comparing indicators of sexual sadism as predictors of recidivism among adult male sexual offenders. *Journal of Consulting and Clinical Psychology, 78*(4), 574–584.

Knight, R. A., Sims-Knight, J., & Guay, J. P. (2013). Is a separate diagnostic category defensible for paraphilic coercion? *Journal of Criminal Justice, 41*(2), 90–99.

Koch, J., Berner, W., Hill, A., & Briken, P. (2011). Sociodemographic and diagnostic characteristics of homicidal and nonhomicidal sexual offenders. *Journal of Forensic Sciences, 56*(6), 1626–1631.

Krafft-Ebing, R. von. (1999). *Psychopathia sexualis*. Bloat Books. Burbank, Calif. ISBN 0-9650324-1-8 (Original work published 1886)

Krueger, R. B. (2010a). The DSM diagnostic criteria for sexual masochism. *Archives of Sexual Behavior, 39*(2), 346–356.

Krueger, R. B. (2010b). The DSM diagnostic criteria for sexual sadism. *Archives of Sexual Behavior, 39*(2), 325–345.

Kurt, H., & Ronel, N. (2017). Addicted to pain: A preliminary model of sexual masochism as addiction. *International Journal of Offender Therapy and Comparative Criminology, 61*(15), 1760–1774.

Lammers, J., & Imhoff, R. (2016). Power and sadomasochism: Understanding the antecedents of a knotty relationship. *Social Psychological and Personality Science, 7*(2), 142–148.

Langevin, R., Ben-Aron, M. H., Wright, P., Marchese, V., & Handy, L. (1988). The sex killer. *Sex Abuse, 1*, 263–301.

Larue, D., Schmidt, A. F., Imhoff, R., Eggers, K., Schönbrodt, F. D., & Banse, R. (2014). Validation of direct and indirect measures of preference for sexualized violence. *Psychological Assessment, 26*(4), 1173–1183.

Lawrence, A. A., & Love-Crowell, J. (2007). Psychotherapists' experience with clients who engage in consensual sadomasochism: A qualitative study. *Journal of Sex & Marital Therapy, 34*(1), 67–85.

Leiser, R. (2018). Surprisingly straight: The pervasiveness of heteronormativity within BDSM and kink communities. In C. Stewart (Ed.), *Lesbian, gay, bisexual, and transgender Americans at risk: Problems and solutions—Adults, Generation X, and Generation Y* (Vol. 2, pp. 135–144). Santa Barbara, CA: Praeger/ABC-CLIO.

Lewandowski, E. (2011). *The complete costume dictionary*. Lanham, MD: Scarecrow Press.

Lindemann, D. (2011). BDSM as therapy? *Sexualities, 14*(2), 151–172. https://doi.org/10.1177/1363460711399038

Longpré, N., Guay, J. P., Knight, R. A., & Benbouriche, M. (2018). Sadistic offender or sexual sadism? Taxometric evidence for a dimensional structure of sexual sadism. *Archives of Sexual Behavior, 47*(2), 403–416.

Looman, J., Dickie, I., & Maillet, G. (2008). Sexual arousal among rapist subtypes. *Journal of Sexual Aggression, 14*(3), 267–279.

Luo, S., & Zhang, X. (2017). Empathy in female submissive BDSM practitioners. *Neuropsychologia, 116*(Part A), 44–51.

Luo, S., & Zhang, X. (2018). Embodiment and humiliation moderation of neural responses to others' suffering in female submissive BDSM practitioners. *Frontiers in Neuroscience, 12*, 463.

Lykins, A., & Hucker, S. J. (2014). Treatment of sexual masochism. In W. T. O'Donohue (Eds.), *Case studies in sexual deviance: Toward evidence-based practice* (pp. 102–116). New York, NY: Routledge.

Marshall, W. L., Hucker, S. J., Nitschke, J., & Mokros, A. (2017). Assessment of sexual sadism. In D. P. Boer, A. R. Beech, T. Ward, L. A. Craig, M. Rettenberger, L. E. Marshall, & W. L. Marshall (Eds.), *The Wiley handbook on the theories, assessment, and treatment of sexual offending* (Vols. 1–3, pp. 849–862). Malden, MA: Wiley-Blackwell.

Martin, R. J. (2012). *Powerful exchanges: Ritual and subjectivity in Berlin's BDSM scene*. Doctoral dissertation, Princeton University, Princeton, NJ (ProQuest Dissertations, Accession No. 3481620).

Martinez, K. (2012). *Bound in theory and practice: A mixed-methods exploration of consensual sadomasochism*. Doctoral dissertation (Accession No. 3468405).

Martinez, K. (2018). BDSM role fluidity: A mixed-methods approach to investigating switches within dominant/submissive binaries. *Journal of Homosexuality, 65*(10), 1299–1324.

McGrath, M., & Turvey, B. E. (2008). Sexual asphyxia. In B. E. Turvey (Ed.), *Criminal profiling: An introduction to behavioral evidence analysis* (3rd ed., pp. 605–628). San Diego, CA: Elsevier.

McLawsen, J. E., Jackson, R. L., & Vannoy, S.D. (2012). Perspectives on sexual sadism—The role of diagnostic experience. In J. McLawsen, R. L. Jackson, & S. D. Vannoy (Eds.), *The sex offender: Current trends in policy and treatment practice* (Vol. 7, pp. 1–20). Kingston, NJ: Civic Research Institute.

McLawsen, J. E., Jackson, R. L., Vannoy, S. D., Gagliardi, G. J., & Scalora, M. J. (2008). Professional perspectives on sexual sadism. *Sexual Abuse, 20*(3), 272–304.

Mendelsohn, R. (2014). Revisting the sadomasochistic marriage: the paranoid-masochistic relationship. *Psychoanalytic Review, 101*(5), 647–673. doi:10.1521/prev.2014.101.5.647

Merrick, W. A. (2016). Changes in DSM-5 diagnostic criteria for paraphilic disorders. *Archives of Sexual Behavior, 45*(8), 2173–2179.

Mokros, A., Osterheider, M., Hucker, S. J., & Nitschke, J. (2011). Psychopathy and sexual sadism. *Law and Human Behavior, 35*(3), 188–199.

Mokros, A., Schilling, F., Eher, R., & Nitschke, J. (2012). The Severe Sexual Sadism Scale: Cross-validation and scale properties. *Psychological Assessment, 24*(3), 764–769.

Mokros, A., Schilling, F., Weiss, K., Nitschke, J., & Eher, R. (2014). Sadism in sexual offenders: Evidence for dimensionality. *Psychological Assessment, 26*(1), 138–147.

Müller, J. L. (2011). Are sadomasochism and hypersexuality in autism linked to amygdalohippocampal lesion? *Journal of Sexual Medicine*, *8*(11), 3241–3249.

Myers, W. C., Bukhanovskiy, A., Justen, E., Morton, R. J., Tilley, J., Adams, K., . . . Hazelwood, R. R. (2008). The relationship between serial sexual murder and autoerotic asphyxiation. *Forensic Science International*, *176*(2–3), 187–195.

Myers, W. C., Chan, H. C., Vo, E. J., & Lazarou, E. (2010). Sexual sadism, psychopathy, and recidivism in juvenile sexual murderers. *Journal of Investigative Psychology and Offender Profiling*, *7*(1), 49–58.

Newmahr, S. (2010). Power struggles: Pain and authenticity in SM play. *Symbolic Interaction*, *33*(3), 389–411.

Nitschke, J., Blendl, V., Ottermann, B., Osterheider, M., & Mokros, A. (2009). Severe sexual sadism—An underdiagnosed disorder? Evidence from a sample of forensic inpatients. *Journal of Forensic Sciences*, *54*(3), 685–691.

Nitschke, J., Istrefi, S., Osterheider, M., & Mokros, A. (2012). Empathy in sexually sadistic offenders: An experimental comparison with non-sadistic sexual offenders. *International Journal of Law and Psychiatry*, *35*(3), 165–167.

Nitschke, J., Mokros, A., Osterheider, M., & Marshall, W. L. (2013). Sexual sadism: Current diagnostic vagueness and the benefit of behavioral definitions. *International Journal of Offender Therapy and Comparative Criminology*, *57*(12), 1441–1453.

Nitschke, J., Osterheider, M., & Mokros, A. (2009). A cumulative scale of severe sexual sadism. *Sexual Abuse*, *21*(3), 262–278.

Novick, K. K., & Novick, N. J. (2012). Some suggestions for engaging with the clinical problem of masochism. In D. Holtzman & K. Nancy (Eds.), *The clinical problem of masochism* (pp. 51–75). Northvale, NJ: Aronson.

Olson, I. (2017). Abduction in the public sphere: Sadomasochism, surveillance, and counterpublics. *Sexuality & Culture: An Interdisciplinary Quarterly*, *21*(3), 795–812.

Palermo, G. B. (2013). The various faces of sadism. *International Journal of Offender Therapy and Comparative Criminology*, *57*(4), 399–401.

Pflugradt, D., & Allen, B. (2012). A grounded theory analysis of sexual sadism in females. *Journal of Sexual Aggression*, *18*(3), 325–337.

Pitagora, D. (2016a). Intimate partner violence in sadomasochistic relationships. *Sexual and Relationship Therapy*, *31*(1), 95–108.

Pitagora, D. (2016b). The kink-poly confluence: Relationship intersectionality in marginalized communities. *Sexual and Relationship Therapy*, *31*(3), 391–405.

Powls, J., & Davies, J. (2012). A descriptive review of research relating to sadomasochism: Considerations for clinical practice. *Deviant Behavior*, *33*(3), 223–234.

Reed, R. A. (2015). *The validity of the sex and aggression version of the implicit association test as a measure of sexual sadism*. Doctoral dissertation, Fairleigh Dickinson University, Hackensack, NJ (ProQuest Dissertations, Accession No. 3580185).

Reiersøl, O., & Skeid, S. (2006). The ICD diagnoses of fetishism and sadomasochism. *Journal of Homosexuality*, *50*, 243–262.

Ressler, R. K., Burgess, A. W., & Douglas, J. E. (1988). *Sexual homicide: patterns and motives*. Lexington, MA: Lexington Books.

Richards, H., & Jackson, R. L. (2011). Behavioral discriminators of sexual sadism and paraphilia nonconsent in a sample of civilly committed sexual offenders. *International Journal of Offender Therapy and Comparative Criminology*, *55*(2), 207–227.

Richters, J., De Visser, R. O., Rissel, C. E., Grulich, A. E., & Smith, A. M. (2008). Demographic and psychosocial features of participants in bondage and discipline, "sadomasochism" or dominance and submission (BDSM): Data from a national survey. *Journal of Sexual Medicine*, *5*(7), 1660–1668.

Robertson, C. A. (2018). *Psychopathic and sexually sadistic cognitions, traits, and behaviors: Relations with biomarkers and stress responses*. Doctoral dissertation, Brandeis University, Waltham, MA (ProQuest Dissertations, Accession No. 10240709).

Robertson, C. A., & Knight, R. A. (2014). Relating sexual sadism and psychopathy to one another, non-sexual violence, and sexual crime behaviors. *Aggressive Behavior*, *40*(1), 12–23.

Rodemaker, D. (2008). *Altsex: The clinician's guide to BDSM*. Doctoral dissertation, Chicago School of Professional Psychology, Chicago, IL (ProQuest Dissertations, Accession No. 3436690).

Roush, J. F., Brown, S. L., Mitchell, S. M., & Cukrowicz, K. C. (2017). Shame, guilt, and suicide ideation among bondage and discipline, dominance and submission, and sadomasochism practitioners: Examining the role of the interpersonal theory of suicide. *Suicide and Life-Threatening Behavior, 47*(2), 129–141.

Sacher-Masoch, Leopold, Ritter von. (1932). *The Rahnghild edition of Venus in furs*. New York, NY: Faro.

Sacher-Masoch, W. (1990). *The confessions of Wanda Von Sacher-Masoch*. San Francisco, CA: Re/Search. (Original work published 1906)

Sagarin, B. J., Cutler, B., Cutler, N., Lawler-Sagarin, K. A., & Matuszewich, L. (2009). Hormonal changes and couple bonding in consensual sadomasochistic activity. *Archives of Sexual Behavior, 38*(2), 186–200.

Seto, M. C., Lalumière, M. L., Harris, G. T., & Chivers, M. L. (2012). The sexual responses of sexual sadists. *Journal of Abnormal Psychology, 121*(3), 739–753.

Shindel, A. W., & Moser, C. A. (2011). Why are the paraphilias mental disorders? *Journal of Sexual Medicine, 8*(3), 927–929.

Shipley, S. L., & Arrigo, B. A. (2015). Sexual homicide: A clinical and investigative analysis. In S. L. Shipley & B. A. Arrigo (Eds.), *The Routledge international handbook of biosocial criminology* (pp. 530–543). New York, NY: Routledge.

Simula, B. L. (2012). Does bisexuality "undo" gender? Gender, sexuality, and bisexual behavior among BDSM participants. *Journal of Bisexuality, 12*(4), 484–506.

Sprott, R. A., Randall, A., Davison, K., Cannon, N., & Witherspoon, R. G. (2017). Alternative or Nontraditional Sexualities and Therapy: A Case Report. *Journal of Clinical Psychology, 73*, 929–937. doi:10.1002/jclp.22511

Stefanska, E. B., Higgs, T., Carter, A. J., & Beech, A. R. (2017). When is a murder a sexual murder? Understanding the sexual element in the classification of sexual killings. *Journal of Criminal Justice, 50*, 53–61.

Stein, D. (2002). *Safe, sane, consensual. The making of a shibboleth*. GMSMA

Stiles, B. L., & Clark, R. E. (2011). BDSM: A subcultural analysis of sacrifices and delights. *Deviant Behavior, 32*(2), 158–189.

Stone, M. H. (2010). Sexual sadism: A portrait of evil. *Journal of the American Academy of Psychoanalysis and Dynamic Psychiatry, 38*(1), 133–157.

Terry, L. L., & Vasey, P. L. (2011). Feederism in a woman. *Archives of Sexual Behavior, 40*(3), 639–645.

Tomassilli, J. C., Golub, S. A., Bimbi, D. S., & Parsons, J. T. (2009). Behind closed doors: An exploration of kinky sexual behaviors in urban lesbian and bisexual women. *Journal of Sex Research, 46*(5), 438–445.

Trapold, J. (2013). *Identifying sexually violent interests in various types of sex offenders using items on the Structured Risk Assessment: Forensic Version Light*. Doctoral dissertation, Alliant International University, California School of Forensic Studies, Irvine, CA (ProQuest Dissertations, Accession No. 3512754).

Turley, E. L. (2016). "Like nothing I've ever felt before": Understanding consensual BDSM as embodied experience. *Psychology & Sexuality, 7*(2), 149–162.

Weierstall, R., & Giebel, G. (2017). The sadomasochism checklist: A tool for the assessment of sadomasochistic behavior. *Archives of Sexual Behavior, 46*(3), 735–745.

Weinberg, J. (2016). *Regulating legal consent: Policing good and bad pain*. Northwestern University, Evanston, IL (ProQuest Dissertations, Accession No. 3705397).

Wilkinson, E. (2009). Perverting visual pleasure: Representing sadomasochism. *Sexualities, 12*(2), 181–198.

Williams, D. J. (2009). Deviant leisure: Rethinking "the good, the bad, and the ugly." *Leisure Sciences, 31*(2), 207–213.

Williams, D. J., Prior, E. E., Alvarado, T., Thomas, J. N., & Christensen, M. C. (2016). Is bondage and discipline, dominance and submission, and sadomasochism recreational leisure? A descriptive exploratory investigation. *Journal of Sexual Medicine, 13*(7), 1091–1094.

Wilson, D., & Brookes, M. (2011). Making sense of the sexual sadist between the wars: The case of Harold Jones. *Journal of Forensic Psychiatry & Psychology, 22*(4), 535–550.

Wilson, G. D. (2010). The sex fantasy questionnaire: An update. *Sexual and Relationship Therapy, 25*(1), 68–72.

Wismeijer, A. A., & Van Assen, M. A. (2013). Psychological characteristics of BDSM practitioners. *Journal of Sexual Medicine, 10*(8), 1943–1952.

World Health Organization. (2004). *International classification of diseases* (10th revision, 2nd ed.). Geneva, Switzerland: Author.

Wortis, J. (1954). *Fragments of an analysis with Freud* (Chapter 3). Oxford, UK: Simon & Schuster, p. 153.

Wright, S. (2010). Depathologizing consensual sexual sadism, sexual masochism, transvestic fetishism, and fetishism. *Archives of Sexual Behavior, 39*(6), 1229–1230.

Wurmser, L. (2013). Trauma, archaic superego, and sadomasochism: Discussion of the case of Mariah. In H. I. Basseches, P. L. Ellman, & N. R. Goodman (Eds.), *Battling the life and death forces of sadomasochism: Clinical perspectives* (pp. 213–226). London, UK: Karnac.

Wylie, R. A., & Wylie, K. R. (2016). Sexual masochism disorder. In R. Balon (Ed.), *Practical guide to paraphilia and paraphilic disorders* (pp. 107–122). Cham, Switzerland: Springer.

Yang, D. O., & Youn, G. (2012). Effects of exposure to pornography on male aggressive behavioral tendencies. *The Open Psychology Journal, 5*(1), 1–10.

Yates, P. M., Hucker, S. J., & Kingston, D. A. (2008). Sexual sadism: Psychopathology and theory. In R. D. Laws & W. T. O'Donohue (Eds.), *Sexual deviance: Theory, assessment, and treatment* (2nd ed., pp. 213–230). New York, NY: Guilford.

Yost, M. R. (2010). Development and validation of the Attitudes About Sadomasochism Scale. *Journal of Sex Research, 47*(1), 79–91.

8

Transvestic Disorder

You can tell a lot about a person by who his or her heroes are.

—Steve Jobs (2004)

Introduction

The Fifth edition of the *Diagnostic and Statistical Manual of Mental Disorders* (DSM-5; American Psychiatric Association [APA], 2013) defines *transvestic disorder* as a condition in which there is persistent (at least 6 months), recurrent, and intense sexual arousal from wearing clothes associated with the opposite gender as evidenced by fantasies, urges, or behaviors. The category B criteria mandate that to be a disorder, the condition must cause clinically significant distress or impairment in social, occupational, or other important areas of functioning.

The DSM-5 includes two specifiers: "with fetishism" if the person is aroused by fabrics, materials, or garments; and "with autogynephilia" if the person is aroused by thoughts or images of being a female. As with most other DSM-5 paraphilias, two other specifiers are available: "in a controlled environment" is intended to be used in situations in which the person does not meet the criteria due to being in an environment in which cross-dressing is not permitted, and "in full remission" is used for people who have had no distress or impairment in social, occupational, or other areas of functioning for at least 5 years in an uncontrolled environment (APA, 2013, p. 702).

These diagnostic criteria are changed from earlier versions of the DSM in which the person was required to be both male and heterosexual in order to be diagnosed with transvestic fetishism. Inclusion of those criteria in earlier versions of the DSM was likely due to the fact that most people with transvestism are heterosexual men. Nevertheless, the fact that women can be aroused by wearing men's clothing and that people with homosexual orientation can be aroused by cross-dressing makes the DSM-5 criteria more accurate and useful.

There are some obvious problems with the DSM-5 criteria. For example, transvestism is defined by wearing clothes associated with the opposite gender, so the "fetish" specifier involving fabrics, material, or garments will always be applicable. In addition, it is important that a distinction is made between acts, intents, and motivations. Many people choose to wear clothing that is not gender-specific and for a variety of reasons. Gender fashions are culturally specific. Therefore, it would be wrong to diagnose a Scottish man who chooses to wear a kilt as a transvestite. However, if the same man also persistently chooses to wear women's lingerie to enhance his gender identity as a woman, he may have gender dysphoria if this causes distress, if he wears the lingerie for the purpose of achieving or enhancing sexual arousal, then and only then is a designation of transvestism appropriate. In this chapter, the term *transvestism* is used in recognition that most people with transvestic interests never seek or require psychiatric care. This chapter discusses transvestic disorder, which is a paraphilia, but not gender dysphoria, which is a nonsexually motivated condition. One interesting condition associated with cross-dressing is *autogynephilia*, which is characterized by sexual arousal from the fantasy of being a woman (Lawrence, 2011). People with gender dysphoria have understandably been concerned that gender dysphoria (due to issues involving gender identity) may be confused with a paraphilia such as transvestic disorder (which is a condition due to issues related to sexual interest in women's clothing).

Case Report 8.1

A soldier in uniform came for an appointment. He was embarrassed to say why he had come for an assessment. He explained it was his wife's idea. She had discovered a collection of panties in the glove compartment of his car. She thought he was having an affair, but he confessed to her that he was a "cross-dresser" and used the panties to masturbate while he was in the garage.

In interview, he was anxious to relate a story from Halloween when he was a child. His older sister had dressed him as a girl. He remembered feeling sexually aroused and concluded that this incident had "caused" his transvestic interests. In further discussion, he admitted that he would not have sought treatment if he was single.

Case Report 8.1 illustrates several characteristics of men with transvestic disorder. Many are fascinated by "dressing up" and gender roles. Many select occupations that involve wearing uniforms, and many choose stereotypically "hypermasculine" professions such as soldier or firefighter. They are often ashamed of their transvestic interests and have been worried about whether they might be gay. In order to keep their "shameful secret" under cover, they may resort to acts such as masturbating in their garage, stealing lingerie, and in some cases autoerotic self-asphyxia (AES). They are often ashamed of their transvestic interests and have been worried about their sexual orientation. In order to keep their "shameful secret" under cover, they may resort to acts such as masturbating in their garage, stealing lingerie, and, in some cases, AES. Many resort to childhood events such as Halloween to explain the onset of their interests. Importantly, most seek treatment due to concerns of their partners.

Variations

Transvestic fetishism appears to be an ideal condition for studies about paraphilias because it concerns interests that do not necessarily involve potentially illegal acts. However, the condition also presents unique research problems. The first is in identifying true transvestism. Some men wear women's clothes to entertain themselves and others (e.g., "drag queens"). Some attempt to "pass" as women in order to facilitate sexual relations with heterosexual men or lesbian women. Some do so in order to facilitate sexual relations with men who are sexually attracted to so-called she-males. Others wear women's clothes due to a nonsexual wish to assume a female gender role or identity. A failure to distinguish between motivations due to gender, orientation, and sexual interest has resulted in acrimonious disputes by subgroups of cross-dressers who believe they have been mislabeled and/or misunderstood.

This issue is further complicated by the fact that the categories listed previously can change. For example, many men are sexually aroused by scantily clad women. There are entire industries that play to this interest in the form of women wearing revealing lingerie. For some men, the interest becomes fetishistic in the sense that the lingerie becomes more sexually interesting that the woman wearing the lingerie. This can progress to a wish to be more intimate with the lingerie by touching, smelling, or wearing it. These acts are often highly sexualized, accompanied by masturbation and fantasies that can include taking the role of the woman. Men with transvestic fetishism often masturbate while wearing lingerie and often watch themselves in the mirror while imagining they are a woman having sex. Fedoroff (1988) published a case report of a man whose sexual interest in lingerie was enough to cause his wife to complain he was not sexually interested in her. His fetishistic interest in lingerie disappeared when he was treated with the serotonergic modulator buspirone, to the point that his wife noticed he no longer "tuned out" when they had sex.

Aging Transvestites

In some cases, the sexual arousal from cross-dressing is replaced by a sense of reduced anxiety when wearing women's clothes. Sessions in which cross-dressing is accompanied by masturbation are gradually replaced by increasingly lengthy sessions in which the man cross-dresses while assuming his view (often stereotypic) of a female gender role. The Sexual Behaviors Clinic at Johns Hopkins Hospital referred to men who presented in this way as "aging transvestites" because the change in interests and behaviors was associated with a reduction in sex drive and a process by the man of coming to terms with his comfort in assuming a female gender role and, in some cases, female gender identity.

Autoerotic Self-Asphyxia

An important subgroup of individuals with transvestic disorder are people who cross-dress and self-asphyxiate. This syndrome has been labeled AES and is often also associated with sexual masochism (Blanchard & Hucker, 1991). Why transvestic fetishism, sexual masochism, and AES often co-occur is unknown.

Autoerotic Self-Asphyxia as Role Playing

One theory is that men with AES have sadistic fantasies and are aroused by the idea of women in bondage, including being strangled. The act of cross-dressing and self-strangulation therefore represents enactment of a sadistic fantasy. However, this theory does not explain why people with sexual sadism rarely self-asphyxiate. It does support the hypothesis that sadism and masochism are in fact closely related (see Chapter 7, this book). It is also important to note that many people (including women) self-asphyxiate independently of any transvestic interests.

Cross-Contamination and Dissociation

A second explanation is that some people who associate sexual arousal with cross-dressing are confronted with "cross-contamination" of issues involving sexual arousal, sexual interest, sexual orientation, and gender identity. These are people who have progressed from having a simple fetish to a situation in which they take the role of the object of their desire. When they masturbate while fantasizing about being a woman, they are confronted by the fact that they have a penis. This can make it more difficult to maintain the fantasy and lead to attempts to further dissociate. Breath-holding and self-asphyxia can facilitate dissociation.

Sympathetic Sexual Enhancement

Orgasm in men typically follows the process of obtaining an erection that is primarily facilitated by parasympathetic arousal. Orgasm itself occurs in the context of a surge in sympathetic arousal. One of the best ways to induce a wave of sympathetic stimulation is anoxia. Therefore, it may be that some people with transvestic fetishism stumble onto AES as a means to facilitate or accentuate orgasm, which becomes a self-reinforcing behavior. People who resort to anoxia to facilitate orgasm may be those with a "sticky switch" in terms of switching from primary parasympathetic to sympathetic sexual arousal.

Every person diagnosed with transvestic disorder should be asked about any attempts to enhance orgasm, including self-asphyxia. This is especially important because people who self-strangle can easily misjudge their ability to revive themselves once they lose consciousness from anoxia. Anyone who self-asphyxiates is in danger of accidental death. It is also important for clinicians to ask about other methods of inducing anoxia, including chest compression, "wraps," gags, bags, and drowning. All of these activities are dangerous. An evolving problem in the United States is breath-holding contests and underwater swimming. This is because people can condition themselves to overcome the instinct to breathe when carbon dioxide rises but can lose consciousness before the urge to breath due to decreased oxygen kicks in.

Assessment and Treatment Recommendations

Assessment should begin by assuring patients that their problems are not unusual. They should be interviewed concerning other paraphilic interests and any sexual dysfunctions that may have led to unconventional sexual behaviors such as AES. Phallometric testing can be of assistance, primarily to obtain objective evidence of possible homosexuality or, more importantly to help assure the patient they are not gay. Importantly, assurance that the person is not gay should be presented with the reminder that being gay is not a problem in itself, only guilt about being gay, especially if the person is basing the worry on the false premise that gay men wear women's clothing.

It is always helpful to know what caused the person to seek treatment at this time. Often, it is due to being caught or almost caught by a spouse. If this is the case, the nature and health of the relationship should be explored.

In the Sexual Behaviours Clinic (SBC), selective serotonergic reuptake inhibitors (SSRIs) have been found to be very successful in the consensual treatment of men who feel dependent on cross-dressing to the point that it is interfering with their sexual relations. It is important to prescribe SSRIs at low doses in order to avoid inducing delayed orgasm. See Chapter 2 for further treatment suggestions.

Prognosis

People with transvestic fetishism often collect lingerie and then have episodes in which they impulsively dispose of their collection. After some time, the urge to cross-dress returns, and they begin to collect lingerie again. Some men with transvestic fetishism experience a complete resolution of their urges to cross-dress when treated with low-dose SSRIs. It is of interest that in Fedoroff's (1988) previously discussed case report, the who responded to buspirone (which is a 5-hydroxytryptamine autoreceptor partial agonist), together with his wife, elected to stop taking buspirone. He said that once his wife knew his fetishistic interest in lingerie was due to a "chemical imbalance," she was comfortable incorporating lingerie into their sexual activities.

As with many of the paraphilias that do not involve criminal acts if acted on, the need to change the interest often changes when the person understands that their paraphilic interest is not in itself dangerous. This is particularly true if there are no relationship difficulties. Sometimes, concerns about a paraphilic interest are raised when in fact it is the relationship that is in trouble. It is helpful to ask the partner when they first became aware of the paraphilia and what their understanding of its meaning is to them.

Case Report 8.2

A man was transported to the SBC in prison clothes and handcuffs. He was accompanied by several armed guards. The court had ordered an assessment after he had been arrested for breaking into a woman's house while she was asleep in her bed. Fortunately, she heard him coming into the house and was able to call 911. She did not know the intruder, but a month before she had called the police to report a break and enter. That thief had taken her laptop. Of more concern to her (and the police) was that he had also stolen some of her lingerie.

The prisoner was cooperative with the assessment, which included a full psychiatric interview and phallometric testing. On phallometric testing, he showed sexual arousal in response to pictures of panties. He also responded to audiotapes describing cross-dressing but not to other audiotapes describing coercive sexual scenarios. When interviewed, he admitted that he had engaged in voyeuristic acts (going out at night to search for women undressing who had forgotten to draw the blinds to their bedroom). He had a list of addresses that he frequented for this purpose. He suspected that some of the women he spied on knew he was watching and "put on a show" for him on purpose. He said then when he thought a woman knew he was watching, he lost interest and would scratch her off his list of voyeuristic sites to visit. He also admitted to a fetishistic interest in women's lingerie that had progressed to him wearing lingerie when he masturbated. He did not engage in AES. He said that he had spied on the woman whose house he broke into and had sexual fantasies about her. He knew she would not be interested in him, so he decided to steal some of her lingerie as a substitute. He said he had never previously broken into anyone's house but admitted stealing lingerie from laundromats. If fact, he said he preferred unwashed lingerie. He said he had never even considered purchasing lingerie because "that would be too embarrassing."

He had previously been diagnosed as having an autistic spectrum disorder that included a solitary lifestyle and eccentric thinking. He had never had a girlfriend, and he identified himself as a "virgin."

Men such as the one described in Case Report 8.2 are often cited by experts who believe that people with fetishes and/or transvestic disorder are prone to "deterioration" from paraphilias that do not involve thoughts about criminal acts leading to paraphilias associated with crimes. There have been several famous cases involving sexual homicide by men who also had fetishes or so-called courtship disorder paraphilias. Although sexual homicide certainly occurs, most people with transvestic disorder never engage in any criminal acts. It is also important to note that most serial sexual offenders are neither cross-dressers nor people with transvestic disorder or fetishes.

The reason that myths persist about the potential dangerousness of people with transvestic fetishism likely results from selective recall by investigators. They recall the rare cases in which a criminal had a fetish, and they forget all the cases in which the criminal did not have a fetish. There is a rumor that some detectives developed a similar belief about *Star Trek* movies and *Star Trek* paraphernalia after several raids on men who had child pornography in their homes. During the searches, it was discovered many also had *Star Trek* videos. For some time, search warrants included the expectation that *Star Trek* materials would also be found. This observation overlooked the fact that the same people who viewed child pornography—unemployed, single, Caucasian men—belonged to a larger group who also liked *Star Trek*. However, there is no causal link between child pornography and *Star Trek*.

A similar logical mistake has been noted concerning the widespread belief that people who have been sexually abused are more likely to become abusers themselves. In fact, there is no direct association. However, investigators are prone to recall cases in which an offender is discovered to have previously been sexually assaulted (Fedoroff & Pinkus, 1996).

Transvestism is exemplary as a condition that attracts attention when it is discovered. There is a widespread mistaken belief that men with transvestic disorder are somehow prone to criminality due to the disorder. This view is likely due to the *Star Trek* phenomenon described previously in which a notable finding (e.g., a man wearing women's clothing) is recalled and mistakenly elevated from the status of correlation to causation. Although many men have committed break and enter offenses due to transvestic interests, most break and enters are committed by men who do not have transvestic interests.

Conclusion

Transvestism, defined as sexual arousal from wearing women's clothes, especially lingerie, is likely a common phenomenon. There are legitimate concerns about labeling men with this interest as people with a psychiatric disorder. However, men with this sexual interest should be eligible to receive profession counseling concerning its character and prognosis. They should also be assessed for the possibility of interest in the potentially life-threatening activity of AES. In addition, it is important to assist men with transvestism to avoid letting the interest interfere with their ability to engage in healthy, meaningful, and fulfilling sexual interactions with consenting partners.

Review of the Literature

The following table summarizes the literature that has been published on "transvestic disorder" or "transvestic fetish*" from 2008 to 2018 based on PsycINFO and PubMed searches. Cultural experiences of cross-dressing have also been included to highlight the differences between transvestic fetishism disorder and cross-dressing that has or has not been pathologized. Also note that there is considerable controversy concerning the appropriate terminology for people in this group. Terminology in this section reflects the terminology used in the articles cited.

Summary	Reference
Etiology	
Descriptive analysis and quantitative comparison of 192 adolescents referred for gender identity disorder and 137 boys referred for transvestic fetishism. Males with transvestic fetishism and males with gender identity disorder self-reported similar behaviors.	Zucker et al. (2012)
Assessed 571 males with transvestism. The authors found that transvestic fetishism usually begins during adulthood and is lifelong. Also, age, ethnicity, and sexual orientation were statistically significant predictors for transvestic fetishism.	Nuttbrock et al. (2011)
Discusses Blanchard's hypothesis of erotic target location errors and erotic target identity inversion, and its manifestations as paraphilic interests, such as transvestic fetishism.	Lawrence (2009a)
Discusses erotic target location errors as proposed by Blanchard and Hucker in 1991, and its manifestation as transvestism.	Lawrence (2009b)
Discusses the differences between transvestic fetishism and transsexualism, and their relation to autogynephilia.	Lawrence (2009c)
Insights into Transvestic Fetishistic Behaviors	
From a contemporary Finnish cohort, self-report data of 5,990 male and female twins between the ages of 18 and 32 years were analyzed for paraphilias and sexually coercive behavior. Transvestic fetishism was the only paraphilia not associated with sexual coercion, whereas other paraphilias had moderate to strong associations with sexually coercive behaviors.	Baur et al. (2016)

Summary	Reference
This study investigated paraphilias and their associations with the Big Five and Dark Triad personality traits. It was found that transvestism was associated with greater openness to experience.	Lodi-Smith, Shepard, & Wagner (2014)
Case study of a 36-year-old man who was found dead in his bedroom, dressed in his mother's clothes. This case study involves autoerotic asphyxia and anal self-stimulation.	Atanasijević, Jovanović, Nikolić, Popović, & Jašović-Gašić (2009)
Society and Culture	
Festive transvestism is cross-dressing by young Ghanians during festive events. The author challenges Western perceptions of sexual orientations.	Geoffrion (2013)
"Spontaneous transvestism" occurs in the Spring Fiestas in Spain, when women dress in costumes that were designed for men. The article discusses how this activity has received negative reactions from local authorities.	Cano-López (2011)
Examines Argentinean television programs from 1993 to 2010 concerning how transvestic individuals were represented. The author found that television programs often portray transvestic individuals as having a need for social inclusion and having to fight for their human rights.	Soich (2016)
During World War I, cross-dressing was viewed as entertainment. This article discusses how impersonating women allowed men a "pleasurable dissociation."	Sigel (2016)
Analyzes how the French used "transvestic" characters in comedy.	Quemener (2012)
Analyzes the language used by a European-American drag queen while she was on stage.	Mann (2011)
Discusses a "male-to-female transvestism" culture.	Allen (2014)
Interviewed 27 drag kings and found that they do not overtly challenge the gender status quo but, rather, use drag as an outlet to explore female masculinity and transsexuality.	Baker & Kelly (2016)
Interviewed drag queens regarding how they experience and cope with being alienated yet admired as performers.	Berkowitz & Belgrave (2010)
Diagnosis	
DSM Criticisms	
The World Professional Association for Transgender Health (WPATH) states its recommendations for the DSM-5 concerning transvestic fetishism. Along with changes in diagnostic criteria, the authors advocate changing the name of the diagnosis to transvestic disorder.	Gijs & Carroll (2011)

Summary	Reference
The authors propose changes for the DSM-5 criteria for transvestic disorder and critique a previously submitted draft.	De Cuypere, Knudson, & Bockting (2011)
Response to WPATH's recommendations on transvestic fetishism, after the WPATH did not reach a consensus about whether transvestic fetishism should be in the DSM-5.	Knudson, De Cuypere, & Bockting (2011)
Proposes changes to the diagnostic criteria for the DSM-5 to include new specifiers.	Blanchard (2010)
Discusses the idea that consensual paraphilias, such as transvestic fetishism, should be depathologized.	Wright (2010)
Variations	
Case study of a 4-year-old boy who cross-dressed and hoped to be a female like his older sister but was afraid of castration. The author follows a Freudian framework to understand the child's experiences and manifestations.	Scharff (2017)
Case study of a 25-year-old man with bipolar disorder type I with paraphilic behaviors (including transvestism), attention-deficit/hyperactivity disorder, and oppositional behaviors.	Kamalzadeh, Alavi, & Salehi (2015)
Case series of three persons with transvestism. Two of the cases had other paraphilias. The last case had transvestism and obsessive–compulsive disorder but was treated using a selective serotonin reuptake inhibitor.	Anupama, Gangadhar, Shetty, & Dip (2016)
Case study of a man with transvestic fetishism, mental retardation, and psychosis.	Velayudhan et al. (2014)
Case series of transgendered persons with breast cancer. One of the male-to-female individuals was identified as a transgendered person with transvestic fetishism.	Brown (2015)
Investigated the characteristics of 13 participants who cross-dressed and who also had learning disabilities.	Parkes, Hall, & Wilson (2009)
Review of the literature for autogynephilia (sexual arousal from the thought or image of oneself as a woman). The author discusses supporting evidence for autogynephilia and its controversy.	Lawrence (2017)
Examined gynandromorphophilic (GAMP) men (sexual attraction to gyandromorphs—an attraction to males with breasts and penises). The two studies compared 314 GAMP men, 211 non-homosexual men without GAMP, and homosexual men. It was found that GAMP men were more likely to respond to the gyandromorph stimuli.	Rosenthal (2017)

Summary	Reference
Assessment	
Found five group factors underlying autogynephilia. The new assessment had good internal consistency, reliability, and validity. It was also found that the scale was able to differentiate between autogynephilic men and heterosexual men.	Hsu, Rosenthal, & Bailey (2015)
Treatment	
Case study of clinical treatment for a cross-dressing client, and strategic marriage therapy for him and his spouse.	Gallo (2016a)
Discusses transvestism, the diagnostic history, and how to improve therapeutic practices. The author advocates for a nonjudgmental atmosphere and notes that clients are usually disinterested in ceasing to cross-dress.	Gallo (2016b)
Examined the post-treatment experiences of patients who had undergone treatment for homosexuality and transvestism between 1949 and 1992. Seven male participants responded to the study. All reported that the treatments to change their sexual desires and behaviors were unsuccessful. Instead, the former patients reported that the treatments did more harm than good.	Dickinson, Cook, Plyle, & Hallett (2012)
Case study of a 9-year-old boy with transvestic fetishism who was successfully treated with sertraline.	Guney, Ceylan, & Sener (2011)
Literature review of anti-androgens used to treat paraphilias, including transvestic fetishism.	Guay (2009)
Book Chapters	
Baez-Sierra, D., Balgobin, C., & Wise, T. N. (2016). Treatment of paraphilic disorders. In R. Balon (Ed.), *Practical guide to paraphilia and paraphilic disorders* (pp. 43–62). Cham, Switzerland: Springer.	
Balon, R. (2016). Transvestic disorder. In R. Balon (Ed.), *Practical guide to paraphilia and paraphilic disorders* (pp. 171–185). Cham, Switzerland: Springer.	
Greaves, C. C., & Reicherter, D. (2015). Gender dysphoria. In L. W. Roberts & A. K. Louie (Eds.), *Study guide to DSM-5* (pp. 317–334). Arlington, VA: American Psychiatric Publishing.	
Newring, K. A. B., Wheeler, J., & Draper, C. (2008). Transvestic fetishism: Assessment and treatment. In D. R. Laws & W. T. O'Donohue (Eds.), *Sexual deviance: Theory, assessment, and treatment* (2nd ed., pp. 285–304). New York, NY: Guilford.	
Wheeler, J., Newring, K. A. B., & Draper, C. (2008). Transvestic fetishism: Psychopathology and theory. In D. R. Laws & W. T. O'Donohue (Eds.), *Sexual deviance: Theory, assessment, and treatment* (2nd ed., pp. 272–284). New York, NY: Guilford.	

References

Allen, S. (2014). Whither the transvestite? Theorising male-to-female transvestism in feminist and queer theory. *Feminist Theory, 15*(1), 51–72.

American Psychiatric Association. (2013). *Diagnostic and statistical manual of mental disorders* (5th ed.). Arlington, VA: American Psychiatric Publishing.

Anupama, M., Gangadhar, K. H., Shetty, V. B., & Dip, P. B. (2016). Transvestism as a symptom: A case series. *Indian Journal of Psychological Medicine, 38*(1), 78–80. doi:10.4103/0253-7176.175131

Atanasijević, T., Jovanović, A. A., Nikolić, S., Popović, V., & Jašović-Gašić, M. (2009). Accidental death due to complete autoerotic asphyxia associated with transvestic fetishism and anal self-stimulation-case report. *Psychiatria Danubina, 21*(2), 246–251.

Baez-Sierra, D., Balgobin, C., & Wise, T. N. (2016). Treatment of paraphilic disorders. In R. Balon (Ed.), *Practical guide to paraphilia and paraphilic disorders* (pp. 43–62). Cham, Switzerland: Springer.

Baker, A. A., & Kelly, K. (2016). Live like a king, y'all: Gender negotiation and the performance of masculinity among Southern drag kings. *Sexualities, 19*(1–2), 46–63.

Balon, R. (2016). Transvestic disorder. In R. Balon (Ed.), *Practical guide to paraphilia and paraphilic disorders* (pp. 171–185). Cham, Switzerland: Springer.

Baur, E., Forsman, M., Santtila, P., Johansson, A., Sandnabba, K., & Långström, N. (2016). Paraphilic sexual interests and sexually coercive behavior: A population-based twin study. *Archives of Sexual Behavior, 45*(5), 1163–1172.

Berkowitz, D., & Belgrave, L. (2010). "She works hard for the money": Drag queens and the management of their contradictory status of celebrity and marginality. *Journal of Contemporary Ethnography, 39*(2), 159–186.

Blanchard, R., & Hucker, S. J. (1991). Age, transvestism, bondage, and concurrent paraphilic activities in 117 fatal cases of autoerotic asphyxia. *British Journal of Psychiatry, 159* (3), 371–377. doi:10.1192/bjp.159.3.371

Blanchard, R. (2010). The DSM diagnostic criteria for transvestic fetishism. *Archives of Sexual Behavior, 39*(2), 363–372.

Brown, G. R. (2015). Breast cancer in transgender veterans: A ten-case series. *LGBT Health, 2*(1), 77–80.

Cano-López, M. (2011). Welcome to La Huerta: The attempts to curb cross-dressing during the Spring Fiestas in Murcia. *Journal of Gender Studies, 20*(2), 183–192.

De Cuypere, G., Knudson, G., & Bockting, W. (2011). Second Response of the World Professional Association for Transgender Health to the Proposed Revision of the Diagnosis of Gender Dysphoria for DSM 5. *International Journal of Transgenderism, 13*(2), 51–53. doi:10.1080/15532739.2011.624047

Dickinson, T., Cook, M., Playle, J., & Hallett, C. (2012). "Queer" treatments: Giving a voice to former patients who received treatments for their "sexual deviations." *Journal of Clinical Nursing, 21*(9–10), 1345–1354.

Fedoroff, J. P. (1988). Buspirone hydrochloride in the treatment of transvestic fetishism. *Journal of Clinical Psychiatry, 49*, 408–409.

Fedoroff, J. P., & Pinkus, S. (1996). The genesis of pedophilia: Testing the abuse to abuser hypothesis. *Journal of Offender Rehabilitation, 23*, 85–101.

Gallo, M. (2016a). A case study of cross-dressing: Using a strategic therapy lens in couple's counseling. *The Family Journal, 24*(1), 77–84.

Gallo, M. (2016b). Treating transvestism: A counselor's look at diagnosing and treatment of cross-dressers. *The Family Journal, 24*(2), 195–199.

Geoffrion, K. (2013). Ghanaian youth and festive transvestism. *Culture, Health & Sexuality, 15*(Suppl. 1), 48–61.

Gijs, L., & Carroll, R. (2010). Should Transvestic Fetishism Be Classified in DSM 5? Recommendations from the WPATH Consensus Process for Revision of the Diagnosis of Transvestic Fetishism. *International Journal of Transgenderism, 12*(4), 189–197. doi:10.1080/15532739.2010.550766

Greaves, C. C., & Reicherter, D. (2015). Gender dysphoria. In L. W. Roberts & A. K. Louie (Eds.), *Study guide to DSM-5* (pp. 317–334). Arlington, VA: American Psychiatric Publishing.

Guay, D. R. (2009). Drug treatment of paraphilic and nonparaphilic sexual disorders. *Clinical Therapeutics, 31*(1), 1–31.

Guney, E., Ceylan, M. F., & Sener, S. (2011). Successful treatment of transvestic fetishism with sertralin in a prepubertal child. *Yeni Symposium: Psikiyatri, noroloji ve davranis bilimleri dergisi, 49*(3), 181–184.

Hsu, K. J., Rosenthal, A. M., & Bailey, J. M. (2015). The psychometric structure of items assessing autogynephilia. *Archives of Sexual Behavior, 44*(5), 1301–1312.

Jobs, S. (2004, October 12).The seed of Apple's innovation [Interview]. *Bloomberg*. Retrieved from http://www.bloomberg.com

Kamalzadeh, L., Alavi, K., & Salehi, M. (2015). Comorbidity of bipolar disorder and multiple paraphilias: A case report. *Iranian Journal of Psychiatry and Clinical Psychology, 21*(1), 69–74.

Lawrence, A. A. (2009a). Anatomic autoandrophilia in an adult male. *Archives of Sexual Behavior, 38*(6), 1050–1056.

Lawrence, A. A. (2009b). Erotic target location errors: An underappreciated paraphilic dimension. *Journal of Sex Research, 46*(2–3), 194–215.

Lawrence, A. A. (2009c). Transgenderism in nonhomosexual males as a paraphilic phenomenon: Implications for case conceptualization and treatment. *Sexual and Relationship Therapy, 24*(2), 188–206.

Lawrence, A. A. (2011). Autogynephilia: An underappreciated paraphilia. *Advances in Psychosomatic Medicine, 31*, 135–48. doi:10.1159/000328921

Lawrence, A. A. (2017). Autogynephilia and the typology of male-to-female transsexualism. *European Psychologist, 22*(1), 39–54.

Lodi-Smith, J., Shepard, K., & Wagner, S. (2014). Personality and sexually deviant behavior. *Personality and Individual Differences, 70*, 39–44.

Mann, S. L. (2011). Drag queens' use of language and the performance of blurred gendered and racial identities. *Journal of Homosexuality, 58*(6–7), 793–811.

Newring, K. A. B., Wheeler, J., & Draper, C. (2008). Transvestic fetishism: Assessment and treatment. In D. R. Laws & W. T. O'Donohue (Eds.), *Sexual deviance: Theory, assessment, and treatment* (2nd ed., pp. 285–304). New York, NY: Guilford.

Nuttbrock, L., Bockting, W., Mason, M., Hwahng, S., Rosenblum, A., Macri, M., & Becker, J. (2011). A further assessment of Blanchard's typology of homosexual versus non-homosexual or autogynephilic gender dysphoria. *Archives of Sexual Behavior, 40*(2), 247–257.

Parkes, G., Hall, I., & Wilson, D. (2009). Cross dressing and gender dysphoria in people with learning disabilities: A descriptive study. *British Journal of Learning Disabilities, 37*(2), 151–156.

Quemener, N. (2012). Mockery or fantasy? Transvestite characters, cross-dressing and subaltern sexualities in sketches in French talk shows. *Sexualities, 15*(1), 80–92.

Rosenthal, A. M. (2017). *Who are the gynandromorphophilic men? Two studies of men with sexual interest in transgender women*. Doctoral dissertation, Northwestern University, Evanston, IL (ProQuest Dissertations, Accession No. 10160454).

Scharff, J. S. (2017). Case study: Analysis of a traumatized hemophiliac boy. *International Journal of Psychoanalysis, 98*(1), 71–90.

Sigel, L. Z. (2016). "Best love": Female impersonation in the Great War. *Sexualities, 19*(1–2), 98–118.

Soich, M. (2016). The collective need to be inside, the individual spectacle of the outer: Critical discourse analysis of the construction of discursive representations about transvestites on Argentinean television. *Discourse & Society, 27*(2), 215–238

Velayudhan, R., Khaleel, A., Sankar, N., Kumar, M., Kazhungil, F., & Raghuram, T. M. (2014). Fetishistic transvestism in a patient with mental retardation and psychosis. *Indian Journal of Psychological Medicine, 36*(2), 198–200. doi:10.4103/0253-7176.130995

Wheeler, J., Newring, K. A. B., & Draper, C. (2008). Transvestic fetishism: Psychopathology and theory. In D. R. Laws & W. T. O'Donohue (Eds.), *Sexual deviance: Theory, assessment, and treatment* (2nd ed., pp. 272–284). New York, NY: Guilford.

Wright, S. (2010). Depathologizing consensual sexual sadism, sexual masochism, transvestic fetishism, and fetishism. *Archives of Sexual Behavior, 39*(6), 1229–1230. http://dx.doi.org/10.1007/s10508-010-9651-y

Zucker, K. J., Bradley, S. J., Owen-Anderson, A., Kibblewhite, S. J., Wood, H., Singh, D., & Choi, K. (2012). Demographics, behavior problems, and psychosexual characteristics of adolescents with gender identity disorder or transvestic fetishism. *Journal of Sex & Marital Therapy, 38*(2), 151–189.

9
Voyeuristic Disorder

Any photographer who says he is not a voyeur is either stupid or a liar.
—Helmut Newton (2009)

Introduction

Voyeuristic disorder is perhaps the most misdiagnosed of the disorders in the Fifth edition of the *Diagnostic and Statistical Manual of Mental Disorders* (DSM-5; American Psychiatric Association [APA], 2013) and the 10th revision of the *International Classification of Diseases* (ICD-10; World Health Organization, 2004). The reason is that it involves a behavior (observation) that is virtually ubiquitous in courtship behavior. Many commentators fail to note that voyeurism involves sexual arousal not from observation but, rather, from the person's belief that the observation is happening without the observed person's knowledge.

The DSM-5 defines voyeuristic disorder as a condition in which a person experiences persistent (at least 6 months), recurrent, and intense sexual arousal from observing an unsuspecting person "who is naked, in the process of disrobing, or engaging in sexual activity, as manifested by fantasies, urges or behaviors" (APA, 2013, p. 686). The B criteria require that the person has acted on the voyeuristic urges with a non-consenting person or the condition has caused "clinically significant distress or impairment in social, occupational or other important areas of functioning." The C criteria specify that the person must be at least 18 years old.

The proposed ICD-11 criteria are essentially the same ("Voyeuristic Disorder," n.d.):

> Voyeuristic Disorder is characterized by a sustained, focused and intense pattern of sexual arousal—as manifested by persistent sexual thoughts, fantasies, urges, or behaviours—that involves observing an unsuspecting individual who is naked, in the process of disrobing, or engaging in sexual activity. In addition, in order for Voyeuristic Disorder to be diagnosed, the individual must have acted on these thoughts, fantasies or urges or be markedly distressed by them.

The ICD-11 adds an important exclusion: "Voyeuristic Disorder specifically excludes consensual voyeuristic behaviours that occur with the consent of the person or persons being observed."

The DSM-5 estimates the prevalence of true voyeuristic disorder to be as high as 12% in men and 4% in women.

Variations

Many people mistakenly self-diagnose or are mislabeled as "voyeuristic" because they are aroused by looking at pornography, which is better described as scoptophilia. Scoptophilia is an example of a sexual characteristic that is both common and nonpathologic. Similarly, sexual arousal in response to a chance glimpse of a naked or seminaked person is insufficient to be diagnosed as a voyeuristic disorder any more than arousal from seeing an attractive person in tight jeans constitutes a sexual fetish. In the case of voyeurism, it is also important to avoid labeling a person who enjoys going to strip clubs as voyeuristic, as Case Report 9.1, illustrates (this case has previously been described; Fedoroff, 2003). In that case, a man was advised to seek treatment after he had been beaten up in an alley. He had been caught standing on the hood of his vehicle and peeking in the window of a strip club from which position he could spy on exotic dancers in their change room. Asked why he had put himself is such a predicament when he could have gone in the front door of the establishment and gotten a better view and a drink, he explained that his arousal came from the idea that he was seeing women who did not know they were being watched. It is this non-consensual aspect of true voyeurism that is essential for the diagnosis.

In the same way that people with exhibitionism do not enjoy nude beaches (because everyone is consensually nude), people with true voyeurism do not enjoy strip clubs, where the dancers know they are being watched. If people with voyeurism view pornography, they prefer sites that suggest the subjects of the images were explicitly non-consenting either to the images being posted (e.g., so-called revenge porn sites in which people post naked pictures of ex-spouses/ex-partners) or to the images being taken (e.g., "upskirt" sites). A useful question to ask during assessment of a person caught peeking in a window is if the person has ever gone out a night with the specific intention of searching for someone to spy upon. A man who took a second look when he noticed a woman in a window while he was walking his dog is less likely to have voyeuristic disorder than a man with a history of intentionally seeking windows in which he could spy, especially if there is an indication of sexual motivation such as masturbating during the act. Men with voyeurism often have previous charges such as "trespass by night."

The Sexual Behaviours Clinic (SBC) has recently had a surge of referrals involving men arrested for taking pictures with their cell phones focusing on the genital areas of women wearing skirts. In some cases, these are orchestrated collections of images taken by men who intentionally position themselves at the foot of public staircases or who create elaborate devices in which their cell phone is placed on a wheeled platform facing up or even using fiber-optic cables allowing pictures to be taken from the tip of the shoe when they discretely slide their foot under the dress of the woman in front of them in line, for example, at a grocery store checkout. These men almost invariably describe voyeuristic interests centered on some variation of the theme of spying on the women's genitals without the women's knowledge or consent.

However, a new group of men charged with the same offense are now being referred more frequently. These men typically have apparently serendipitously found themselves in a situation in which it would be easy to "snap a picture" (e.g., a woman in a skirt standing on a ladder while stocking a shelf). These men are similar to men who happen to notice a woman undressing in a window but who keep walking. The reason they are becoming more frequent is not an increase in the frequency of voyeurism but, rather, an increase in the number of men who have cell phones that are capable of taking pictures. In the past, most people did not walk around with cameras. It is notable that the interest in photographing women without consent does not seem to be shared by women, in terms of photographing either men or women (for further comments, see Chapter 11, this book).

In a recent review of the origins of clinical opinion concerning people with voyeurism (Janssen, 2018), it was noted that early descriptions of people with voyeurism included men who frequented houses of prostitution that provided "peek holes" that allowed the patrons to spy on others having sex. It was noted that the same men who spied would also engage in sex with the prostitutes, presumably with the knowledge that they may be watched by other men through the same peek holes. This combination of voyeurism with exhibitionism has been conceptualized as a disorder of courtship (Freund & Blanchard, 1986).

There are several cases on record of male gynecologists who took surreptitious photographs of their patients during vaginal examinations. In these cases, the women clearly consented to being examined but of course did not consent to being photographed for the sexual pleasure of their doctor. Some may wonder why a man who medically examines women's genitals on a daily basis, as part of his work as a gynecologist, would have any interest in making a collection consisting of photographs of the same women he has seen in person. Although motivations undoubtedly vary, a common reason is because people with voyeurism are aroused primarily by the fact that they are making observations of women who do not know they are being observed for a sexual purpose. Some textbooks claim that voyeurs do not spy on their own wives, but the SBC has had several referrals involving men doing exactly that. When asked why they were spying on a person who would have consented to being observed, again the answer typically is that seeing their wife "with her guard down" is especially sexually arousing to a person with voyeurism. In fact, for many, the fact that the person who is being spied on is known to the person with voyeurism makes the voyeuristic act more exciting. For others, the less they know about the victim, the better. It is important for the assessor to investigate the degree to which the person with voyeurism knows the victim because the act may be part of an erotomanic disorder or part of a larger pattern of stalking behavior (Menzies, Fedoroff, Green, & Isaacson, 1995). Assessors should always ask about fantasies the person may have in terms of their relationship with the victim.

Case Report 9.1

An elderly bachelor was referred after being arrested for "trespassing." He was a cartographer and polyglot. On assessment, he was found to be a virgin and a loner who had never had a girlfriend. He admitted that his only source of sexual arousal was from peeking at women who were undressing. He admitted masturbating while looking at the women or while recalling women he had seen. On further examination, he was found to have a lifelong distrust of women and a rudimentary knowledge about sex in general.

He loved maps and languages and said he could understand most of the major languages of the world, as well as Latin. Asked what he got from voyeuristic activities, he said it was similar to what he got from maps and languages. He explained that he had always thought of countries as women. He believed that by learning a country's geography and language, he learned its "essence." He had not explicitly sexualized his interest in maps and language but admitted having masturbated to the point of ejaculation onto maps. In the case of women, he believed that seeing them without them having the ability to put up guards or to otherwise "deceive" him brought him closer to their "essence."

Treatment in this case began with basic sex education. He was also taught about the difference between fantasy and reality, and he was introduced to legal adult pornography that he had previously conceptualized as "evil." Importantly, he was also educated about the harm he caused by acting on his voyeuristic fantasies.

Candaulism

Case Report 9.2

A woman was stopped by a border guard at a custom's checkpoint. She voluntarily provided the password to her phone. The guard discovered a collection of photographs and videos of the woman engaging in one-to-one sexual acts with several different men. The woman explained that her husband enjoyed seeing her with different men (a condition known as candaulism). Candaulism was originally named by Richard von Krafft-Ebing based on the legend of Candaules, King of Lydia, who arranged for another man to see his wife naked.

The woman admitted that the men did not know they were being watched and photographed.

In Case Report 9.2, the woman's husband would meet the diagnostic criteria for voyeurism except for the fact that his wife was aware she was being watched. Her husband would technically meet diagnostic criteria for voyeurism if he in fact was primarily aroused by spying on the men. Candaulism-by-proxy refers to a practice in which the husband allows a third person to re-post pictures of his wife so that he voluntarily gives up control over what happens to the pictures. Although this may sound like an unlikely scenario, it has been speculated that many of the amateur pornographic pictures posted on the internet are in fact posted by people who have candaulism-by-proxy and are aroused by the idea that people are looking at pictures of their sexual partner. The fantasy that others are being sexually aroused by one's spouse without the spouse's knowledge may also meet diagnostic criteria for voyeurism-by-proxy, which in turn approximates exhibitionism (see Chapter 3, this book).

For completeness, if the border guard mentioned in Case Report 9.2 had a pattern of secretly keeping copies of the woman's photographs or if he shared the pictures with any of his colleagues who did so, this would also suggest that the guard or his colleagues had voyeurism. It is of interest that people with paraphilias often seek occupations compatible with their paraphilic interests; for example, voyeurs may be window washers. Again, in assessing variations of voyeurism or exhibitionism, it is important to determine whether the person is engaging in the act due to a sexual motivation or some other motivation, such as opportunity or revenge.

Prognosis

Of the paraphilias involving sexual interests that would be criminal if acted on, voyeurism and exhibitionism are the most difficult to treat. The likely reasons for this difficulty are because it is easy for people with these disorders to avoid thinking about the consequences of their actions. It is common for men arrested for voyeurism to complain that there would have been no problem if they had not been caught. In the case of a person with voyeurism who is caught without the victim's knowledge, an ethical question arises about whether the victim should be informed by the legal authorities. Some victims of voyeurism state that although they are happy the offender was caught, they wish they had not been told. The effect on victims of voyeurism is exacerbated if there is evidence the offender may have posted their pictures on the internet or social media outlets.

In contrast to classical voyeurs who actively seek out women to spy on, opportunistic offenders who take pictures with their cell phones typically respond very well to therapy and education about why voyeurism is against the law. However, people with voyeuristic disorder certainly deserve treatment aimed at changing their dependence on non-consensual acts to interest in consenting sexual relations. This can be done most effectively in group treatment in which social skills can become one of the focuses of treatment (see Chapter 2, this book).

Review of the Literature

The following table summarizes the literature that has been published on "voyeur*," "voyeurism," or "voyeuristic disorder" from 2008 to 2018 based on PsycINFO and PubMed searches.

Summary	Reference
History	
Reviews the history of the term "voyeurism" and how it became a medical term.	Janssen (2018)
Insights into Voyeuristic Behaviors	
In a survey of 871 undergraduate students in Nigeria, the most common paraphilia reported was voyeurism.	Abdullahi, Jafojo, & Udofia (2015)
Case study of a man who took upskirt videos of his colleagues.	Challinor & Duff (2017)
Phenomenological study of men who engaged in voyeuristic behaviors and who self-identify as "sexual addicts."	Shagaga (2016)
Suggests sex-specific profiles for exhibitionism, voyeurism, and those who have committed both.	Hopkins, Green, Carnes, & Campling (2016)
Reports that 16.4% of 1,049 high school students had been victims of voyeurism in locker rooms.	Joing & Vors (2015)
Examines possible models of the "heterosexual male script" based on the so-called centerfold syndrome, and possible treatment methods.	Elder, Brooks, & Morrow (2012)
Diagnosis	
DSM Criticisms	
Discusses the criteria for paraphilic disorders in the DSM-5.	Balon (2016a)
Argument for why exhibitionism, voyeurism, and frotteurism should not be in the DSM.	Hinderliter (2010)
Reviews the empirical literature from 1980 to 2008 on voyeurism, exhibitionism, and frotteurism, finding little support for any changes in the DSM-IV-TR criteria.	Langstrom (2010)
Variations	
Describes individuals with Klinefelter syndrome and its relation to paraphilias (finding a higher frequency of voyeuristic fantasies).	Fisher et al. (2015)
Case study of a 19-year-old male who's voyeuristic behaviors were linked to cyclothymia.	Ramadas (2017)

Summary	Reference
Treatment	
Voyeuristic behaviors in a 16-year-old boy were treated with sertraline. The behaviors decreased and remitted in 3 months.	Yalcin, Guney, & Saripinar (2014)
A case study using psychoanalysis to treat voyeurism.	Blechner (2016)
Book Chapters	
Balon, R. (2016). Voyeuristic disorder. In R. Balon (Ed.), *Practical guide to paraphilia and paraphilic disorders* (pp. 63–75). Cham, Switzerland: Springer.	
Hocken, K., & Thorne, K. (2012). Voyeurism, exhibitionism and other non-contact sexual offences. In B. Winder & P. Banyard (Eds.), *A psychologist's casebook of crime: From arson to voyeurism* (pp. 243–263). New York, NY: Palgrave Macmillan.	
Krueger, R. B., & Kaplan, M. S. (2016). Noncontact paraphilic sexual offenses. In A. Phenix & H. M. Hoberman (Eds.), *Sexual offending: Predisposing antecedents, assessments, and management* (pp. 79–102). New York, NY: Springer.	
Quayle, E., & Hayes, E. (2015). Interventions with an internet sexual offender. In D. T. Wilxoc, T. Garrett, & L. Harkins (Eds.), *Sex offender treatment: A case study approach to issues and interventions* (pp. 163–180). Malden, MA: Wiley-Blackwell.	
Stuyvesant, R. P., Mercier, D. G., & Haidle, A. (2014). Voyeurism: A case study. In W. T. O'Donohye (Ed.), *Case studies in sexual deviance: Toward evidence-based practice* (pp. 117–148). New York, NY: Routledge.	

References

Abdullahi, H., Jafojo, R. O., & Udofia, O. (2015). Paraphilia among undergraduates in a Nigerian university. *Sexual Addiction & Compulsivity*, *22*(3), 249–257.

American Psychiatric Association. (2013). *Diagnostic and statistical manual of mental disorders* (5th ed.). Arlington, VA: American Psychiatric Publishing.

Balon, R. (2016a). Lack of clarity in the DSM-5 criteria of voyeuristic disorder. *Journal of Sex & Marital Therapy*, *42*(5), 391–392.

Balon, R. (2016b). Voyeuristic disorder. In R. Balon (Ed.), *Practical guide to paraphilia and paraphilic disorders* (pp. 63–75). Cham, Switzerland: Springer.

Blechner, M. J. (2016). Psychoanalysis and sexual issues. *Contemporary Psychoanalysis*, *52*(4), 502–546.

Challinor, L. E., & Duff, S. (2017). Sexual offending hierarchies, personality attributions, and the clinical implications. *Journal of Forensic Practice*, *19*(3), 190–197.

Elder, W. B., Brooks, G. R., & Morrow, S. L. (2012). Sexual self-schemas of heterosexual men. *Psychology of Men & Masculinity*, *13*(2), 166–179.

Fedoroff, J. P. (2003). The paraphilic world. In S. B. Levine (Ed.), *Handbook of clinical sexuality for mental health professionals*. New York, NY: Brunner/Routledge.

Fisher, A., Castellini, G., Casale, H., et al. (2015). Hypersexuality, Paraphilic Behaviors, and Gender Dysphoria in Individuals with Klinefelter's Syndrome. *The Journal of Sexual Medicine*, *12*(12), 2413–2424.

Freund, K., & Blanchard, R. (1986). The concept of courtship disorder. *Journal of Sex & Marital Therapy, 12*(2), 79–92. doi:10.1080/00926238608415397

Hinderliter, A.C. (2010). Disregarding science, clinical utility, and the DSM's definitio of mental disorder: The case of exhibitionism, voyeurism, and frotteurism. *Archives of Sexual Behavior, 39*(6), 1235–1237.

Hocken, K., & Thorne, K. (2012). Voyeurism, exhibitionism and other non-contact sexual offences. In B. Winder & P. Banyard (Eds.), *A psychologist's casebook of crime: From arson to voyeurism* (pp. 243–263). New York, NY: Palgrave Macmillan.

Hopkins, T. A., Green, B. A., Carnes, P. J., & Campling, S. (2016). Varieties of intrusion: Exhibitionism and voyeurism. *Sexual Addiction & Compulsivity, 23*(1), 4–33.

Janssen, D. F. (2018). "Voyeuristic disorder": Etymological and historical note. *Archives of Sexual Behavior, 47*(5), 1307–1311.

Joing, I., & Vors, O. (2015). Victimisation and the social climate at secondary school: Changing rooms in PE and sport. *Déviance et Société, 39*(1), 51–71.

Krueger, R. B., & Kaplan, M. S. (2016). Noncontact paraphilic sexual offenses. In A. Phenix & H. M. Hoberman (Eds.), *Sexual offending: Predisposing antecedents, assessments, and management* (pp. 79–102). New York, NY: Springer.

Langstrom, N. (2010). The DSM diagnostic criteria for exhibitionism, voyeurism, and frotteurism. *Archives of Sexual Behavior, 39*(2), 317–324.

Menzies, R. P. D., Fedoroff, J. P., Green, C., & Isaacson, K. (1995). Prediction of dangerousness in male erotomania. *British Journal of Psychiatry, 166*, 529–536.

Newton, H. (2009). *Helmut Newton*. Practical Photography. Retrieved November 3, 2018, from http://photoquotations.com/a/511/Helmut+Newton

Quayle, E., & Hayes, E. (2015). Interventions with an internet sexual offender. In D. T. Wilxoc, T. Garrett, & L. Harkins (Eds.), *Sex offender treatment: A case study approach to issues and interventions* (pp. 163–180). Malden, MA: Wiley-Blackwell.

Ramadas, S. (2017). A peep into "Peeping Tom": Successful management of cyclothymia presenting as voyeuristic disorder. *The Primary Care Companion for CNS Disorders, 19*(3). doi:10.4088/PCC.16l02070

Shagaga, K. (2016). *Through the eyes of the voyeur: The lived subjective experience of males who self-identify as sexual addicts.* Doctoral dissertation, Chicago School of Professional Psychology, Chicago, IL (ProQuest Dissertations, Accession No. 3716735).

Stuyvesant, R. P., Mercier, D. G., & Haidle, A. (2014). Voyeurism: A case study. In W. T. O'Donohye (Ed.), *Case studies in sexual deviance: Toward evidence-based practice* (pp. 117–148). New York, NY: Routledge.

Voyeuristic disorder. (n.d.). World Health Organization. Retrieved July 11, 2018, from https://icd.who.int/browse11/l-m/en#/http://id.who.int/icd/entity/1832861162

World Health Organization. (2004). *International classification of diseases* (10th revision, 2nd ed.). Geneva, Switzerland: Author.

Yalcin, O., Guney, E., & Saripinar, E. G. (2014). Dramatic improvement with sertraline in a male adolescent with voyeurism. *Bulletin of Clinical Psychopharmacology, 24*(3), 292–294.

10
Other Specified Paraphilic Disorders

The only thing that is constant is change.

—Heraclitus (Plato 401d)

Introduction

The Fifth edition of the *Diagnostic and Statistical Manual of Mental Disorders* (DSM-5; American Psychiatric Association [APA], 2013) has a category of disorders termed *other specified paraphilic disorders* (OSPD). The DSM-5 diagnostic criteria for these disorders are contradictory, on the one hand referring to symptoms "characteristic of a paraphilic disorder" and on the other hand referring to symptoms that "do not meet the full criteria for any of the disorders in the paraphilic disorders class" (p. 705). The DSM-5 lists six specific paraphilias involving persistent sexual interest (6 months or longer): telephone scatalogia (obscene phone calls), necrophilia (corpses), zoophilia (animals), coprophilia (feces), klismaphilia (enemas), and urophilia (urine). The DSM-5 offers no explanation for why these six disorders are specified but does indicate there are others. The most likely explanation for their inclusion is because they were listed in previous versions of the DSM and the authors of the DSM-5 were instructed to make changes only if there was evidence to justify doing so.

Box 10.1 lists some of the paraphilias that have been described in the literature. It is a revised and expanded version of a previously published list (Fedoroff, 2003). There are several lists in existence that can be easily accessed on the Internet. However, some lists include sexual dysfunctions (physical problems having sex), gender dysphoric conditions, and even variations in sexual orientation, none of which are true paraphilias.

For good measure, the DSM-5 also includes a category termed *unspecified paraphilic disorder*, which is truly a wastebasket category for conditions with "symptoms characteristic of a paraphilic disorder . . . but do not meet criteria for any of the disorders in the paraphilic disorders diagnostic class" for situations in which "the clinician chooses *not* to specify the reason the criteria are not met" (APA, 2013, p. 705, italics in original).

Box 10.1 Paraphilias Described in the Literature

Other Specified Paraphilic Disorders

- Literature review on paraphilias not otherwise specified (Kafka, 2010b).
- After adding sertraline to an adolescent female's medical routine for 6 weeks, it was found that her paraphilias improved; these included "hypersexuality," urophagia, and coprophagia (Mendhekar & Duggal, 2005).

Abasiophilia

Definition: Sexual attraction to those who cannot walk (whether temporarily or permanently).

- A woman with abasiophilia and autoabasiophilia (Money, 1990b).

Acarophilia

Definition: Sexual arousal from scratching.

Acousticophilia

Definition: Sexual arousal from auditory stimulus, including those that are not intended to be erotic.

Acrophilia

Definition: Sexual arousal from heights.

Acrotomophilia

Definition: Sexual attraction to amputees.

- Two articles were found for acrotomophilia: one female with acrotomophilia and apotemnophilia (Money, 1990b) and one male with both paraphilias (Money & Simco, 1984).

Adult Baby Syndrome

Definition: Identification as a baby, not necessarily sexual.

- Case study of 38-year-old male with adult baby syndrome with gender identity issues (Kise & Nguyen, 2011).
- Explored the different sexual behaviors that members of the Adult Baby/Diaper Lover community engage in and its associations with their attachment styles and gender (Hawkinson & Zamboni, 2014).
- See also Paraphilic Infantilism.

Agalmatophilia

Definition: Sexual attraction to a statue, mannequin, or doll.

- Two papers examine agalmatophilia. One describes it as common in "ancient times" (Scobie & Taylor, 1975), and the other reports only one documented case of it (White, 1978).

Agonophilia

Definition: Sexual arousal from a partner pretending to resist before being overpowered, and consequently engaging in sexual acts.

Agrexophilia

Definition: Sexual arousal from knowing or discovering that one is engaging in sexual acts.

Algolagnia

Definition: Sexual arousal from receiving and giving pain (sadomasochism). For more details, see Chapter 7.

Amaurophilia

Definition: Sexual arousal from one's partner being unable to see.

Anasteemaphilia

Definition: Sexual arousal to a partner who is either significantly shorter or taller than oneself.

Andromimetophilia/Genemimetophilia/Transvestophilia

Definition: Sexual attraction to a transsexual person(s). For more details, see Chapter 8.

Anililagnia

Definition: Sexual attraction to "older" women.

Anthropophagy

Definition: Sexual arousal from eating human flesh.

Apodysophilia

Definition: See Exhibitionism.

Apotemnophilia

Definition: Sexual arousal by an able-bodied person to have a limb amputated or to become disabled.

- Literature reviews of apotemnophilia and its etiology. Other names associated with apotemnophilia are *body integrity identity disorder* and *xenomelia* (Baubet et al., 2007; Donix & Reuster, 2007; Everaerd, 1983; Godlewski & Szalankiewicz, 1987; Sedda & Bottini, 2014).
- According to the literature on body integrity identity disorder (BIID), BIID is also found in non-Western cultures, including Japan and China (Blom et al., 2016).
- The right parietal lobe is associated with body image disorders, and damage to it might be the cause of some disorders. McGeoch et al. (2011) state that the term *xenomelia* appropriately describes this phenomenon, rather than BIID and apotemnophilia, because its origins are from brain damage. Apotemnophilia was also previously found to be a neurological disorder linked to the right parietal lobe (Brang, McGeoch, & Ramachandran, 2008).
- The ethics of amputating a limb when presented with apotemnophilia are discussed by Dua (2010) and Ryan (2009); there was no known treatment method for it previously (Money, Jobaris, & Furth, 1977).
- Cognitive–behavioral therapy to treat apotemnophilia (Braam, Visser, Cath, & Hoogendijk, 2006).

Aquaphilia

Definition: Sexual arousal from people being underwater and/or sexual acts in water.

Arachnophilia

Definition: A sexual attraction to spiders.

Aretifism

Definition: Sexual attraction to people who are barefoot (see also Podophilia).

Asphyxiophilia

Definition: Sexual arousal from restricting oxygen. Usually referring to self-suffocation to sexual arousal. Also called "autoerotic self-asphyxiation."

- Incidence of asphyxiation was found to be 0.5–2 cases per 1 million inhabitants in Scandinavia per year (Innala & Ernulf, 1989).
- Case studies of autoerotic asphyxiation (Cooper, 1996; Cosgray, Hanna, Fawley, & Money, 1991; Quackelbeen, Nobus, & Temmerman, 1997; Williams, Phillips, & Ahmed, 2000; Zaviacic, 1993).
- Article on asphyxiophilia, which discusses the epidemiology, characteristics, and familial effects (Innala & Ernulf, 1987).
- Considers whether erotic asphyxiation is an addiction (Ernoul, Orsat, Mesu, Garre, Jean-Bernard, & Richard-Devantoy, 2012).

- Discussion of sexual asphyxia (Book & Perumal, 1993).
- Treatment of autoerotic asphyxiation in an autistic male using a behavioral and psychoeducational program (Thompson & Beail, 2002).

Autagonistophilia

Definition: Sexual arousal from being sexually viewed (see also Chapter 3).

Autassassinophilia

Definition: Sexual arousal from the thought or risk of being killed.

- Discusses the phenomenology of autassassinophilia (Downing, 2004).

Autoandrophilia/Autogynephilia

Definition: Sexual arousal from idea of being the other gender (see also Chapter 8).

- Study included 51 women who were asked if they have been aroused by thinking of themselves as a woman (3% could be classified as utogynephilic; Moser, 2009).

Autoerotic Self-Asphyxia

Definition: See Asphyxiophilia.

Autohemofetishism

Definition: Sexual arousal from making oneself bleed.

- Autohemofetishism and "injection masochism" associated with intravenous drug users. Explained as due to classical conditioning (Bartholomew, 1973).

Autonepiophilia

Definition: Sexual arousal from dressing and role playing as an infant; also called paraphilic infantilism.

- Case study of an 80-year-old man with paraphilic infantilism (Pandita-Gunawardena, 1990).
- Treated paraphilic disorders (including transsexual fetishism, pedophilic disorder, and paraphilic infantilism) with depo-medroxyprogesterone (Lehne & Money, 2000).

Autophagiophilia

Definition: Sexual arousal from self-ingestion.

Biastophilia

Definition: Sexual arousal from sexually assaulting another person (without consent).

- Discussion of biastophilia and erotophonophilia and the legal system (Money, 1990a).

Candaulism

Definition: Sexual arousal from exposing a female sexual partner to others.

- Out of 95 swingers, 42% reported arousal from candaulism (Houngbedji & Guillem, 2016).

Capnolagnia

Definition: Sexual arousal from seeing and/or smelling another person smoking.

Catherophilia

Definition: Sexual arousal from catheterization.

Celebriphilia

Definition: Sexual arousal from celebrities.

Chremastistophlia

Definition: Sexual attraction by being robbed, detained, or charged for sexual services. See also Harpaxophilia.

Chronophilia

Definition: Sexual attraction to specific age ranges.

- Pedophilia is described as a chronophilia, which is "a sexual orientation for age" (Seto, 2017). Several comments have been published in response to Seto that support his theories (Beier & Amelung, 2017; Janssen, 2017; Miletski, 2017; Mokros, 2017). However, Fedoroff (2018) and Baily and Hsu (2017) challenge several claims in the article by Seto, suggesting that sexual orientation should not be conflated with sexual interest. Others argue for more research (Bailey & Hsu, 2017; Imhoff, Banse, & Schmidt, 2017).

Coprophagia

Definition: Sexual arousal from consuming feces.

- Case study of a man with depression and substance use-related problems with this paraphilia (Wise & Goldberg, 1995).

Coprophilia

Definition: Sexual arousal from feces and defecating.

- Case study of a man with intellectual disability who argues the coprophilia was a response to a "limited institutional environment" (Hingsburger, 1989).
- Case study of a man with Gilles de la Tourette syndrome who also developed coprophilia (Marneros, 1984).
- Case study of coprophilia that manifested with other symptoms, such as reduced human contact and increased attachment to pets (Xavier, 1955).

Crush Fetish

Definition: Sexual arousal from seeing an object being crushed.

Dacnolagnomania

Definition: Sexual arousal from murdering another person. Also known as *erotophonophilia*.

- Articles that examine dacnolagnomania (also known as "lust murder") (Arrigo & Purcell, 2001; McClellan, 2008; Money, 1990a; Purcell, 2000).

Dacryphilia

Definition: Sexual arousal from seeing tears or hearing crying.

- Compassion, dominance and submission, and curled lips were found to be related to dacryphilia and the dacryphilic experience (Greenhill & Griffiths, 2016).
- Case study of a woman who pathologizes her dacryphilia (Greenhill & Griffiths, 2016).

Dendrophilia

Definition: Sexual arousal from and/or sexual attraction to trees.

Dermatophilia

Definition: Sexual arousal from skin, leather, and/or fur.

Devotee

Definition: Sexual attraction to disabled person(s).

- Discusses the devotee community and the responses of disabled person(s) to devotees (Aguilera, 2000).
- Article that includes the debate of being attracted to those who are disabled and whether this redefines beauty standards (Solvang, 2007).

Dippoldism

Definition: Sexual arousal from the use of corporal punishment (see also Chapter 7).

Doraphilia

Definition: Sexual attraction to disfigured bodies.

Ecouteurism

Definition: Sexual arousal from the sound of sex, especially overhearing others having sex.

Emetophilia

Definition: Sexual arousal from vomiting or seeing others vomit.

Entomophilia

Definition: Sexual attraction to insects. See also Formicophilia.

Ephebophilia

Definition: Sexual attraction to mid- to late adolescence (ages 15–19 years); see also Chronophilia.

- Most, if not all, research articles on ephebophilia tend to include cases involving the Roman Catholic clergy (Brehob, 2006; Cartor, Cimbolic, & Tallon, 2008; Cimbolic & Cartor, 2006; Gerard, Jobes, Cimbolic, Ritzler, & Montana, 2003; Gerard-Sharp, 2000; Lee, 2007; Musser, Cimbolic, & Rossetti, 1995; Noonan-Karstens, 2009; Pallone, 2002; Rossetti, Anthony, Cimbolic, & Wright, 1996).
- Theories of ephebophilia (Lothstein, 1990).
- Treatment: 12-step recovery program was used on two men with ephebophilia (Nu Ez, 2003).

Eproctophilia

Definition: Sexual arousal from flatulence.

- Case study of a male who began engaging in "eproctophile acts" at approximately age 16 or 17 years (Griffiths, 2013).

Erotic asphyxiation

Definition: See Asphyxiophilia.

Erotophonophilia

Definition: See Dacnolagnomania.

Exhibitionism

Definition: Sexual arousal from exposing oneself to non-consenting people. See Chapter 3.

Faunoiphilia

Definition: Sexual arousal from observing animals mating.

Feederism

Definition: Sexual attraction to weight gain, feeding, and overweight person(s).

- Case study of a female with feederism (Terry & Vasey, 2011).
- Found that people from the general population rated visual stimuli of feeding to be more sexually arousing than neutral stimuli (Terry, Suschinsky, Lalumiere, & Vasey, 2012).
- Feederism is described as a "communal behavior" (Prohaska, 2014).

Formicophilia

Definition: Sexual arousal from having small insects crawling or "nibbling" on one's body.

- Case of a Buddhist male with formicophilia, who was treated with counseling and behavior therapy (Dewaraja, 1987) and anti-androgenic hormones (Dewaraja & Money, 1986).

Frotteurism

Definition: Sexual arousal from touching non-consenting person(s). See Chapter 5.

Gerontophilia

Definition: Sexual attraction to elderly person(s).

- Case study of a man who attempted to sexually assault four women in their 70s and 80s (Oules, Boscredon, & Bataille, 1977).

Gonophilia

Definition: Sexual arousal due to knees.

Gynemimetophilia

Definition: Sexual arousal toward men with breasts (often including a female body type aside from genitalia: "she-males").

Harpaxophilia

Definition: Sexual arousal from being robbed. See also Chremastistophlia.

Hebephilia

Definition: Sexual attraction to early adolescence (ages 11–14 years). Also see Chronophilia, Ephebophilia, and Pedophilia.

- Hebephilia is often grouped with pedophilia in research studies (Beier, Amelung, Grundmann, & Kuhle, 2015; Stephens, Cantor, Goodwill, & Seto, 2017).
- When evaluating the construct validity of hebephilia, it was found that there was much overlap between pedophilia and hebephilia. The divergent validity between pedophilia and hebephilia was found to be poor (Stephens, Seto, Goodwill, & Cantor, 2017).
- However, individuals with hebephilia report more distress and "deviant" personality characteristics compared to individuals with pedophilia (Beier et al., 2013; Beier, Amelung, Kuhle, et al., 2015). Also, it was found that phallometric testing could detect hebephilia with 70.0% sensitivity and 90.7% specificity compared to pedophilia, which had 46.9% sensitivity and 100% specificity (Blanchard et al., 2009; Cantor & McPhail, 2015).
- It was also attempted to demonstrate differences between pedophilia and hebephilia using the Abel Assessment for Sexual Interest-2 (Burke, 2014).
- It is explained that hebephilia was not included in the DSM-5 because the evidence for it being a disease is unconvincing (Good & Burstein, 2012; Hames & Blanchard, 2012; Singy, 2015a). Also, including it would have legal and research consequences (Franklin, 2010).

Hematophilia

Definition: Sexual arousal due to blood.

Heterophilia

Definition: Sexual attraction toward the other gender.

Hierophilia

Definition: Sexual arousal associated with religious objects.

Hodophilia

Definition: Sexual arousal from traveling to new places.

Homeovestism

Definition: Sexual arousal from wearing clothes that are congruent with one's gender role.

- Homeovestism is often associated with fetishism and transvestism (Zavitzianos, 1972, 1977).

Homilophilia

Definition: Sexual arousal from religious speeches and/or sermons.

Hoplophilia

Definition: Sexual arousal associated with firearms.

Hybristophilia

Definition: Sexual arousal from a partner committing a transgression within the partnership and/or one's partner committing a crime.

- Hyberistophilia was once known as enclitophilia (Benezech, 2016).

Hygrophilia

Definition: Sexual arousal from fabrics.

Iatronudia

Definition: Sexual attraction to doctors and/or those in the medical profession.

Incest

Definition: Sexual attraction to relative(s).

- A preliminary search on PsycINFO using the term "incest" with additional limitations that results would show publications between 2008 and 2018 yielded 289 results. Because of the extant research on this specific paraphilia and in consideration for space, the search was further limited to include only literature and clinical reviews (Abu-Baker, 2013; Anonymous, 2008; Lapointe & Le Bosse, 2010; Panagakis, 2012; Yates, 2017) and meta-analyses (Pullman, Sawatsky, Babchishin, McPhail, & Seto, 2017; Seto, Babchishin, Pullman, & McPhail, 2015; Ventus, Antfolk, & Salo, 2017).
- Literature review on incest with siblings (Panagakis, 2012; Yates, 2017).
- Meta-analysis found that sociolegal incest offenders have more antisocial features compared to biological incest offenders. However, biological incest offenders have more mental health problems (Pullman et al., 2017).
- Meta-analysis found that victims of intrafamilial abuse were younger than victims of extrafamilial abuse (Ventus et al., 2017).
- A literature review found that there was limited research on whether it was more beneficial or harmful for children to have contact with the parent who abused them. However, it was found that it is usually more harmful (Anonymous, 2008).
- Literature review of resilience after incest (Lapointe & Le Bosse, 2010).
- Review of how non-Western cultures respond to incest (Abu-Baker, 2013).

Infantophilia

Definition: Sexual attraction to infants (between ages 0 and 4 years).

- A comparison of infantophilia with pedophilia found no significant differences in characteristics between the two groups (Greenberg, Bradford, & Curry, 1995).

Katoptronophilia

Definition: Sexual arousal from the use of mirrors, such as watching oneself having sex and/or one's partner(s).

Kleptolagnia

Definition: Sexual arousal from committing theft.

- Study examined 224 participants who committed sexually motivated burglaries. It was found that sexually motivated burglars differed from regular burglars in their response to opportunistic situational cues (Pedneault, Beauregard, Harris, & Knight, 2015).
- Found three types of sexual burglars: non-contact burglars that did not involve theft, violence, and weapon; versatile contact, involving sexual assault, theft, violence, and weapon; and sexual assault without theft, violence, or weapon (Brankley, Goodwill, & Reale, 2014).
- A case study written in French (Van Renynghe De Voxvrie & Massion-Verniory, 1964).

Klismaphilia

Definition: Sexual arousal from enemas.

- Discussion of why klismaphilia is physiologically gratifying (Agnew, 1982)
- Two cases of men with klismaphilia (Denko, 1973).
- Person(s) with klismaphilia typically does not want treatment (Denko, 1976).

Lactaphilia

Definition: Sexual arousal from breastfeeding or breast-sucking.

Lust Murder

Definition: See Dacnolagnomania and/or Erotophonophilia.

Macrophilia

Definition: Sexual arousal from the idea of sexual relations with giants.

Maiesiophilia
Definition: Sexual attraction to pregnant women.

Maschalagnia
Definition: Sexual arousal to armpits.

Mask Fetishism
Definition: Sexual arousal to masks and/or removing masks.

Masochism
Definition: Sexual arousal from experiencing pain and/or humiliation. See Chapter 7.

Mechanophilia
Definition: Sexual attraction to vehicles.

Melissophilia
Definition: Sexual attraction to bees.

Melolagnia
Definition: Sexual arousal associated with music.

Menophilia
Definition: sexual arousal from menstruation and/or tampons.

Microphilia
Definition: Sexual arousal associated with people with a small stature.

Morphophilia
Definition: Sexual arousal from differences in body size.

Mucophilia
Definition: Sexual arousal from mucous.

Mysophilia
Definition: Sexual arousal from objects that are soiled or filthy. An example is used underwear. See also Salirophilia.

- Case of mysophilia in a male who also had urophilia, fetishism, and masochism (Rousal & Brinchcin, 1971).
- Comments on a case of mysophilia (Fraenkel, 1954).

Nanophilia

Definition: Sexual attraction toward a short partner. See also Anasteemaphilia and Microphilia.

Narratophilia

Definition: Sexual arousal from storytelling that uses erotic language.

Nasophilia

Definition: Sexual arousal from noses.

Necrobestialism

Definition: Sexual arousal from dead animals and/or sexual interest in engaging in sexual acts with dead animals.

Necrophilia

Definition: Sexual arousal from engaging in sexual acts with dead bodies.

- Articles that were published between 2008 and 2018 on necrophilia (Fitzgerald, 2011; Giordano, White, & Lester, 2012; Higgs, Stefanska, Carter, & Browne, 2017; Lemma, 2013; Lester, White, King, & Drive, 2011; Pettigrew, 2017, 2019; Stein, Schlesinger, & Pinizzotto, 2010; Troyer, 2008).
- Necrophilia could be related to Asperger's syndrome (Fitzgerald, 2011; Lester et al., 2011).
- Study that examined cannibals and whether necrophilia was present (Giordano et al., 2012).
- Although sexual murderers may engage in sexual acts with a dead body, it does not necessarily mean they have necrophilia. However, they may have sadism (Higgs et al., 2017).
- The United States has no laws specifically against necrophilia (Troyer, 2008).

Case Studies

- Case study of patient treated for eczema who described necrophilic fantasies during treatment (Lemma, 2013).
- Case study examining the relationship between necrophilia and somnophilia (Pettigrew, 2017).
- Case study on the development of necrophilia (Pettigrew, 2019).
- Case review of necrophilia that resulted in sexual homicides (Stein, Schlesinger, & Pinizzotto, 2010).

Nosophilia

Definition: Sexual attraction to a person who has a terminal illness.

Odaxelagnia
Definition: Sexual arousal from being bitten or from biting.

Olfactophilia
Definition: Sexual arousal from body odors.

Omorashi
Definition: Sexual arousal from the sensation of needing to urinate. See also Urolagnia/Urophilia.

Paraphilic Infantilism
Definition: Sexual arousal to newborns (aged 0–2 years). See also Autonepiophilia.

Partialism
Definition: Sexual arousal from a specific body part (excluding genitals).

- Articles published usually report that partialism is concurrent with other paraphilias (Chan & Beauregard, 2016; Chan, Beauregard, & Myers, 2015).
- Suggests that the distinction between partialism and fetishism is no longer relevant (Kafka, 2010a).

Pecattiphilia
Definition: Sexual arousal from performing what one believes are "sinful" acts.

Pedophilia
Definition: Sexual attraction to children. See also Chapter 6.

Pedovestism
Definition: Sexual arousal from wearing children's clothes.

Phobophilia
Definition: Sexual arousal from fear.

Pictophilia
Definition: Sexual arousal from photographs (i.e., pornography).

Piquerism
Definition: Sexual arousal from picking and/or stabbing.

Plushophilia
Definition: Sexual arousal from stuffed animals.

Podophilia

Definition: Sexual arousal from feet.

Pseudozoophilia

Definition: Sexual arousal from one's partner posing as an animal.

Public Masturbation

Definition: Sexual arousal from masturbating in public without being seen. Also see Exhibitionism and Chapter 3.

- Most case studies involve individuals who are on the autism spectrum and have intellectual disabilities and/or developmental disabilities (Cook, Altman, Shaw, & Blaylock, 1978; Gill, 2012; Hurley & Sovner, 1983; Lundervold & Young, 1992; Lunsky, Frijters, Griffiths, Watson, & Williston, 2007).
- It was found that men with intellectual disabilities who had committed sex offenses (e.g., public masturbation) did not significantly differ in the amount of sexual knowledge they had compared to individuals with intellectual disabilities who did not commit any sexual offenses (Lunsky et al., 2007).
- Social skills training was found to help men with developmental disabilities who had offended (Lundervold & Young, 1992).
- 10.5% of individuals began having interest in exhibitionism and/or public masturbation following a traumatic brain injury (Simpson, Sabaz, & Daher, 2013).
- Children who engaged in public masturbation treated with behavioral therapy (Cook et al., 1978; Dufrene, Watson, & Weaver, 2005; Ferguson & Rekers, 1979; Hurley & Sovner, 1983; Janzen & Peacock, 1978; Wagner, 1968).
- Case study of a man treated with functional analytic psychotherapy and acceptance and commitment therapy for exhibitionism and public masturbation (Paul, Marx, & Orsillo, 1999).

Pygophilia

Definition: Sexual arousal from buttocks.

Pyrophilia

Definition: Sexual arousal from fire and/or fire-setting.

Retifism

Definition: Sexual arousal from shoes.

- Case study of a male with a foot fetishist—notably, the authors reported their patient as having retifism instead of podophilia (Kunjukrishnan, Pawlak, & Varan, 1988).

Rhabdophilia

Definition: Sexual arousal from self-flagellation.

Sadism

Definition: Sexual arousal from having control. See Chapter 7.

Saliromania

Definition: Sexual arousal from degradation of appearance.

Salirophilia

Definition: Sexual arousal from soiling the sexual partner(s) or from perspiration. See Mysophilia and Coprophilia.

Scopophilia/Scoptophilia

Definition: Sexual arousal from looking at erotic objects.

- The history of scopophilia (Allen, 1974).
- Case studies of men with scopophilia with voyeurism (Almansi, 1979; Stoylen, 1985), in which one was treated with cognitive–behavioral therapy (Stoylen, 1985).
- Case study of scopophilia, wherein the author believes sadism may be involved (Fenichel, 1937).
- Discussion of pornography and scopophilia and its associations (de Giorgio, 1985).

Scoptic Syndrome

Definition: Sexual arousal from being castrated (male).

Somnophilia

Definition: Sexual arousal due to an unconscious person.

- Discussions of the similarities between somnophilia and necrophilia (Knafo, 2015; Pettigrew, 2017).
- Case study of somnophilia in which the victim was drugged (Lauerma, 2016).

Sthenolagiophilia

Definition: Sexual arousal from female bodybuilders.

Sthenolagnia

Definition: Sexual arousal from seeing muscles or a show of strength.

Stigmatophilia

Definition: Sexual arousal from piercings, tattoos, and/or uniforms.

Stitophilia

Definition: Sexual arousal from food.

Symphorophilia

Definition: Sexual arousal from staging and/or watching response to a disaster.

Tamakeri

Definition: Sexual arousal from causing pain to a man's testes, typically by kicking or stepping on the testes.

Taphophilia

Definition: Sexual arousal from being buried alive.

Telephone Scataologia

Definition: Sexual arousal from making obscene telephone calls.

- Studies that examined telephone scatologia. Notably, most were published prior to 2008 (Dalby, 1988; Ginsburg, Ogletree, & Silakowski, 2003; Goldberg & Wise, 1985; Lande, 1993; Pakhomou, 2006; Price, Gutheil, Commons, Kafka, & Dodd-Kimmey, 2001a, 2001b; Price, Kafka, Commons, Gutheil, & Simpson, 2002; Saunders & Awad, 1991).
- Case study of telephone scatologia with schizophrenic symptoms and other psychiatric disorders (Altintas, Oguz, Oguz, & Inanc, 2016).
- Psychodynamic treatment was used to treat telephone scataologia in one case study (Goldberg & Wise, 1985).

Teratophilia

Definition: Sexual arousal from deformed bodies. See also Doraphilia.

Thesauromania

Definition: Sexual arousal from collecting women's clothing.

Timophilia

Definition: Sexual arousal from wealth and/or status.

Toucherism

Definition: Sexual arousal from touching a non-consenting person. See Chapter 5.

Transvestism

See Chapter 8.

Transvestophilia

Definition: Sexual arousal toward people with transvestism and/or cross-dressing.

Trichophilia

Definition: Sexual arousal related to hair.

Troilism

Definition: Sexual arousal from situations involving three people. See also Candaulism.

- Examined troilism with gay men (Lehmiller, Ley, & Savage, 2018).

Undinism

Definition: Sexual arousal from water and/or urine.

- Case history of a 17-year-old boy with udinism/urolagnia (Denson, 1982).

Urolagnia/Urophilia

Definition: Sexual arousal from drinking urine or from urination ("golden showers"). Also known as urophilia.

- Theory of urophilia's manifestation (Christoffel, 1934).
- Urolagnia is typically treated as a fetishism or masochism in Germany (Klimmer, 1968).
- Four cases of urolagnia (Massion-Verniory & Dumont, 1958).

Urophagia

Definition: Sexual arousal from drinking urine. See also Urolagnia/Urophili.

Vampirism

Definition: Sexual arousal from drinking blood.

- Theory on the etiology of vampirism (Gubb, Segal, Khota, & Dicks, 2006; Prins, 1985).

- Discussion of Renfield's syndrome, which is an "obsession" (not necessarily sexual) to drink blood (Olry & Haines, 2011; Oppawasky, 2010).
- Cases of cannibalism and vampirism (Benezech, Bourgeois, Boukhabza, & Yesavage, 1981; Fellion, Duflot, Anglade, & Fraillon, 1980).
- Reviews of vampirism (Jaffe & DiCataldo, 1994; McCully, 1964; Vanden Bergh & Kelly, 1964).
- Treatment of vampirism and other psychiatric disorders using carbamazepine and fluvoxamine (Cro, Peronti, & Bersani, 1997).

Vomerophilia

Definition: Sexual arousal from vomit or vomiting. See also Emetophilia.

Vorarephilia

Definition: Sexual arousal from consuming or being consumed by another person or creature.

- Case study of a man with a "submissive" vorarephilic fantasy (Lykins & Cantor, 2014).

Voyeurism

Definition: Sexual arousal from watching others undressing, nude, and/or engaging in sexual activity. See Chapter 9.

Wannabe

Definition: Sexual arousal from the wish to have a paraphilia, especially related to becoming disabled. See Apotemnophilia and Devotee.

Zoophilia and Bestiality

Definitions: zoophilia: Sexual arousal from engaging in sexual relations with non-human animals; *bestiality*: Legal term for human having sex with a non-human animal.

- Literature review on bestiality (Holoyda, Sorrentino, Friedman, & Allgire, 2018).
- Studies on zoophilic practices that were published from 2008 to 2018 (de Cassio Zequi et al., 2012; Earls & Lalumiere, 2009; Eichenberg & Surangkanjanajai, 2012; Maratea, 2011; Sendler, 2018).
- The prevalence of bestiality in juvenile sex offenders is underreported (Schenk, Cooper-Lehki, Keelan, & Fremouw, 2014).
- Some people with zoophilia claim it is their "orientation" (Sendler, 2018).
- An online survey of zoophilia (Eichenberg & Surangkanjanajai, 2012).

- Those who engaged in childhood bestiality were found to have a higher risk of committing "interpersonal crimes" as adults (Hensley, Tallichet, & Dutkiewicz, 2010).
- Imitating dog behaviors is not the same as zoophilia (Wignall & McCormack, 2017).

Case studies

- Case study of a patient with zoophilia and autism (Chandradasa & Champika, 2017).
- Case study of a patient who reported zoophilia as part of the early development of psychosis (Lesandric, Orlovic, Peitl, & Karlovic, 2017).
- Case study of a man with schizophrenia and zoophilia (Amoo, Abayomio, & Olashore, 2012).
- Case study in which zoophilic behaviors ceased once mania was treated (Eroglu, Caliskan, & Topbas, 2015).
- Case study of a man with "hypersexuality" who engaged in zoophilic behaviors (Othman, Razak, & Zakaria, 2014).
- Case study of a man who exhibited zoophilic behaviors as his Parkinson's disease progressed (Almeida, de Oliveira Filho, Lopes Nery, Guimaraes Silva, & Campos Sousa, 2013).

Zoosadism

Definition: Sexual arousal from performing cruel/sadistic acts to animals.

- Some Swiss children and adolescents with aggression problems engaged in zoosadism (Wochner & Klosinski, 1988).

Books and Book Chapters

Otherwise Specified Paraphilic Disorder

Briken, P., Klein, V., & von Franque, F. (2016). Other specified paraphilic disorders. In R. Balon (Ed.), *Practical guide to paraphilia and paraphilic disorders* (pp. 187–196). Cham, Switzerland: Springer.

Asphyxiophilia

Hucker, S. (2016). Autoerotic asphyxia and asphyxiophilia. In B. A. Sharpless (Ed.), *Unusual and rare psychological disorders: A handbook for clinical practice and research* (pp. 149–163). New York, NY: Oxford University Press.

Money, J., Wainwright, G., & Hingsburger, D. (1991). *The breathless orgasm: A lovemap biography of asphyxiophilia*. Amherst, MA: Prometheus.

Bestiality

de Cassio Zequi, S. (2014). The medical consequences of sex between humans and animals. In G. H. Allez (Ed.), *Sexual diversity and sexual offending: Research, assessment, and clinical treatment in psychosexual therapy* (pp. 185–202). London, UK: Karnac.

Coprophilia
London, L. S., & Caprio, F. S. (1950). Coprophilia. In L. S. London & F. S. Caprio (Eds.), *Sexual deviations* (pp. 557–575). Washington, DC: Linacre Press.

Ephebophilia
Lothstein, L. M. (1990). Psychological theories of pedophilia and ephebophilia. In S. J. Rossetti(Ed.), *Slayer of the soul: Child sexual abuse and the Catholic Church* (pp. 19–43). Mystic, CT: Twenty-Third Publications.

Hebephilia
Singy, P. (2015b). Danger and difference: The stakes of hebephilia. In S. Demazeux & P. Singy (Eds.), *The DSM-5 in perspective: Philosophical reflections on the psychiatric Babel* (pp. 113–124). New York, NY: Springer.
Stephens, S., & Seto, M. C. (2016). Hebephilic sexual offending. In A. Phenix & H. M. Hoberman (Eds.), *Sexual offending: Predisposing antecedents, assessments, and management* (pp. 29–43). New York, NY: Springer.

Necrophilia
West, S. G., & Resnick, P. J. (2017). Necrophilia. In B. A. Sharpless (Ed.), *Unusual and rare psychological disorders: A handbook for clinical practice and research* (pp. 124–135). New York, NY: Oxford University Press.

Scopophilia
Allen, D. W. (Ed.). (1974). *The fear of looking or scopophilic—Exhibitionistic conflicts.* Charlottesville, VA: University of Virginia Press.

Telephone Scatologia
Newring, K. A. B. (2014). Telephone scatologia. In W. T. O'Donohue (Ed.), *Case studies in sexual deviance: Toward evidence-based practice* (pp. 168–194). New York, NY: Routledge.

Urolagnia
London, L. S., & Caprio, F. S. (1950). Urolagnia. In L. S. London & F. S. Caprio (Eds.), *Sexual deviations* (pp. 576–587). Washington, DC: Linacre Press.

The fact that most paraphilias fall under the OSDP criteria is a problem, suggesting the DSM-5 has defaulted to simply providing a list rather than a useful, evidence-based classification system. But the problem is worse than it seems. Although the list of paraphilias provided includes more than 100 paraphilias in the OSDP category, it is an underestimation of the true number. Accepting that fetishes are conditions in which sexual arousal is provoked by an inanimate object, the number of potential fetishes is limited only by the number of objects that can be named. Furthermore, virtually every paraphilia has an opposite. Obvious examples are exhibitionism (exposing) and voyeurism (spying) or sadism (non-consensual control) and masochism (loss of control) (see Chapter 7, Figures 7.1 and 7.2).

The statement that every paraphilia has an opposite may seem surprising. However, patients often report that their unconventional sexual interest(s) in many ways is caused by a sense of anxiety leading to opposing interests. Examining this more closely, it is clear that sexual feelings are normal and vital not only to individual health but also to the survival of the species. Despite this, many people have feelings of guilt about sex. One way to deal with this problem is to develop sexual feelings that are the opposite of conventional sexual interests. A person who feels guilty about engaging in sex with a person they love may divert their interests toward a person or thing or situation in which sex and love do not coexist.

As a result, for all the paraphilias listed in Box 10.1, there is a paraphilia that seems opposite. It is fascinating that people often have opposite paraphilias—for example, people with voyeurism (spying) often also have exhibitionism (being seen). This fact can assist both in assessment and in treatment. A person with a sexual interest in children may also have a sexual interest in older people that with treatment can replace the pedophilic interest. In some cases, paraphilic interests take the form of counterphobic interests. In the same way that some people with acrophobia (fear of heights) become parachutists, some people with a fear of intimacy develop sexual interests in inanimate objects or in unavailable sexual partners.

In addition, every paraphilia can be directed toward a target of any gender or be self-directed. This means that any list of paraphilias will never be comprehensive.See Chapter 11 for comments on this issue.

The DSM-5 lists six specific paraphilias in the text for OSPD that provide a basis for a broader view of the paraphilias in general.

Telephone Scatologia

This condition is characterized by the practice of making obscene phone calls to non-consenting people. It is a paraphilia that has been classified as a type of "courtship disorder" because it involves a short-circuiting of conventional courtship behavior. Its prevalence appears to have been significantly diminished by telephone "call display," which allows victims to quickly identify the caller. Surprisingly, even people who should know better continue to be arrested. A case in point is the president of American University, whose obscene phone calls were traced to his private university office (Berendzen, 1993). His autobiography, in which he presents his theory regarding why he engaged in the acts that led to his dismissal, in fact suggests that his acts were actually a substitution for other paraphilic interests. Clinicians assessing patients presenting with OSPD paraphilias should consider the possibility that these are a substitution for a potentially more serious paraphilic interest.

Variations of telephone scatologia now include people who post sexual photographs to social media sites or to individuals who are non-consenting. An important variation are men who, while masturbating, call rape crisis lines. In most cases, these men are taking advantage of the fact that the operators are accustomed to speaking about sex-related issues. Men who are sexually aroused by talking to strangers while masturbating can be further subclassified on the basis of the sexual topics they choose to describe. In a manner analogous to men who masturbate in their parked cars while watching women but who have no wish to be seen, some men engage in nonsexual banter while they masturbate. These variations, which are paraphilic because they are sexually motivated, need to be distinguished from antisocial acts committed by men who are motivated by anger or opportunism.

Necrophilia

This condition is characterized by a persistent sexual interest in death or dead people. People with this condition do not like the idea of being watched (true spectatoring) and are motivated by the fact that any sexual activity with a dead person will not be witnessed. Reasons for not wanting to be seen while having sex can include social phobia, embarrassment, guilt, and shame. Another common motivating theme is the fact that the dead person cannot end the relationship. This idea was described in detail concerning a serial sexual killer, Dennis Nilsen, in a book that summarized his stated motivation, *Killing for Company* (Masters, 1985). Three more motivations for necrophilia are the ability to carry out illegal acts without being witnessed (e.g., a man who targets dead children), arousal by the taboo nature of sexual relations with a corpse, and arousal by the idea of being in total control of a situation in which anything may happen. This latter motivation is often found in women with necrophilia. These variations need to be distinguished from people who are motivated by the idea of hunting and killing the target or by sadistic interests and from people who are motivated by the idea of cannibalism.

Zoophilia

Zoophilia, characterized by persistent sexual interest in animals, is a paraphilia that typically induces feelings of revulsion when people first hear of it. This contributes to commentators endorsing theories that reflect more their emotional reaction to the syndrome than to actual data. At the end of a presentation on the topic of zoophilia, Dr. S. Hatter Friedman asked for a show of hands from the audience concerning how many believed zoophilia (sexual interest in animals) and bestiality (sex with animals) should be illegal on the basis of cruelty to animals under any circumstances. Most raised their hands. Then she asked how many in the audience were vegetarians. She had dramatically demonstrated that it is the fact that zoophilic acts involve sex with animals that raises concern, rather than issues of nonconsent and harm to animals that are raised by examination of practices in the food industry.

Case Report 10.1

An athletic young man was referred by a psychiatrist due to "atypical grief and relationship problems." The man agreed with his psychiatrist's assessment. He explained that he was suffering grief due to the death of a cow on a farm where he worked as a farmhand. Asked why he had come to the Sexual Behaviours Clinic, he admitted that he had engaged in ongoing penile–vaginal sex with the cow. He quickly added that every sexual encounter had been "consensual" and accompanied by what he described as mutual feelings of love. He added that he knew other men who treated cows "like animals with no respect for their feelings." He said he had always been "monogamous" with his cow but also admitted to looking at zoophilic pornography. With some reluctance, he agreed to attend group therapy. He was worried about coming into contact with "sex offenders." He did not know that the group was attended by two other men with variants of zoophilia (different animals, different sex acts, and different degrees of "affection"). The focus of therapy in the social skills group he attended was to improve social skills supportive of relationships with consenting adults.

Acceptance of behaviors involving sex between people and animals varies between cultures and venues. For example, one survey of 47 men living in Cordoba, Columbia, reported that 32 of the participants had sex with an animal (primarily donkeys) sometime between ages 7 and 30 years. Of these, 18 said they would want their sons to have the same experience. The authors concluded that there is a cultural belief in this area that sex with animals helps "correct" nonculturally accepted behaviors such as "homosexuality and drug use" (Medina-Pérez, Garcia-Vega, & Villard, 2018).

Coprophilia

This condition is defined as a sexual interest in feces and/or defecation. It can present in numerous variations often involving themes of submission or humiliation of oneself or one's partner(s). It may also involve a fetishistic interest in feces, especially involving odor. The theme of coprophilia is surprisingly common. One survey of American college students found that 17% of men and 4% of women reported repeated internet viewing of pornography involving urine and/or feces (Prentky et al., 2010). Interest in themes such as this likely reflects a tendency for people to be interested in viewing things that are "gross" or taboo.

Klismaphilia

This is a paraphilia based on sexual arousal involving enemas (Denko, 1973). Again, multiple variations are possible, including whether the arousal arises from giving or receiving the enema, the nature of the enema, and whether the activity occurs in private or with a sexual partner(s) (Denko, 1976). Variations can also occur in terms of how sexually motivating are themes of submission and humiliation. In some cases, the arousal is due to the physical sensations induced by the enema, which can induce autonomic arousal.

Urophilia and Omorashi

Urophilia is similar to coprophilia, involving urine instead of feces. Like coprophilia, which can be related to klismaphilia, urophilia can be associated with sexual arousal from catheterization and/or urethral probing. The theme of taking control of an autonomic process is prominent in the paraphilia known as omorashi, which involves sexual arousal associated with the sensation of needing to urinate due to a full bladder. Behaviors involving overstimulation of the autonomic nervous system are suggestive of "boosting" seen in paraplegic or tetraplegic athletes who improve their athletic performance by acts such as clamping their catheters, sitting on tacks, and even intentionally breaking a toe (Harris, 1994).

Review of the Literature

The following table summarizes the literature that has been published on "other specified" paraphilias. The table is based on a previously published list (Fedoroff, 2010). For paraphilias with no known updates in English language literature since 2008, only brief definitions of the paraphilias are provided.

Paraphila	Breif Definition	Reference(S)
General: Paraphilias Otherwise specified	Review	Kafka, 2010 Briken et al, 2016
Abasiophilia	Impaired mobility	Money, 1990
Acarophilia	Scratching	Aggrawal, 2019
Acousticophilia	Sounds	Lehne, 2009
Acrophilia	Heights	Lehne, 2009
Acrotomphilia	Amputees	Money, 1990; Money & Simco, 1984
Adult baby see also Infantilism	Being a baby; not necessarily sexual. Not pedophilia.	Kise & Nguyen, 2011 Hawkinson & Zamboni, 2014
Agalmatophilia	Statues or dolls	Scobie, & Taylor, 1975 White, 1979 (disputes prevalence)
Agonophilia; sometimes used to describe arousal from combat sports	"Rape fantasy", overpowering a victim who becomes consensual	Cheney, 2004
Agrexophilia	Poorly defined: Self-spectatoring or observing; not voyeurism	Cheney, 2004
Algolagnia	Pain (as opposed to sadism)	MacCulloch et al., 2000

Paraphila	Breif Definition	Reference(S)
Amaurophilia arousal by sightless partner, may be related to dominance and/or poor self-perception	Blindness	Aggrawal (2009);
Anasteemaphilia	Height discrepancy	Lehne, 2008
Andromimetophilia/Genemimetophilia/ Transvestophilia	Attraction to gender transition	See chapter 8 Transvestic Disorder
Anililagnia	Older women	Pocknell, 2017
Anthropophagy	Sexually motivated cannibalism (critically reviewed)	Rehn &may Borgerson, 2005
Apodysophilia (exhibitionism) May be confused with consensual nudity	Public nudity	See Chapter 3: Exhibitionistic Disorder
Apotemnophilia; body integrity disorder (BID), xenomelia	Becoming an amputee	Baubet et al., 2007; Donix & Reuster, 2007; Everaerd, 1983; Godlewski & Szalankiewicz, 1987; Sedda & Bottini, 2014
Apotemnophilia vs BID		Blom et al, 2016
Apotemnophilia due to brain damage (right parietal)		McGeoch et al., 2011; Brang, McGeoch, & Ramachandran, 2008
Apotemnophilia (ethics)		Dua, 2010; Ryan, 2009; Money, Jobaris, & Furth, 1977
Apotemnophilia cognitive-behavioural treatment		Braam, Visser, Cath, & Hoogendijk, 2006
Aquaphilia (not the physics term for water attraction)	Sex and water	See asphyxiophilia/Breath Play
Arachnophilia (similar to other counter-phobic arousals)	Spiders	See chapter 4: Fetishistic Disorder

Asphyxiophilia: sexual arousal from restricting oxygen. Usually referring to self-suffocation to sexual arousal. Also called "auto-erotic self-asphyxiation." Incidence of asphyxiation was found to be at about 0.5-2 cases per one million inhabitants in Scandinavia per year (Innala & Ernulf, 1989) Case studies of auto-erotic asphyxiation (Cooper, 1996; Cosgray, Hanna, Fawley, & Money, 1991; Quackelbeen, Nobus, & Temmerman, 1997; Williams, Phillips, & Ahmed, 2000; Zaviacic, 1993) Paper on asphyxiophilia, which discusses the epidemiology, characteristics, and familial effects (Innala & Ernulf, 1987) Considers whether erotic asphyxiation is an addiction (Ernoul, Orsat, Mesu, Garre, Jean-Bernard, & Richard-Devantoy, 2012)	Oxygen restriction	Innala & Ernulf, 1989; Cooper, 1996; Cosgray, Hanna, Fawley, & Money, 1991; Quackelbeen, Nobus, & Temmerman, 1997; Williams, Phillips, & Ahmed, 2000; Zaviacic, 1993; Innala & Ernulf, 1987; Ernoul, Orsat, Mesu, Garre, Jean-Bernard, & Richard-Devantoy, 2012; Book & Perumal, 1993; Hucker, S. (2016). Thompson, 2002: Money, J., Wainwright, G., & Hingsburger, D. (1991).
Discussion of sexual asphyxia (Book & Perumal, 1993); Hucker (2016)		
Treatment of auto-erotic asphyxiation in an autistic male using a behavioural and psycho-educational programme (Thompson, 2002) Book-length case report (Money et al)		

Paraphila	Breif Definition	Reference(S)
Autoandrophilia/Autogynephilia (see also Chapter 9: transvestic fetishism)	Having opposite sex body parts	Moser, 2009; Lawrence, A., 2011
Autassassinophilia	Being killed	Downing, 2004
Autagonistophilia	Being seen	Chapter 3: Exhibtionistic Disorder
Autoerotic self-asphyxia see asphyxiophilia Can co-occur with sadism/masochism and transvestic fetishism and Chapter 9: transvestic fetishism	Self-asphyxia	See Chapters 7 and 8 Sadomasochism Disorders and Transvestic Disorder
Autohemofetishism	Self-bleeding	Bartholomew, 1973
Autonepiophilia: sexual arousal from the idea of being an infant different from pedophilia	Being an infant	Pandita-Gunawardena, 1990
Autophagiophilia	Self-ingestion	None
Bestiality: legal term. See Zoophilia	Animals	See zoophilia
Biastophilia	Rape	Money, 1990
Breath Play: not a paraphilia but indicative of asphyxiophilia	Asphyxia	See Asphyxia
Candaulism	Partner infidelity	Houngbedji & Guillem, 2016; Chapter 10
Capnolagnia	Smoking	Aggrawal, 2019
Catherophilia	Catheterization	See chapter 4: Fetishistic Disorder
Celebriphilia not erotomania. Often involves famous criminals.	Celebrities	Guinn, 2013
Chremastistophlia (also related to compulsive money exchange). See also Harpaxophilia	Being robbed	See Madonna-Whore syndrome, Chapter 7: Sadomasochistic disorders

Chronophilia Pedophilia is described as a chronophilia which is described as "a sexual orientation for age" (Seto, 2017). Several comments have been published in response to Seto which support his theories (Beier & Amelung, 2017; Janssen, 2017; Miletski, 2017; Mokros, 2017). However, Fedoroff (2018) and Baily & Hsu, 2017challenge several claims in the article suggesting that sexual orientation should not be conflated with sexual interest. Others argue for more research (Bailey & Hsu, 2017; Imhoff, Banse, & Schmidt, 2017).	Age discrepancy	Seto, 2017; Beier & Amelung, 2017; Janssen, 2017; Miletski, 2017; Mokros, 2017 Fedoroff 2018; Baily & Hsu, 2017; Imhoff, Banse, & Schmidt, 2017 See also Chapter 6: Pedophilic Disorder
Coprophagia: Case study of a man with depression and substance use-related problems with this paraphilia (Wise & Goldberg, 1995)	Feces consumption	Wise & Goldberg, 1995 See also Chapter 4: Fetishistic Disorder
Coprophilia: Case study of a man with intellectual disability (Hingsburger, 1989) who argues the coprophilia was a response to a "limited institutional environment". Review: London, L.S., & Caprio, F.S. (1950). Case study of a man with Gilles de la Tourette Syndrome who also developed coprophilia (Marneros, 1984)	Feces and defecation	Hingsburger, 1989; Marneros, 1984; Xavier, 1955; London, L.S., & Caprio, F.S. (1950). See also Chapter 4: Fetishistic Disorder

Paraphila	Breif Definition	Reference(S)
Case study of coprophilia that manifested with other symptoms, such as reduced human contact and increased attachment to pets (Xavier, 1955)		
Crush fetish: often incorporates high heels; "crushed objects" can be animate or inanimate	Crushing	Popular on the Internet but not studied. See also Chapter 4: Fetishistic Disorder
Dacnolagnomania see also *erotophonophilia*	Lust murder	Arrigo & Purcell, 2001; Mcclellan, 2008; Money, 1990; Purcell, 2001 See also Chapter 7: Sadomasochistic disorders
Dacryphilia: Case study of a woman who pathologizes her dacryphilia (Greenhill & Griffiths, 2016) Compassion, dominance and submission, and curled-lips were found to be related to dacryphilia and the dacryphilic experience (Greenhill & Griffiths, 2015)	Tears or crying	Greenhill & Griffiths, 2015 Greenhill & Griffiths, 2016 See also Chapter 4: Fetishitic Disorder and Chapter 7: Sadomasochistic Disorder
Dendrophilia (see also arbophilia): important to distinguish true sexual arousal from other motivations such as avoidance of social relationships	Trees	Popular on the Internet. No studies. See Chapter 4: Fetishistic Disorders
Dermatophilia	Skin, leather or fur	See Chapter 4: Fetishistic Disorders
Devotee Discusses the devotee community and the responses of disabled person(s) to devotees (Aguilera, 2000)	Disability	Aguilera, 2000; Solvang, 2007 See also Chapter 7: Sadomasochistic Disorders

Paper which includes the debate of being attracted to those who are disabled and whether this re-defines beauty standards (Solvang, 2007)		
Dippoldism: See Chapter 7: *Sexual masochism and sadism*	Corporal punishment	See also Chapter 7: Sadomasochistic Disorders
Doraphilia see Dermatophilia	Animal skin	See Chapter 4: Fetishistic Disorders
Ecouteurism	Hearing sex	See Chapter 4: Fetishistic Disorders
Emetophilia	Vomit	See Chapter 4: Fetishistic Disorders
Entomophilia. See also formicophilia	Insects	See Chapter 4: Fetishistic Disorders
Ephebophilia: Poorly defined with variable age and developmental descriptions. Most, if not all research papers on ephebophilia have included cases involving the Roman Catholic clergy (Brehob, 2006; Cartor, Cimbolic, & Tallon, 2008; Cimbolic & Cartor, 2006; Gerard, Jobes, Cimbolic, Ritzler, & Montana, 2003; Gerard-Sharp, 2000; Lee, 2007; Musser, Cimbolic, & Rossetti, 1995; Noonan-Karstens, 2009; Pallone, 2002; Rossetti, Anthony, Cimbolic, & Wright, 1996) Theories of ephebophilia (Lothstein, 1990) Treatment: 12-step recovery program was used on two men with ephebophilia (Nu Ez, 2003)	Adolescentce	Brehob, 2006; Cartor, Cimbolic, & Tallon, 2008; Cimbolic & Cartor, 2006; Gerard, Jobes, Cimbolic, Ritzler, & Montana, 2003; Gerard-Sharp, 2000; Lee, 2007; Musser, Cimbolic, & Rossetti, 1995; Noonan-Karstens, 2009; Pallone, 2002; Rossetti, Anthony, Cimbolic, & Wright, 1996; Lothstein, 1990; Nu Ez, 2003 See also Chapter 6: Pedophilic Disorder
Eproctophilia	Flatualnce	Griffiths, 2013 See Chapter 4: Fetishistic Disorders

Paraphila	**Breif Definition**	**Reference(S)**
Erotophonophilia see *dacnolagnomania*	Lust murder	See Chapter 7: Sadomasochistic Disorders
Exhibitionism see Chapter 5 *Exhibitonistic dosorder*	Exposing	Chapter 3: Exhibitionistic Disorders
Faunoiphilia	Seeing animals mating	Aggrawal, A (2011)
Feederism Case study of a female with feederism (Terry & Vasey, 2011)		
Found that people from the general population rated visual stimuli of feeding to be more sexually arousing than neutral stimuli (Terry, Suschinsky, Lalumiere, & Vasey, 2012) Feederism is described as a "communal behaviour" (Prohaska, 2014)	Weight gain, often imposed	Terry & Vasey, 2011; Terry, Suschinsky, Lalumiere, & Vasey, 2012; Prohaska, 2014 See also Chaptrer 7: Sadomasochistic Disorders
Formicophilia: sexual arousal from having small insects crawling or "nibbling" on one's body. Case of a Buddhist male with formicophilia, who was treated with counseling and behaviour therapy (Dewaraja, 1987), and antiandrogenic hormones (Dewaraja & Money, 1986)	Insects	Dewaraja, 1987; Dewaraja & Money, 1986 See also Chapter 4: Fetishistic Disorders
Frotteurism	Touching or rubbing	Chapter 5: Frotteuristic Disorders

Gerontophilia: Poorly defined. A good example of a paraphilia in which interest is contextual and prone to change (the concept of old changes as people age). Case study of a man who attempted to sexually assault four women in their 70s and 80s (Oules, Boscredon, & Bataille, 1977)	Elderly	Oules, Boscredon, & Bataille, 1977
Gonophilia: see fetishes and partialism	Knees	Chapter 4: Fetishistic Disorders
Gynemimetophilia: sexual arousal toward men with breasts (often including a female body type aside from genitalia: "she-males").	Men with female breasts	Chapter 8: Transvestic Disorder
Harpaxophilia. See also *Chremastistophlia*	Being robbed	Chapter 7: Sadomasochistic Disorders
Hebephilia: poorly defined as early adolescence. Also see *chronophilia, ephebophilia* and *pedophilia.* Hebephilia is often grouped with pedophilia in research studies (Beier, Amelung, Grundmann, & Kuhle, 2015; Stephens, Cantor, Goodwill, Alasdair, & Seto, 2017) When evaluating the construct validity of hebephilia, it was found that there was much overlap between pedophilia and hebephilia. The divergent validity between pedophilia and hebephilia was found to be poor (Stephens, Seto, Goodwill, & Cantor, 2017)	Youth	Beier, Amelung, Grundmann, & Kuhle, 2015; Stephens, Cantor, Goodwill, Alasdair, & Seto, 2017; Stephens, Seto, Goodwill, & Cantor, 2017; Beier et al., 2013; Beier et al., 2015; Blanchard et al., 2009; Cantor & McPhail, 2015; Burke, 2014; Good & Burstein, 2012; Hames & Blanchard, 2012; Singy, 2015; Franklin, 2010 See also Chapter 6: Pedophilic Disorder

Paraphila	Breif Definition	Reference(S)
However, individuals with hebephilia report more distress and "deviant" personality characteristics when compared to individuals with pedophilia (Beier et al., 2013; Beier et al., 2015). Also, it was found that phallometric testing could detect hebephilia with 70.0% sensitivity and 90.7% specificity when compared to pedophilia, which had a 46.9% sensitivity and 100% specificity (Blanchard et al., 2009; Cantor & McPhail, 2015) Differences between pedophilia and hebephilia were also attempted to be demostrated using the Abel Assessment for Sexual Interest-2 (Burke, 2014) It is explained that hebephilia was not included in the DSM-5, because the evidence of it being a disease is unconvincing (Good & Burstein, 2012; Hames & Blanchard, 2012; Singy, 2015). Also, including it would have legal and research consequences (Franklin, 2010)		
Hematophilia	Blood	Chapter 4: Fetishistic Disorder

Heterophilia. A good example of blending gender and interest.	Opposite sex	See Chapter 1: Perspectives and Paradigms
Hierophilia	Religious objects	Chapter 4: Fetishistic Disorder
Hodophilia	Foreign places	Chapter 4: Fetishistic Disorder
Homeovestism: sexual arousal from wearing clothes that are congruent with one's gender role. Homeovestism is often associated with fetishism and transvestism (Zavitzianos, 1972; Zavitzianos, 1977)	Same gender clothes	Zavitzianos, 1972; Zavitzianos, 1977 See also: Chapter 7 Transvestic Disorder
Homilophilia: sexual arousal from religious speeches and/or sermons.	Sermons	Chapter 4: Fetishistic Disorder
Hoplophilia	Firearms	Chapter 4: Fetishistic Disorder
Hybristophilia: sexual arousal from a partner committing a transgression within the partnership and/or one's partner committing a crime. Hyberistophilia was once known as enclitophilia (Benezech, 2016)	Criminal partner	Benezech, 2016 See also: Chapter 7 Sadomasochistic Disorders
Hygrophilia	Fabrics	Chapter 4: Fetishistic Disorder
Iatronudia	Doctors	Chapter 4: Fetishistic Disorder

Paraphila	Breif Definition	Reference(S)
Incest paraphilia Refers *to* sexual attraction to relative(s) (not necessarily involing children). A preliminary search on PsycINFO using the term "incest" with additional limitations that results would show publications between 2008 and 2018 yielded 289 results. Because of the extant research on this specific paraphilia and in consideration for space, the search was further limited to include only literature and clinical reviews (Abu-Baker, 2013; Anonymous, 2008; Lapointe & Le Bosse, 2010; Panagakis, 2012; Yates, 2017), and meta-analyses (Pullman, Sawatsky, Babchishin, McPhail, & Seto, 2017; Seto, Babchishin, Pullman, Lesleigh, & McPhail, 2015; Ventus, Antfolk, & Salo, 2017) Literature review on incest with siblings (Panagakis, 2012; Yates, 2017) Meta-analysis found that sociolegal incest offenders have more antisocial features when compared to biological incest offenders. However, biological incest offenders have more mental health problems (Pullman et al., 2017)	Relatives	Abu-Baker, 2013; Anonymous, 2008; Lapointe & Le Bosse, 2010; Panagakis, 2012; Yates, 2017; Pullman, Sawatsky, Babchishin, McPhail, & Seto, 2017; Seto, Babchishin, Pullman, Lesleigh, & McPhail, 2015; Ventus, Antfolk, & Salo, 2017; Panagakis, 2012; Yates, 2017; Lapointe & Le Bosse, 2010 See also: Chapter 6 Pedophilic Disorder

Meta-analysis found that intrafamilial abuse had younger victims when compared to extrafamilial abuse (Ventus et al., 2017) A literature review found that there was limited research on whether it was more beneficial or harmful for children to have contact with the parent who abused them. However, it was found that it is usually more harmful (Anonymous, 2008) Literature review of resilience after incest (Lapointe & Le Bosse, 2010) Review of how non-western cultures responds to incest (Abu-Baker, 2013)		
Infantophilia: Poorly defined. Can range from newborn to 4. A comparison of infantophilia with pedophilia found no significant differences in characteristics between the two groups (Greenberg, Bradford, & Curry, 1995)	Infants	Greenberg, Bradford, & Curry, 1995 See also: Chapter 6 Pedophilic Disorder
Katoptronophilia: sexual arousal from the use of mirrors, such watching oneself having sex and/or one's partner(s).	Mirrors	Chapters 3 and 9: Exhibitionistic and Voyeuristic Disorders.

Paraphila	Breif Definition	Reference(S)
Kleptolagnia: Study examined 224 participants who committed sexually motivated burglaries. It was found that sexually motivated burglars differed than regular burglars in their response to opportunistic situational cues. Pedneault, Beauregard, Harris, & Knight (2015) Found three types of sexual burglars: noncontact burglars that did not involve theft, violence and weapon; versatile contact, involving sexual assault, theft, violence, and weapon; sexual assault without theft, violence or weapon. Brankley, Goodwill, & Reale (2014) A case study written in French (Van Renynghe De Voxvrie & Massion-Verniory, 1964)	Theft	Pedneault, Beauregard, Harris, & Knight (2015; Brankley, Goodwill, & Reale (2014); Van Renynghe De Voxvrie & Massion-Verniory, 1964 Chapter 4: Fetishistic Disorder
Klismaphilia: Discussion of why klismaphilia is physiologically gratifying (Agnew, 1982) Two cases of men with klismaphilia (Denko, 1973) Person(s) with klismaphilia typically do not want treatment (Denko, 1976)	Enemas	Agnew, 1982; Denko, 1973, 1976 Chapter 4: Fetishistic Disorder

Lactaphilia	Breast-feeding or lactation	Chapter 4: Fetishistic Disorder
Lust murder: see *dacnolagnomania* and/or *erotophonophilia*.	Killing	See dacnolagnomania See also Chapter 7: Sadomasochistic Disorders
Macrophilia: popular theme in fiction	Giants	Chapter 4: Fetishistic Disorder
Maiesiophilia: opposite of Madonna-Whore syndrome	Pregnancy	See Madonna-Whore syndrome See also: Chapter 7 Sadomasochistic Disorders
Maschalagnia	Armpits	Chapter 4: Fetishistic Disorder
Mask fetishism: sexual arousal to masks and/or removing masks.	Masks	Chapter 4: Fetishistic Disorder
Masochism: variable definitions	Submission	Chapter 7: Sadomascochistic disorder
Mechanophilia	Vehicles	Chapter 4: Fetishistic Disorder
Melissophilia	Bees	Chapter 4: Fetishistic Disorder
Melolagnia	Music	Chapter 4: Fetishistic Disorder
Menophilia: sexual arousal from menstruation and/or tampons.	Menstruation	Chapter 4: Fetishistic Disorder
Microphilia	Small stature	Chapter 4: Fetishistic Disorder
Morphophilia: different or changing size	Size or shape	Chapter 4: Fetishistic Disorder
Mucophilia	Mucous	Chapter 4: Fetishistic Disorder
Mysophilia: sexual arousal from objects that are soiled or filthy. An example is used underwear. See also *salirophilia*. Case of mysophilia in a male who also had urophilia, fetishism, and masochism (Rousal & Brinchcin, 1971) Comments on a case of mysophilia (Fraenkel, 1954)	Filth	Rousal & Brinchcin, 1971; Fraenkel, 1954 Chapter 4: Fetishistic Disorder

Paraphila	Breif Definition	Reference(S)
Nanophilia: sexual attraction towards a short partner. See also *anasteemaphilia* and *microphilia*	Short partner	Chapter 4: Fetishistic Disorder
Narratophilia: sexual arousal from storytelling that uses erotic language. Questionable if this is a paraphilia	Narrative	Non-specific
Nasophilia	Noses	Chapter 4: Fetishistic Disorder
Necrobestialism: sexual arousal from dead animals and/or sexual interest in engaging in sexual acts with dead animals. (also termed necrozoophilia)	Dead animals	Chapter 4: Fetishistic Disorder
Necrophilia: sexual arousal from engaging in sexual acts with dead bodies. Papers and chapters published between 2008 to 2018 on necrophilia: West, S.G., & Resnick, P.J. (2017). Necrophilia. In B.A. Sharpless (Ed.), *Unusual and rare psychological disorders: A handbook for clinical practice and research* (pp. 124-135). New York, NY: Oxford University Press. (Fitzgerald, 2011; Giordano, White, & Lester, 2012; Higgs, Stefanska, Carter, & Browne, 2017; Lemma, 2013; Lester & White, 2011; Pettigrew, 2017; Pettigrew, 2018; Stein, Schlesinger, & Pinizzotto, 2010; Troyer, 2008)	Dead bodies	West, S.G., & Resnick, P.J. (2017 Fitzgerald, 2011; Giordano, White, & Lester, 2012; Higgs, Stefanska, Carter, & Browne, 2017; Lemma, 2013; Lester & White, 2011; Pettigrew, 2017; Pettigrew, 2018; Stein, Schlesinger, & Pinizzotto, 2010; Troyer, 2008; See also: Chapter 7 Sadomasochistic Disorder

Necrophilia could be related to Asperger's Syndrome (Fitzgerald, 2011; Lester & White, 2011) Study which examined cannibals and whether necrophilia was present (Giordano, White, & Lester, 2012) Although sexual murderers may engage in sexual acts with a dead body, it does not necessarily mean they have necrophilia. Relation of necrophilia to sadism (Higgs et al., 2017) The US has no laws specifically against necrophilia (Troyer, 2008) *Selected Case studies* Case study of patient treated for eczema who described necrophilic fantasies during treatment (Lemma, 2013) Case study examining the relationship between necrophilia and somnophilia (Pettigrew, 2017) Case study on the development of necrophilic interests (Pettigrew, 2018) Case review of necrophilia that resulted in sexual homicides (Stein, Schlesinger, & Pinizzotto, 2010)		
Nosophilia: sexual attraction to a person who has a terminal illness.	Terminal illness	Chapter 4: Fetishistic Disorder

Paraphila	Breif Definition	Reference(S)
Odaxelagnia: sexual arousal from being bitten or from biting.	Biting	Chapter 4: Fetishistic Disorder
Olfactophilia: sexual arousal from body odours.	Odours	Chapter 4: Fetishistic Disorder
Omorashi: sexual arousal from the sensation of needing to urinate. See also *urolagnia* and *urophilia*	Bladder pressure	Chapter 4: Fetishistic Disorder
Partialism: sexual arousal from a specific body part (excluding genitals). Questions remain about why genitals are excluded. Papers published usually report partialism is concurrent with other paraphilias (Chan & Beauregard, 2016; Chan, Beauregard, & Myers, 2015) Suggests that the distinction between partialism and fetishism is no longer relevant (Kafka, 2010)	A body part	Chan & Beauregard, 2016; Chan, Beauregard, & Myers, 2015; Kafka, 2010 Chapter 4: Fetishistic Disorder
Pecattiphilia: sexual arousal from performing what one believes are "sinful" acts.	Sin	Chapter 4: Fetishistic Disorder
Pedophilia	Children	See Chapter 6: Pedophilic disorder
Pedovestism: sexual arousal from wearing children's clothes.	Children's clothes	Chapter 4: Fetishistic Disorder
Phobophilia	Fear	Chapter 4: Fetishistic Disorder
Piquersim: sexual arousal from picking and/or stabbing.	Stabbing	Chapter 4: Fetishistic Disorder
Plushophilia	Stuffed animals	Chapter 4: Fetishistic Disorder

Podophilia (not pedophilia)	Feet	Chapter 4: Fetishistic Disorder
Pseudozoophilia: sexual arousal from one's partner posing as an animal. (attraction to "furies"	Furies	Chapter 4: Fetishistic Disorder
Public masturbation: Definition: sexual arousal from masturbating in public without being seen. Most case studies involve individuals who are on the autism spectrum, have intellectual disabilities and/or developmental disabilities (Cook, Altman, Shaw, & Blaylock, 1978; Gill, 2012; Hurley & Sovner, 1983; Lundervold & Young, 1992; Lunsky, Frijters, Griffiths, Watson, & Williston, 2007) It was found that men with intellectual disabilities who had committed sex offences (such as public masturbation) did not significantly differ in the amount of sexual knowledge they had when compared to individuals with intellectual disabilities who did not commit any sexual offences (Lunsky et al., 2007) Social skills training was found to help men with developmental disabilities who had offended (Lundervold & Young, 1992) 10.5% of individuals began having interests in exhibitionism and/or public masturbation following a traumatic brain injury (Simpson, Sabaz, & Daher, 2013)	Masturbation in public without being seen	Cook, Altman, Shaw, & Blaylock, 1978; Gill, 2012; Hurley & Sovner, 1983; Lundervold & Young, 1992; Lunsky, Frijters, Griffiths, Watson, & Williston, 2007; Lundervold & Young, 1992; Simpson, Sabaz, & Daher, 2013; Dufrene, Watson, & Weaver, 2005; Ferguson & Rekers, 1979; Hurley & Sovner, 1983; Janzen & Peacock, 1978; Wagner, 1968); Paul, Marx, & Orsillo, 1999) See also: Chapter 3 Exhibitionistic Disorder

Paraphila	Breif Definition	Reference(S)
Children who engaged in public masturbation treated with behavioural therapy (Cook, Altman, Shaw, & Blaylock, 1978; Dufrene, Watson, & Weaver, 2005; Ferguson & Rekers, 1979; Hurley & Sovner, 1983; Janzen & Peacock, 1978; Wagner, 1968) Case study of a man treated with Functional Analytic Psychotherapy and Acceptance and Commitment Therapy for exhibitionism and public masturbation (Paul, Marx, & Orsillo, 1999)		
Pygophilia: Fetish/Partialism (question why this is designated a paraphilia while sexual interest in genitals is excluded	Buttocks	Chapter 4: Fetishistic Disorder
Pyrophilia: sexual arousal from fire and/or fire-setting.	Fire-setting	Chapter 4: Fetishistic Disorder
Retifism: sexual arousal from shoes. Case study of a male with a foot fetishist – notably, the authors reported their patient as having retifism instead of podophilia (Kunjukrishnan, Pawlak, & Varan, 1988)	Shoes	Kunjukrishnan, Pawlak, & Varan, 1988 Chapter 4: Fetishistic Disorder
Rhabdophilia: sexual arousal from self-flagellation.	Self-flagellation	Chapter 7: Sadomasochistic disorders
Sadism: multiple types and defintions	Control	Chapter 7: Sexual masochism and sadism disorder.

Saliromania: sexual arousal from degradation of appearance.(self-or others)	Degraded appearance	Chapter 7: Sexual masochism and sadism disorder.
Scopophilia/Scoptophilia: not voyeurism. sexual arousal from looking at erotic objects. The history of scopophilia (Allen, 1974) Case studies of men with scopophilia with voyeurism (Almansi, 1979; Stoylen, 1985), in which one was treated with cognitive-behavioural therapy (Stoylen, 1985) Case study of scopophilia, wherein the author believes sadism may be involved (Fenichel, 1937) Discussion of pornography and scopophilia and its associations (de Giorgio, 1985)	Looking	Allen, 1974; Almansi, 1979; Stoylen, 1985; Fenichel, 1937; de Giorgio, 1985 See also Chapter 9 Voyeuristic Disorder
Scoptic syndrome: sexual arousal from being castrated (male). Described in Fedoroff & Fedoroff, 1992	Castration	Coleman & Cesnik (1990) Fedoroff & Fedoroff, 1992
Somnophilia (not sexsomnia): sexual arousal due to an unconscious person. Case study of somnophilia in which the victim was drugged (Lauerma, 2016) Discussions of the similarities between somnophilia and necrophilia (Knafo, 2015; Pettigrew, 2017) Fedoroff et al: Case controlled series of men with sleeping victims	Sleeping person	Fedoroff et al, 1997; Knafo, 2015; Pettigrew, 2017); Lauerma, 2016

Paraphila	**Breif Definition**	**Reference(S)**
Sthenolagnia	Muscles or strenght	Chapter 4: Fetishistic Disorder
Sthenolagiophilia: arousal from female bodybuilders. A variation of arousal from fitness.	Female body builders	Chapter 4: Fetishistic Disorder
Stigmatophilia: sexual arousal from piercings, tattoos, and/or uniforms.	Tatoos	Chapter 4: Fetishistic Disorder
Stitophilia: not feederism	Food	Chapter 4: Fetishistic Disorder
Symphorophilia: sexual arousal from staging and/or watching response to a disaster. Arousal typically related to excitement from sense of control over others	Disaster	Chapter 7: Sadomasochistic Disorder
Tamakeri sexual arousal from causing pain to a man's testes, typically by kicking or stepping on the testes. (see also Crush fetish)	Testicular harm	Chapters 4 and 7: Fetish and sadomasochistic disorders
Taphophilia: sexual arousal from being buried alive. Often related to self-asphyxia from chest compression.	Being buried alive	See asphyxophilia Also Chapter 7: Sadomasochistic Disorder

Telephone scataologia: sexual arousal from making obscene telephone calls. Papers concerning telephone scatologia. Notably, most were published prior to 2008 (Dalby, 1988; Ginsburg, Ogletree, & Silakowski, 2003; Goldberg & Wise, 1985; Lande, 1993; Pakhomou, 2006; Price, Gutheil, Commons, Kafka, & Dodd-Kimmey, 2001; Price, Gutheil, Commons, Kafka, & Dodd-Kimmey, 2001; Price, Kafka, Commons, Gutheil, & Simpson, 2002; Saunders & Awad, 1991); Newring, K.A.B. (2014). Case study of telephone scatologia with schizophrenic symptoms and other psychiatric disorders (Altintas, Oguz, Oguz, & Inanc (2016) Psychodynamic treatment was used to treat telephone scatalogia in one case study (Goldberg & Wise, 1985)	Obscene phone calls	Dalby, 1988; Ginsburg, Ogletree, & Silakowski, 2003; Goldberg & Wise, 1985; Lande, 1993; Pakhomou, 2006; Price, Gutheil, Commons, Kafka, & Dodd-Kimmey, 2001; Price, Gutheil, Commons, Kafka, & Dodd-Kimmey, 2001; Price, Kafka, Commons, Gutheil, & Simpson, 2002; Saunders & Awad, 1991; Altintas, Oguz, Oguz, & Inanc (2016); Goldberg & Wise, 1985; Newring, K.A.B. (2014).
Teratophilia: sexual arousal from deformed bodies.	deformity	Chapter 4: Fetishistic Disorder
Thesauromania: sexual arousal from collecting women's clothing.	clothing	Chapter 4: Fetishistic Disorder
Timophilia: sexual arousal from wealth and/ or status. Can also be related to wealth or power discrpency	Status	Chapter 7: Sadomasochistic disorders

Paraphila	Breif Definition	Reference(S)
Toucherism: sexual arousal from touching a non-consenting person.	Touching	Chapter 5: Frotteuristic disorder
Transvestism: arousal from wearing non-gender congruent clothes	Non-gender congruent clothes	See: Chapter 8: Transvestic Disorder.
Transvestophilia: sexual arousal toward people with transvestism and/or cross-dressing.	Arousal by people with Transvestism	See: Chapter 8: Transvestic Disorder.
Trichophilia: sexual arousal related to hair.	Hair	Chapter 4: Fetishistic Disorder
Troilism: sexual arousal from situations involving three people. Questionable is this a paraphilia rather than an activity within normal variations. See also Candaulism. Researched troilism with sample of gay men (Lehmiller, Ley, & Savage, 2017)	Threesomes	Lehmiller, Ley, & Savage, 2017
Undinism: sexual arousal from water and/or urine.(often involving control) Case history of a 17-year-old boy with udinism/urolagnia (Denson, 1982)	Urine control	Denson, 1982 See also Omorashi:
Urolagnia/Urophilia: sexual arousal from drinking urine or from urination ("golden showers"). Also known as urophilia. Theory of urophilia's manifestation (Christoffel, 1935)	Urine	Christoffel, 1935; Klimmer, 1968; Massion-Verniory & Dumont, 1958); London, L.S., & Caprio, F.S. (1950).

Urolagnia is typically treated as a fetishism or masochism in Germany (Klimmer, 1968) 4 cases of urolagnia (Massion-Verniory & Dumont, 1958) Review: London, L.S., & Caprio, F.S. (1950).		
Vampirism: sexual arousal from drinking blood. Theory on the etiology of vampirism (Gubb, Segal, Khota, & Dicks, 2006; Prins, 1985) Discussion of Renfield's syndrome, which is an "obsession" (not necessarily sexual) to drink blood (Olry & Haines, 2011; Oppawasky, 2010) Cases of cannibalism and vampirism (Fellion, Duflot, Anglade, & Fraillon, 1980; Benezech, Bourgeois, Boukhabza, & Yesavage, 1981) Reviews of vampirism (Jaffe & DiCataldo, 1994; McCully, 1964; Vanden Bergh & Kelly, 1964) Treatment of vampirism and other psychiatric disorders using carbamazepine and fluvoxamine (Cro, Peronti, & Bersani, 1997)	Blood-drinking	Gubb, Segal, Khota, & Dicks, 2006; Prins, 1985; Olry & Haines, 2011; Oppawasky, 2010); Fellion, Duflot, Anglade, & Fraillon, 1980; Benezech, Bourgeois, Boukhabza, & Yesavage, 1981); Jaffe & DiCataldo, 1994; McCully, 1964; Vanden Bergh & Kelly, 1964; Cro, Peronti, & Bersani, 1997
Vomerophilia: Sexual arousal from vomit or vomiting. See also *emetophilia*.	Vomiting	See *emetophilia*.
Vorarephilia: sexual arousal from consuming or being consumed by another person or creature. Case study of a man with a "submissive" vorarephilic fantasy (Lykins & Cantor, 2014).	Being eaten	Lykins & Cantor, 2014

Paraphila	Breif Definition	Reference(S)
Voyeurism: sexual arousal from watching others undressing, nude, and/or engaging in sexual activity. See chapter on *voyeuristic disorder*.	Non-consensual spying	Chapter 9 voyeuristic disorder.
Wannabe: sexual arousal from the wish to have a paraphilia, especially related to becoming disabled see *apotemnophilia* and *devotee*.	Becoming disabled	See *apotemnophilia* and *devotee*.
Zoophilia: sexual arousal from engaging in sexual relations with non-human animals; bestiality: legal term for human having sex with a non-human animal Literature review on bestiality (Holoyda, Sorrentino, Friedman, & Allgire, 2018) Studies on zoophilic practices that were published from 2008-2018 (de Cassio Zequi et al., 2012, 2014; Earls & Lalumiere, 2009; Eichenberg & Surangkanjanajai, 2012; Maratea, 2011; Sendler, 2018) The prevalence of bestiality in juvenile sex offenders is underreported (Schenk, Cooper-Lehki, Keelan, & Fremouw, 2014) Some people with zoophilia claim it is their "orientation" (Sendler, 2018) An on-line survey of zoophilia (Eichenberg & Surangkanjanajai, 2012). Those who engaged in childhood bestiality were found to have a higher risk of committing "interpersonal crimes" as an adult (Hensley, Tallichet, & Dutkiewicz, 2010).	Animals	Holoyda, Sorrentino, Friedman, & Allgire, 2018; de Cassio Zequi et al., 2012, 2014; Earls & Lalumiere, 2009; Eichenberg & Surangkanjanajai, 2012; Maratea, 2011; Sendler, 2018; Schenk, Cooper-Lehki, Keelan, & Fremouw, 2014; Sendler, 2018; Eichenberg & Surangkanjanajai, 2012; Hensley, Tallichet, & Dutkiewicz, 2010; Wignall & McCormack, 2017; Chandradasa & Champika, 2017; Lesandric, Orlovic, Peitl, & Karlovic, 2017; Eroglu, Caliskan, & Topbas, 2015; Othman, Razak, & Zakaria, 2014;; Almeida, de Oliveira Filho, Lopes Nery, Guimaraes Silva, & Campos Sousa, 2013

Imitating dog behaviours is not the same as zoophilia (Wignall & McCormack, 2017) *Case studies* Case study of a with zoophilia and autism (Chandradasa & Champika, 2017) Case study of a patient who reported zoophilia as part of the early development of psychosis (Lesandric, Orlovic, Peitl, & Karlovic, 2017) Case study of a man with schizophrenia and zoophilia (Amoo, Abayomio, & Olashore, 2012) Case study where zoophilic behaviours ceased once mania was treated (Eroglu, Caliskan, & Topbas, 2015) Case study of a man with "hypersexuality" who engaged in zoophilic behaviours (Othman, Razak, & Zakaria, 2014) Case study of a man who exhibited zoophilic behaviours as his Parkinson's Disease progressed (Almeida, de Oliveira Filho, Lopes Nery, Guimaraes Silva, & Campos Sousa, 2013)		
Zoosadism: sexual arousal from performing cruel/sadistic acts to animals Some Swiss children and adolescents with aggression problems engaged in zoosadism (Wochner & Klosinski, 1988).	Harm to animals	Wochner & Klosinski, 1988 Chapter 7: Sadosmasochistic disorders

References

Abu-Baker, K. (2013). Arab parents' reactions to child sexual abuse: A review of clinical records. *Journal of Child Sexual Abuse, 22*(1), 52–71.

Aggrawal, Anil (2009). *Forensic and Medico-legal Aspects of Sexual Crimes and Unusual Sexual Practices* (pp. 369, 375). Boca Raton: CRC Press. ISBN 978-1-4200-4308-2.

Aggrawal, A. (2011). A new classification of zoophilia. *Journal of Forensic and Legal Medicine, 18*, 73–78. doi.org/10.1016/j.jflm.2011.01.004

Aguilera, R. J. (2000). Disability and delight: Staring back at the devotee community. *Sexuality and Disability, 18*(4), 255–261.

Allen, D. W. (Ed.). (1974). *The fear of looking or scopophilic—Exhibitionistic conflicts*. Charlottesville, VA: University of Virginia Press.

Almansi, R. J. (1979). Scopophilia and object loss. *Psychoanalytic Quarterly, 48*(4), 601–619.

Almeida, K. J., de Oliveira Filho, M. C. S., Lopes Nery, P. C., Guimaraes Silva, J. S., & Campos Sousa, R. N. (2013). Zoophilia and Parkinson's disease. *Parkinsonism & Related Disorders, 19*(2), 1167–1168.

Altintas, M., Oguz, M., Oguz, N., & Inanc, L. (2016). Comorbidity of telephone scatologia with multiple psychiatric disorders: A case report. *Journal of Psychiatry and Neurological Sciences, 29*(3), 275–280.

American Psychiatric Association. (2013). *Diagnostic and statistical manual of mental disorders* (5th ed.). Arlington, VA: American Psychiatric Publishing.

Amoo, G., Abayomio, O., & Olashore, A. A. (2012). Zoophilic recidivism in schizophrenia: A case report. *African Journal of Psychiatry, 15*(4), 223–225.

Anonymous. (2008). Incest and parental contact: A psychologist's personal case and literature review. *Journal of Child Sexual Abuse, 17*(1), 1–12.

Arrigo, B. A., & Purcell, C. E. (2001). Explaining paraphilias and lust murder: Toward an integrated model. *International Journal of Offender Therapy and Comparative Criminology, 45*(1), 6–31.

Bailey, J. M., & Hsu, K .J. (2017). Orienting basic research on chronophilias. *Archives of Sexual Behavior, 46*(1), 23–26.

Bartholomew, A. A. (1973). Two features occasionally associated with intravenous drug users: A note. *Australian and New Zealand Journal of Psychiatry, 7*(3), 206–207.

Baubet, T., Gal, B., Dendoncker-Viry, S., Masquelet, A. C., Gatt, M. T., & Moro, M. R. (2007). Apotemnophilia as a contemporary frame for psychological suffering. *L'Encephale, 33*(4 Pt. 1), 609–615.

Beier, K. M., & Amelung, T. (2017). A German sexological perspective on male chronophilias. *Archives of Sexual Behavior, 46*(1), 27–28.

Beier, K. M., Amelung, T., Grundmann, D., & Kuhle, L. F. (2015). Pedophilia and hebephilia in the context of child sexual abuse [in German]. *Sexuologie, 22*(3–4), 137–144.

Beier, K. M., Amelung, T., Kuhle, L., Grundmann, D., Schemer, G., & Neutze, J. (2013). Hebephilia as a sexual disorder [in German]. *Fortschritte der Neurologie, Psychiatrie, 81*(3), 128–137.

Beier, K. M., Amelung, T., Kuhle, L., Grundmann, D., Schemer, G., & Neutze, J. (2015). Hebephilia as a sexual disorder [in German]. *Fortschritte der Neurologie, Psychiatrie, 83*(2), 98.

Benezech, M. (2016). Enclitophilia to hybristophilia [in French]. *Annales Medico-Psychologiques, 174*(6), 509–513.

Benezech, M., Bourgeois, M., Boukhabza, D., & Yesavage, J. A. (1981). Cannibalism and vampirism in paranoid schizophrenia. *Journal of Clinical Psychiatry, 42*(7), 290.

Berendzen, R. (1993). *Come here: A man overcomes the tragic aftermath of childhood sexual abuse*. New York, NY: Villard. ISBN:0-679-41777-X

Blanchard, R., Lykins, A. D., Wherrett, D., Kuban, M. E., Cantor, J. M., Blak, T., . . . Klassen, P. E. (2009). Pedophilia, hebephilia, and the DSM-V. *Archives of Sexual Behavior, 38*(3), 335–350.

Blom, R. M., Vulink, N. C., van der Wal, S. J., Nakamae, T., Tan, Z., Derks, E.M., & Denys, D. (2016). Body integrity identity disorder crosses culture: Case reports in the Japanese and Chinese literature. *Neuropsychiatric Disease and Treatment, 12*, 1419–1423.

Book, R. G., & Perumal, G. (1993). Sexual asphyxia: A lesser epidemic. *Medicine & Law, 12*(6–8), 687–698.

Braam, A. W., Visser, S., Cath, D. C., & Hoogendijk, W. J. G. (2006). Investigation of the syndrome of apotemnophilia and course of a cognitive-behavioural therapy. *Psychopathology, 39*(1), 32–37.

Briken, P., Klein, V., & von Franque, F. (2016). In R. Balon (Ed.), *Practical guide to paraphilia and paraphilic disorders* (pp. 187–196). Cham, Switzerland: Springer International Publishing.

Brang, D., McGeoch, P. D., & Ramachandran, V. S. (2008). Apotemnophilia: A neurological disorder. *Neuroreport, 19*(13), 1305–1306.

Brankley, A. E., Goodwill, A. M., & Reale, K. S. (2014). Escalation from fetish burglaries to sexual violence: A retrospective case study of former col., D. Russell Williams. *Journal of Investigative Psychology and Offender Profiling, 11*(2), 115–135.

Brehob, K. A. (2006). Clinical and statistical classification of sexual disorders: The case of unintegrated sexuality applied to a clergy sample. Doctoral dissertation, Loyola University Maryland, Baltimore, MD (ProQuest Information, UMI No. 3209271).

Burke, S. (2014). Pedophilia and hebephilia: An analysis of deviant sexual interest using the Abel Assessment for Sexual Interest-2. Doctoral dissertation, Alliant International University, California School of Forensic Studies, Irvine, CA (UMI No. 3562268).

Cantor, J. M., & McPhail, I. V. (2015). Sensitivity and specificity of the phallometric test for hebephilia. *Journal of Sexual Medicine, 12*(9), 1940–1950.

Cartor, P., Cimbolic, P., & Tallon, J. (2008). Differentiating pedophilia from ephebophilia in cleric offenders. *Sexual Addiction & Compulsivity, 15*(4), 311–319.

Chan, H. C., & Beauregard, E. (2016). Non-homicidal and homicidal sexual offenders: Prevalence of maladaptive personality traits and paraphilic behaviors. *Journal of Interpersonal Violence, 31*(13), 2259–2290.

Chan, H. C., Beauregard, E., & Myers, W. C. (2015). Single-victim and serial sexual homicide offenders: Differences in crime, paraphilias and personality traits. *Criminal Behaviour and Mental Health, 25*(1), 66–78.

Chandradasa, M., & Champika, L. (2017). Zoophilia in an adolescent with high-functioning autism from Sri Lanka. *Australasian Psychiatry, 25*(5), 486–488.

Cheney, V. (2004). Other paraphilias. In: Sex offenders and their treatments (p. 239). Authorhouse: Blooomington, Indiana.

Christoffel, H. (1934). On the biology of enuresis. *Zeitschrift fur Kinderpsychiatrie, 1*, 76–86.

Cimbolic, P., & Cartor, P. (2006). Looking at ephebophilia through the lens of cleric sexual abuse. *Sexual Addiction & Compulsivity, 13*(4), 347–359.

Coleman, E., & Cesnik, J. (1990). Scoptic syndrome and treatment of an obsessional gender dysphoria with lithium carbonate and psychotherapy. *American Journal of Psychotherapy, 44*, 204–217. doi.org/10.1176/appi.psychotherapy.1990.44.2.204

Cook, J. W., Altman, K., Shaw, J., & Blaylock, M. (1978). Use of contingent lemon juice to eliminate public masturbation by a severely retarded boy. *Behaviour Research and Therapy, 16*(2), 131–134.

Cooper, A. J. (1996). Auto-erotic asphyxiation: Three case reports. *Journal of Sex & Marital Therapy, 22*(1), 47–53.

Cosgray, R. E., Hanna, V., Fawley, R., & Money, M. (1991). Death from auto-erotic asphyxiation in a long-term psychiatric setting. *Perspectives in Psychiatric Care, 27*(1), 21–24.

Cro, F., Peronti, M., & Bersani, G. (1997). A case of auto-vampirism in a patient with borderline personality disorder and chronic multiple substance abuse. *Rivisita di Psichiatria, 32*(4), 165–172.

Dalby, J. T. (1988). Is telephone scatologia a variant of exhibitionism? *International Journal of Offender Therapy and Comparative Criminology, 32*(1), 45–49.

de Cassio Zequi, S., Guimarães, G. C., da Fonseca, F. P., Ferreira, U., de Matheus, W. E., Reis, L. O., . . . Guidoni, L. R. M. (2012). Sex with animals (SWA): Behavioral characteristics and possible association with penile cancer—A multicenter study. *Journal of Sexual Medicine, 9*(7), 1860–1867.

de Cassio Zequi, S. (2014). The medical consequences of sex between humans and animals. In G.H. Allez (Ed.), *Sexual diversity and sexual offending: Research, assessment, and clinical treatment in psychosexual therapy* (pp.185–202). London, England: Karnac Books.

de Giorgio, R. (1985). The pornography of feeling [in Italian]. *Rivista di Psicologia Analitica, 16*(32), 138–146.

Denko, J. D. (1973). Klismaphilia: Enema as a sexual preference. *American Journal of Psychotherapy, 27*(2), 232–250.

Denko, J. D. (1976). Klismaphilia: Amplification of the erotic enema deviance. *American Journal of Psychotherapy, 30*(2), 236–255.

Denson, R. (1982). Undinism: The fetishization of urine. *Canadian Journal of Psychiatry, 27*(4), 336–338.

Dewaraja, R. (1987). Formicophilia, an unusual paraphilia, treated with counseling and behavior therapy. *American Journal of Psychotherapy, 41*(4), 593–597.

Dewaraja, R., & Money, J. (1986). Transcultural sexology: Formicophilia, a newly named paraphilia in a young Buddhist male. *Journal of Sex & Marital Therapy, 12*(2), 139–145.

Donix, M., & Reuster, T. (2007). Apotemnophilia—Diagnostic classification between paraphilia and body integrity identity disorder. *Nervenheilkunde: Zeitschrift fur interdisziplinaere Fortbildung, 26*(6), 477–479.

Downing, L. (2004). On the limits of sexual ethics: The phenomenology of autassassinophilia. *Sexuality & Culture, 8*(1), 3–17.

Dua, A. (2010). Apotemnophilia: Ethical considerations of amputating a healthy limb. *Journal of Medical Ethics, 36*(2), 75–78.

Dufrene, B. A., Watson, T. S., & Weaver, A. (2005). Response blocking with guided compliance and reinforcement for a habilitative replacement behavior: Effects on public masturbation and on-task behavior. *Child & Family Behavior Therapy, 27*(4), 73–84.

Earls, C. M., & Lalumiere, M. L. (2009). A case study of preferential bestiality. *Archives of Sexual Behavior, 38*(4), 605–609.

Eichenberg, C., & Surangkanjanajai, B. (2012). Zoophilia. An online questionnaire study of etiology and the role of the internet [in German]. *Zeitschrift fur Sexualforschung, 25*(2), 131–150.

Ernoul, A., Orsat, M., Mesu, C., Garre, J., & Richard-Devantoy, S. (2012). The fainting game and erotic asphyxiation: From voluntary and temporary asphyxiation to addiction? [in French] *Annales Medico-Psychologiques, 170*(4), 231–237.

Eroglu, M. Z., Caliskan, M., & Topbas, E. (2015). Mania associated with zoophilia: A case report. *Anadolu Psikiyatri Dergisi, 16*(2), 146–149.

Everaerd, W. (1983). A case of apotemnophilia: A handicap as sexual preference. *American Journal of Psychotherapy, 37*(2), 285–293.

Fedoroff, J. P., & Fedoroff, I. (1992). Buspirone and Paraphilic Sexual Behavior. *Journal of Offender Rehabilitation. 18*(3-4), 89–108. doi:10.1300/J076v18n03_09

Fedoroff, J. P. (2003). The paraphilic world. In S. B. Levine (Ed.), *Handbook of clinical sexuality for mental health professionals* (pp. 333–356). New York, NY: Brunner/Routledge.

Fedoroff, J. P. (2010). Paraphilic worlds. In S. B. Levine (Ed.), *Handbook of clinical sexuality for mental health professionals* (pp. 401–424). New York, NY: Routledge.

Fedoroff, J. P. (2018). More puzzles: A response to Seto's (2017) "The puzzle of male chronophilias." *Archives of Sexual Behavior, 47*(8), 2171–2173. doi:10.1007/s10508-016-0889-x

Fedoroff, J. P., Brunet, A., Woods, V., Granger, C., Chow, E., Collins, P., & Shapiro, C. (1997). A case-controlled study of men who sexually assault sleeping victims. In C. Shapiro & A. McCall Smith (Eds.), *Forensic aspects of sleep*. Chichester, UK: John Wiley & Sons.

Fellion, G., Duflot, J. P., Anglade, P., & Fraillon, J. (1980). From fantasy to reality: On criminal and cannibalistic behavior [in French]. *Annales Medico-Psychologiques, 138*(5), 596–602.

Fenichel, O. (1937). The scopophilic instinct and identification. *International Journal of Psychoanalysis, 18*, 6–34.

Ferguson, L. N., & Rekers, G. A. (1979). Non-aversive intervention in public childhood masturbation: A case study. *Journal of Sex Research, 15*(3), 213–223.

Fitzgerald, M. (2011). Necrophilia and autistic psychopathy. *Clinical Neuropsychiatry, 8*(5), 301–303.

Fraenkel, E. (1954). Comments about the case of mysophilia reported by Doctors Hoelen and Fleskens [in French]. *Psyche, Paris, 9*, 194–198.
Franklin, K. (2010). Hebephilia: Quintessence of diagnostic pretextuality. *Behavioral Sciences & the Law, 28*(6), 751–768.
Gerard, S. M., Jobes, D., Cimbolic, P., Ritzler, B. A., & Montana, S. (2003). A Rorschach study of interpersonal disturbance in priest child molesters. *Sexual Addiction & Compulsivity, 10*(1), 53–66.
Gerard-Sharp, S. (2000). A Rorschach study of interpersonal disturbance in priest same-sex ephebophiles. Doctoral dissertation, Catholic University of America, Washington, DC (ProQuest Information & Learning, UMI No. 9969581).
Gill, M. (2012). Sex can wait, masturbate: The politics of masturbation training. *Sexualities, 15*(3–4), 472–493.
Ginsburg, H. J., Ogletree, S. M., & Silakowski, T. D. (2003). Vulgar language: Review of sex differences in usage, attributions, and pathologies. *North American Journal of Psychology, 5*(1), 105–116.
Giordano, B., White, J., & Lester, D. (2012). A typology of criminal cannibalism. *American Journal of Forensic Psychology, 30*(3), 35–44.
Godlewski, J., & Szalankiewicz, M. (1987). Apotemnophilia [in Polish]. *Psychiatria Polska, 21*(2), 141–144.
Goldberg, R. L., & Wise, T. N. (1985). Psychodynamic treatment for telephone scatologia. *American Journal of Psychoanalysis, 45*(3), 291–297.
Good, P., & Burstein, J. (2012). Hebephilia and the construction of a fictitious diagnosis. *Journal of Nervous and Mental Disease, 200*(6), 492–494.
Greenberg, D. M., Bradford, J., & Curry, S. (1995). Infantophilia—A new subcategory of pedophilia? A preliminary study. *Journal of the American Academy of Psychiatry and the Law Online, 23*(1), 63–71.
Greenhill, R., & Griffiths, M. D. (2016). Sexual interest as performance, intellect and pathology: A critical discursive case study of dacryphilia. *Psychology & Sexuality, 7*(4), 265–278.
Griffiths, M. D. (2013). Eproctophilia in a young adult male. *Archives of Sexual Behavior, 42*(8), 1383–1386.
Gubb, K., Segal, J., Khota, A., & Dicks, A. (2006). Clinical vampirism: A review and illustrative case report. *South African Psychiatry Review, 9*(3), 163–168.
Guinn, J. (2013). *The Life and times of Charles Manson*. New York: Simon @ Schuster.
Hames, R., & Blanchard, R. (2012). Anthropological data regarding the adaptiveness of hebephilia. *Archives of Sexual Behavior, 41*(4), 745–747.
Harris, P. (1994). Self-induced autonomic dysreflexia ('boosting') practiced by sme tetraplegic athletes to enhance their athletic performance. *Spinal Cord, 32*, 289–291. doi:10.1038/sc.1994.50
Hawkinson, K., & Zamboni, B. D. (2014). Adult baby/diaper lovers: An exploratory study of an online community sample. *Archives of Sexual Behaviour, 43*(5), 863–877. doi:10.1007/s10508-013-0241-7
Hensley, C., Tallichet, S. E., & Dutkiewicz, E. L. (2010). Childhood bestiality: A potential precursor to adult interpersonal violence. *Journal of Interpersonal Violence, 25*(3), 557–567.
Higgs, T., Stefanska, E. B., Carter, A. J., & Browne, K. D. (2017). The developmental and criminal histories of subgroups of sexual murderers engaging, or not engaging, in post mortem sexual interference, compared to rapists. *Journal of Criminal Justice, 53*, 92–101.
Hingsburger, D. (1989). Motives for coprophilia: Working with individuals who had been institutionalized with developmental handicaps. *Journal of Sex Research, 26*(1), 139–140.
Holoyda, B., Sorrentino, R., Friedman, S. H., & Allgire, J. (2018). Bestiality: An introduction for legal and mental health professionals. *Behavioral Sciences & the Law*, 36(6), 687–697.
Houngbedji, A., & Guillem, E. (2016). Profiles and sexual practices of current and past swingers interviewed on French websites. *Sexologies: European Journal of Sexology and Sexual Health, 25*(1), e1–e4.
Hucker, S. (2016). In B. A. Sharpless (Ed.), *Unusual and rare psychological disorders: A handbook for clinical practice and research* (pp. 149–163). New York, NY: Oxford University Press.

Hurley, A. D., & Sovner, R. (1983). Treatment of sexual deviation in mentally retarded persons. *Psychiatric Aspects of Mental Retardation Newsletter, 2*(4), 13–16.

Imhoff, R., Banse, R., & Schmidt, A. F. (2017). Toward a theoretical understanding of sexual orientation and sexual motivation. *Archives of Sexual Behavior, 46*(1), 29–33.

Innala, S. M., & Ernulf, K. E. (1987). What is asphyxiophilia? [in Swedish]. *Nordisk Sexologi, 5*(3), 108–115.

Innala, S. M., & Ernulf, K. E. (1989). Asphyxiophilia in Scandinavia. *Archives of Sexual Behavior, 18*(3), 181–189.

Jaffe, P. D., & DiCataldo, F. (1994). Clinical vampirism: Blending myth and reality. *Bulletin of the American Academy of Psychiatry & the Law, 22*(4), 533–544.

Janssen, D. F. (2017). "Chronophilia": Appreciating 150 years of puzzle-solving. *Archives of Sexual Behavior, 46*(1), 35–38.

Janzen, W. B., & Peacock, R. (1978). Treatment of public masturbation by behavioral management. *American Journal of Psychotherapy, 32*(2), 300–306.

Kafka, M. P. (2010a). The DSM diagnostic criteria for fetishism. *Archives of Sexual Behavior, 39*(2), 357–362.

Kafka, M. P. (2010b). The DSM diagnostic criteria for paraphilia not otherwise specified. *Archives of Sexual Behavior, 39*(2), 373–376.

Klimmer, R. (1968). Urolagnie: A form of fetishism? *Psychiatrie, Neurologie und Medizinische Psychologie, 20*(6), 219–222.

Knafo, D. (2015). For the love of death: Somnophilic and necrophilic acts and fantasies. *Journal of the American Psychoanalytic Association, 63*(5), 857–886.

Kunjukrishnan, R., Pawlak, A., & Varan, L. R. (1988). The clinical and forensic psychiatric issues of retifism. *Canadian Journal of Psychiatry, 33*(9), 819–825.

Lande, R. G. (1993). Mental responsibility and 900 phone abuse. *Journal of Psychiatry & Law, 21*(1), 109–121.

Lapointe, D., & Le Bosse, Y. (2010). Incest: Is freeing oneself possible? If so, under what conditions? *Revue Quebecoise de Psychologie, 31*(1), 193–206.

Lawrence, A. (2011). Sexual dysfunction: beyond brain-body connection. In: R. Balon (Ed.), *Sexual Dysfunction: Beyond the Brain-Body Connection. Adv Psychosom Med.* (vol. 31, pp. 135–148). Basel, Karger. https://doi.org/10.1159/000328921

Lauerma, H. (2016). Somnophilia and sexual abuse using vaginal administration of triazolam. *Journal of Forensic Sciences, 61*(3), 862–863.

Lee, N. (2007). The impact of psychosocial risk factors on the development of pedophilia and ephebophilia in members of the Roman *Catholic* clergy. Doctoral dissertation, George Mason University, Fairfax, VA (ProQuest Information & Learning, UMI No. 3239469).

Lehmiller, J. J., Ley, D., & Savage, D. (2018). The psychology of gay men's cuckolding fantasies. *Archives of Sexual Behavior, 47*(4), 999–1013.

Lehne, G. K., & Money, J. (2000). The first case of paraphilia treated with Depo-Provera: 40-year outcome. *Journal of Sex Education and Therapy, 25*(4), 213–220.

Lemma, A. (2013). Whose skin is it anyway? Some reflections on the psychic function of necrophilic fantasies. *Rivista di Psicoanalisi, 59*(2), 283–304.

Lesandric, V., Orlovic, I., Peitl, V., & Karlovic, D. (2017). Zoophilia as an early sign of psychosis. *Alcoholism and Psychiatry Research, 53*(1), 27–32.

Lester, D., White, J., King, V., & Drive, F. (2011). Necrophilia in serial killers: Is there evidence for Asperger's syndrome. *Clinical Neuropsychiatry, 8*(6), 367–368.

London, L. S., & Caprio, F. S. (1950a). Coprophilia. In L. S. London & F. S. Caprio (Eds.), *Sexual deviations* (pp. 557–575). Washington, DC: Linacre Press.

London, L. S., & Caprio, F. S. (1950b). Urolagnia. In L. S. London & F. S. Caprio (Eds.), *Sexual deviations* (pp. 576–587). Washington, DC: Linacre Press.

Lothstein, L. M. (1990). Psychological theories of pedophilia and ephebophilia. In S. J. Rossetti (Ed.), *Slayer of the soul: Child sexual abuse and the Catholic Church* (pp. 19–43). Mystic, CT: Twenty-Third Publications.

Lundervold, D. A., & Young, L. G. (1992). Treatment acceptability ratings for sexual offenders: Effects of diagnosis and offense. *Research in Developmental Disabilities, 13*(3), 229–237.

Lunsky, Y., Frijters, J., Griffiths, D. M., Watson, S. L., & Williston, S. (2007). Sexual knowledge and attitudes of men with intellectual disability who sexually offend. *Journal of Intellectual and Developmental Disability, 32*(2), 74–81.

Lykins, A. D., & Cantor, J. M. (2014). Vorarephilia: A case study in masochism and erotic consumption. *Archives of Sexual Behavior, 43*(1), 181–186.

MacCulloch, M., Gray, N., & Watt, A. (2000). Brittain's Sadistic Murderer Syndrome reconsidered: an associative account of the aetiology of sadistic sexual fantasy. *The Journal of Forensic Psychiatry, 11*(2), 401–418. doi:10.1080/09585180050142606

Maratea, R. J. (2011). Screwing the pooch: Legitimizing accounts in a zoophilia on-line community. *Deviant Behavior, 32*(10), 918–943.

Marneros, A. (1984). Gilles de la Tourette's syndrome [in German]. *Fortschritte der Neurologie, Psychiatrie, 52*(7), 250–257.

Massion-Verniory, L., & Dumont, E. (1958). Four cases of urolagnia. *Acta Neurologica et Psychiatrica Belgica, 58*, 446–459.

Masters, B. (1985). *Killing for company: The case of Dennis Nilsen.* London, UK: Cape.

McClellan, J. E. (2008). Profiling violent sexualized homicides: Investigating lust murder. Doctoral dissertation, Northcentral University, San Diego, CA (UMI No. 3318974).

McCully, R. S. (1964). Vampirism: Historical perspective and underlying process in relation to a case of autovampirism. *Journal of Nervous and Mental Disease, 139*(5), 440–452.

McGeoch, P. D., Brang, D., Song, T., Lee, R. R., Huang, M., & Ramachandran, V. S. (2011). Xenomelia: A new right parietal lobe syndrome. *Journal of Neurology, Neurosurgery & Psychiatry, 82*(12), 1314–1319.

Medina-Pérez, Ó. A., García-Vega, L. M., Villard Plaza, J. P., & Ortiz Valencia, J. C. (2018). Characterization of Sex with Animals in Córdoba, Colombia. An Exploratory Study. *Preprints*, 2018090484. doi:10.20944/preprints201809.0484.v1.

Mendhekar, D. N., & Duggal, H. S. (2005). Sertraline for Klüver–Bucy syndrome in an adolescent. *European Psychiatry, 20*(4), 355–356.

Miletski, H. (2017). Zoophilia: Another sexual orientation? *Archives of Sexual Behavior, 46*(1), 39–42.

Mokros, A. (2017). The chronophilia conundrum: Continuum or epiphenomenon? *Archives of Sexual Behavior, 46*(1), 43–45.

Money, J. (1990a). Forensic sexology: Paraphilic serial rape (biastophilia) and lust murder (erotophonophilia). *American Journal of Psychotherapy, 44*(1), 26–36.

Money, J. (1990b). Paraphilia in females: Fixation on amputation and lameness—Two personal accounts. *Journal of Psychology & Human Sexuality, 3*(2), 165–172.

Money, J., Jobaris, R., & Furth, G. (1977). Apotemnophilia: Two cases of self-demand amputation as a paraphilia. *Journal of Sex Research, 13*(2), 115–125.

Money, J., & Simcoe, K. W. (1984). Acrotomophilia, sex and disability: New concepts and case report. *Sexuality and Disability, 7*(1–2), 43–50.

Money, J., Wainwright, G., & Hingsburger, D. (1991). The breathless orgasm: A lovemap biography of asphyxiophilia. In *The breathless orgasm: A lovemap biography of asphyxiophilia.* Amherst, US: Prometheus Books.

Musser, P., Cimbolic, P., & Rossetti, S. (1995). Ephebophilia and the MCMI-II. *Sexual Addiction & Compulsivity, 2*(3), 214–222.

Newring, K. A. B. (2014). Telephone scatologia. In W. T. O'Donohue (Ed.), *Case studies in sexual deviance: Toward evidence-based practice* (pp. 168–194). New York, NY: Routledge/Taylor & Francis Group.

Noonan-Karstens, M. (2009). Psychobiological model of personality and ephebophilia within the Roman Catholic priesthood. Doctoral dissertation, Fielding Graduate University, Santa Barbara, CA (ProQuest Dissertations, UMI No. 3350591).

Nu Ez, J. (2003). Outpatient treatment of the sexually compulsive ephebophile. *Sexual Addiction & Compulsivity, 10*(1), 23–51.

Olry, R., & Haines, D. E. (2011). Renfield's syndrome: A psychiatric illness drawn from Bram Stoker's *Dracula*. *Journal of the History of the Neurosciences, 20*(4), 368–371.

Oppawasky, J. (2010). Vampirism: Clinical vampirism—Renfield's syndrome. *Annals of the American Psychotherapy Association, 13*(4), 58–63.

Othman, Z., Razak, A. A., & Zakaria, R. (2014). Zoophilia in a patient with frontotemporal dementia. *International Medical Journal, 21*(5), 466–467.

Oules, J., Boscredon, J., & Bataille, J. (1977). A case of gerontophilia [in French]. *L'Evolution Psychiatrique, 41*(2), 243–257.

Pakhomou, S. M. (2006). Methodological aspects of telephone scatologia: A case study. *International Journal of Law and Psychiatry, 29*(3), 178–185.

Pallone, N. J. (2002). Sin, crime, arrogance, betrayal: A psychodynamic perspective on the crisis in American Catholicism. *Brief Treatment and Crisis Intervention, 2*(4), 341–372.

Panagakis, M. N. (2012). Sibling incest: An exploration of trauma, impact, and treatment. Doctoral dissertation, Azusa Pacific University, Azusa, CA (ProQuest Dissertations, UMI No. 3472380).

Pandita-Gunawardena, R. (1990). Paraphilic infantilism: A rare case of fetishistic behaviour. *British Journal of Psychiatry, 157*, 767–770.

Paul, R. H., Marx, B. P., & Orsillo, S. M. (1999). Acceptance-based psychotherapy in the treatment of an adjudicated exhibitionist: A case example. *Behavior Therapy, 30*(1), 149–162.

Pettigrew, M. (2017). Comorbid, sequential, or different desires? Exploring the relationship between somnophilia and necrophilia. *Journal of Sexual Aggression, 23*(3), 351–359.

Pettigrew, M. (2019). Fantasy, opportunity, homicide: Testing classifications of necrophilic behaviour. *Journal of Police and Criminal Psychology, 34*, 14–22.

Pocknell, Victoria Charlotte Mary-Rose. (2017). Developmental Factors And Maladjustment Indicators Of Specific Sexual Interests. *Theses and Dissertations*, 2314. https://commons.und.edu/theses/2314

Prentky, R., Dowdell, E., Fedoroff, P., Burgess, A., Malamuth, N., & Schuler, A. (2010). A multi-prong approach to strengthening Internet safety [Monograph]. United States Office of Juvenile Justice and Delinquency Prevention.

Price, M., Gutheil, T. G., Commons, M. L., Kafka, M. P., & Dodd-Kimmey, S. (2001a). Telephone scatologia: Comorbidity and theories of etiology. *Psychiatric Annals, 31*(4), 226–232.

Price, M., Gutheil, T. G., Commons, M. L., Kafka, M. P., & Dodd-Kimmey, S. (2001b). Redefining telephone scatologia: Treatment and classification. *Psychiatric Annals, 31*(5), 282–289.

Price, M., Kafka, M., Commons, M. L., Gutheil, T. G., & Simpson, W. (2002). Telephone scatologia: Comorbidity with other paraphilias and paraphilia-related disorders. *International Journal of Law and Psychiatry, 25*(1), 37–49.

Prins, H. (1985). Vampirism: A clinical condition. *British Journal of Psychiatry, 146*, 666–668.

Prohaska, A. (2014). Help me get fat! Feederism as communal deviance on the internet. *Deviant Behavior, 35*(4), 263–274.

Pullman, L. E., Sawatsky, M. L., Babchishin, K. M., McPhail, I. V., & Seto, M. C. (2017). Differences between biological and sociolegal incest offenders: A meta-analysis. *Aggression and Violent Behavior, 34*, 228–237.

Purcell, C. E. (2000). An investigation of paraphilias, lust murder, and the case of Jeffrey Dahmer: An integrative theoretical model. Doctoral dissertation, California School of Professional Psychology, Los Angeles, CA.

Quackelbeen, J., Nobus, D., & Temmerman, K. (1997). Auto-erotic asphyxiation: A sexual praxis in neurosis and perversion. *Clinical Studies: International Journal of Psychoanalysis, 3*(1), 31–54.

Rehn, A., & Borgerson, J. (2005). Is there a cannibal in organization studies? Notes on anthropophagy and organization (Recipe included). *Culture and Organization, 11*(2), 69–81. doi:10.1080/14759550500091002

Rossetti, S., Anthony, P., Cimbolic, P., & Wright, T. L. (1996). Development and preliminary validation of the MMPI-2 scale for same-sex priest child molesters. *Sexual Addiction & Compulsivity, 3*(4), 341–356.

Rousal, J., & Brichcin, S. (1971). The case of mysophilia [in Czech]. *Ceskoslovenska Psychiatrie, 67*(3), 176–180.

Ryan, C. J. (2009). Out on a limb: The ethical management of body integrity identity disorder. *Neuroethics, 2*(1), 21–33.

Saunders, E. B., & Awad, G. A. (1991). Male adolescent sexual offenders: Exhibitionism and obscene phone calls. *Child Psychiatry and Human Development, 21*(3), 169–178.

Schenk, A. M., Cooper-Lehki, C., Keelan, C. M., & Fremouw, W. J. (2014). Underreporting of bestiality among juvenile sex offenders: Polygraph versus self-report. *Journal of Forensic Sciences, 59*(2), 540–542.

Scobie, A., & Taylor, A. J. W. (1975). Perversions ancient and modern: I. Agalmatophilia, the statue syndrome. *Journal of the History of the Behavioral Sciences, 11*(1), 49–54.

Sedda, A., & Bottini, G. (2014). Apotemnophilia, body integrity identity disorder or xenomelia? Psychiatric and neurologic etiologies face each other. *Neuropsychiatric Disease and Treatment, 10*, 1255.

Sendler, D. J. (2018). Why people who have sex with animals believe that it is their sexual orientation—A grounded theory study of online communities of zoophiles. *Deviant Behavior, 39*(11), 1507–1514.

Seto, M. C. (2017). The puzzle of male chronophilias. *Archives of Sexual Behavior, 46*(1), 3–22.

Seto, M. C., Babchishin, K. M., Pullman, L. E., & McPhail, I. V. (2015). The puzzle of intrafamilial child sexual abuse: A meta-analysis comparing intrafamilial and extrafamilial offenders with child victims. *Clinical Psychology Review, 39*, 42–57.

Simpson, G. K., Sabaz, M., & Daher, M. (2013). Prevalence, clinical features, and correlates of inappropriate sexual behavior after traumatic brain injury: A multicenter study. *Journal of Head Trauma Rehabilitation, 28*(3), 202–210.

Singy, P. (2015a). Hebephilia: A postmortem dissection. *Archives of Sexual Behavior, 44*(5), 1109–1116.

Singy, P. (2015b). Danger and difference: The stakes of hebephilia. In S. Demazeux & P. Singy (Eds.), *The DSM-5 in perspective: Philosophical reflections on the psychiatric Babel* (pp. 113–124). New York, NY: Springer.

Solvang, P. (2007). The amputee body desired: Beauty destabilized? Disability re-valued? *Sexuality and Disability, 25*(2), 51–64.

Stein, M. L., Schlesinger, L. B., & Pinizzotto, A. J. (2010). Necrophilia and sexual homicide. *Journal of Forensic Sciences, 55*(2), 443–446.

Stephens, S., Cantor, J. M., Goodwill, A. M., & Seto, M. C. (2017). Multiple indicators of sexual interest in prepubescent or pubescent children as predictors of sexual recidivism. *Journal of Consulting and Clinical Psychology, 85*(6), 585–595.

Stephens, S., & Seto, M. C. (2016). Hebephilic sexual offending. In A. Phenix & H. M. Hoberman (Eds.), *Sexual offending: Predisposing antecedents, assessments, and management* (pp. 29–43). New York, NY: Springer.

Stephens, S., Seto, M. C., Goodwill, A. M., & Cantor, J. M. (2017). Evidence of construct validity in the assessment of hebephilia. *Archives of Sexual Behavior, 46*(1), 301–309.

Stoylen, I. J. (1985). Voyeurism: Treatment by cognitive behavior therapy in a case of scopophilia [in Norwegian]. *Tidsskrift for Norsk Psykologforening, 22*(10), 561–564.

Terry, L. L., Suschinsky, K. D., Lalumiere, M. L., & Vasey, P. L. (2012). Feederism: An exaggeration of a normative mate selection preference? *Archives of Sexual Behavior, 41*(1), 249–260.

Terry, L. L., & Vasey, P. L. (2011). Feederism in a woman. *Archives of Sexual Behavior, 40*(3), 639–645.

Thompson, A. R., & Beail, N. (2002). The treatment of auto-erotic asphyxiation in a man with severe intellectual disabilities: The effectiveness of a behavioural and educational programme. *Journal of Applied Research in Intellectual Disabilities, 15*(1), 36–47.

Troyer, J. (2008). Abuse of a corpse: A brief history and re-theorization of necrophilia laws in the USA. *Mortality, 13*(2), 132–152.

Van Renynghe De Voxvrie, G., & Massion-Verniory, L. (1964). Regarding a case of kleptolagnia of a homophilic character [in French]. *Acta Neurologica et Psychiatrica Belgica, 64*(7), 753–762.

Vanden Bergh, R. L., & Kelly, J. F. (1964). Vampirism: A review with new observations. *Archives of General Psychiatry, 11*(5), 543–547.

Ventus, D., Antfolk, J., & Salo, B. (2017). The associations between abuse characteristics in child sexual abuse: A meta-analysis. *Journal of Sexual Aggression, 23*(2), 167–180.

Wagner, M. K. (1968). A case of public masturbation treated by operant conditioning. *Child Psychology & Psychiatry & Allied Disciplines*, *9*(1), 61–65.

West, S. G., & Resnick, P. J. (2017). Necrophilia. In B. A. Sharpless (Ed.), *Unusual and rare psychological disorders: A handbook for clinical practice and research* (pp. 124–135). New York, NY: Oxford University Press.

White, M. J. (1978). The statue syndrome: Perversion? Fantasy? Anecdote? *Journal of Sex Research*, *14*(4), 246–249.

Wignall, L., & McCormack, M. (2017). An exploratory study of a new kink activity: "Pup play." *Archives of Sexual Behavior*, *46*(3), 801–811.

Williams, A., Phillips, L., & Ahmed, Z. (2000). Assessment and management of auto-erotic asphyxiation in a young man with learning disability: A multidisciplinary approach to intervention. *British Journal of Learning Disabilities*, *28*(3), 109–112.

Wise, T. N., & Goldberg, R. L. (1995). Escalation of a fetish: Coprophagia in a nonpsychotic adult of normal intelligence. *Journal of Sex & Marital Therapy*, *21*(4), 272–275.

Wochner, M., & Klosinski, G. (1988). Child and juvenile psychiatric features of zoosadists [in German]. *Schweizer Archiv fur Neurologie, Neurochirurgie und Psychiatrie*, *139*(3), 59–67.

Xavier, C. M. (1955). Coprophilia—A clinical study. *British Journal of Medical Psychology*, *28*, 188–190.

Yates, P. (2017). Sibling sexual abuse: Why don't we talk about it? *Journal of Clinical Nursing*, *26*(15–16), 2482–2494.

Zaviacic, M. (1993). Sexual asphyxiophilia. *Cesko-Slovenska Psychiatrie*, *89*(4), 200–208.

Zavitzianos, G. (1972). Homeovestism: Perverse form of behaviour involving wearing clothes of the same sex. *International Journal of Psychoanalysis*, *53*(4), 471–477.

Zavitzianos, G. (1977). The object in fetishism, homeovestism and transvestism. *International Journal of Psychoanalysis*, *58*, 487–495.

11
Putting It All Together
Quo Vadis?

Keep moving forward.

—Muriel Elaine Fedoroff

Introduction

Multiple Perspectives

This book has reviewed ways in which unconventional sexual interests and behaviors have been classified. The system that appeals most to each reader will depend on the reader's background and preferred working paradigm. Those who think of paraphilias from a medical perspective will tend to think of possible anatomic or physiologic pathologies. Those who think of paraphilias from a behavioral perspective will tend to think of learned interests and behaviors due to mechanisms such as unconditioned and conditioned primary and second-order responses, blocking, generalization, punishment, and extinction. Those who think of paraphilias as variations on the range of sexual interests and behaviors shared by diverse population samples of humans will be prone to depathologize paraphilias (in terms of a medical perspective) and to avoid categories. Those who focus on understanding the meaning that the paraphilia has for the person with the paraphilia will tend to think in terms of the person's life history (McHugh & Slavney, 1983; Fedoroff, 2009).

Table 11.1 summarizes the four perspectives described previously and at the beginning of this book. However, this time they are compared with five aspects of sexuality listed in order of mutability from lowest degree of changeability (genes) to highest degree of change (drive). Each table entry provides an example of issues of interest from each perspective. The table is not meant to be comprehensive or definitive but simply to show how the same issue can be addressed from multiple perspectives and via multiple factors. Many of the current disputes about the nature of the paraphilias derive from a failure to be clear about the perspective or factor

Table 11.1 Four Perspectives and Five Factors of Paraphilias

	Disease	Behavioral	Dimensional	Life Story
Genes	Metabolic disorders	Behavioral syndromes	Environmental interactions	Psychotherapies
Gender	Intersex syndromes	Gender roles	Gender identities and roles	Human rights
Orientation	Birth order effects	Self-identity	Kinsey scale	Political rights
Interest	Cortical or limbic damage	Acquired/learned interests	Cultural variations	Individual, couple, family, and group therapies
Drive	Hormones	Sexual activities	Age and opportunity	Couple's therapy

being discussed. For example, a claim that all paraphilias are due to brain damage (a disease perspective) is in danger of mistaking orientation with interest or drive and ignores a variety of interventions (e.g., medications, hormones, education and learning, reframing of the nature of the problem, and a variety of psychotherapeutic interventions). Importantly, it is better to consider all four perspectives and all five factors when deciding if the condition can be modified.

The Danger of Blending Factors and Paradigms

The lovemap paradigm, created and championed by John Money, borrowed from the four perspectives described previously. It also blended concepts derived from genetics, gender, orientation, and sex drive to categorize and explain the paraphilias. The idea that every person has a "lovemap" depathologized people with paraphilias. However, the concept of "vandalized" lovemaps did the opposite.

The lovemap paradigm has proven to be highly persuasive to disparate groups of researchers, clinicians, and people with paraphilias. In part, this is due to the fact that the lovemap paradigm is difficult to disprove because it does not generate testable hypotheses. If a person with pedophilia fails to develop a pedophilic lovemap at age 8 years, it can be explained by stating that the person just did not "realize" their pedophilia until later. If the person with pedophilia changes their lovemap, then the lovemap paradigm advocate simply states that the person obviously did not really have pedophilia in the first place: "They must have had something else or maybe their lovemap was never really vandalized."

As described previously, the lovemap paradigm has unfortunately had some unintended consequences. For example, the blending of love, sexual interest, and gender has fueled acrimonious debates such as the question of whether the desire of some men to live their lives as women is a paraphilia. It has also led to the belief that paraphilias, once "hardwired" or "imprinted" during a "critical period," can never be changed.

Is there a way to move forward more productively? Physics has shown that alternative paradigms can coexist. Newtonian physics and quantum physics present completely different worldviews. However, for most people, Newtonian physics is more than enough, and in many ways better, than quantum physics for everyday tasks such as measuring one's weight and calculating how much exercise and food it will take to avoid getting heavier on planet Earth. Modern physicists do not dismiss Newton as misguided. Instead, they honor his contributions as the basis on which modern physics is built.

Sexologists would do better by adopting the approach of modern physicists. Instead of dismissing alternative paradigms, often by attacking the proponents of the paradigms, they should accept that alternative paradigms and perspectives may "work" better for different people in different situations. For example, a lovemap paradigm may be ideal for teenagers wondering if they are gay (Money, 1986), provided they do not read the literature on "vandalized" lovemaps (Money & Lamacz, 1989).

Sexologists should pay attention to the perspectives they endorse, remembering that multiple perspectives are not only possible but also usually better. Furthermore, they should acknowledge the paradigm they are using, including its strengths and limitations.

Context

Above all else, sexual interest is contextual. The same behavior has completely different significance depending on context. Consider an act: Insertion of a finger into a vagina. If the behavior occurs between two people in the back seat of a car in a secluded parking lot on a moonlit night, it could be part of an exciting romantic interlude between a heterosexual or lesbian couple. However, if the person with the vagina is a child and the person with the finger is an adult, it is behavior indicative of pedophilia. If the finger belongs to a physician, it is still indicative of pedophilia unless the insertion occurs in the physician's office as part of a legitimate medical examination conducted with the voluntary, informed consent of the girl and her parents.

Now suppose the female is an adult but has intellectual disability. What if the person with the finger also has intellectual disability? What if they do not have intellectual disabilities or have unequal disabilities? What if the two people are related? Does it make a difference if they are brother and sister? What if they are related by marriage? Or adoption? Would it make a difference if the genders were reversed and insertion involved a rectum instead of a vagina? The point of all these questions is not to be annoying but to show that the same action can be viewed very differently not only by different people but also by the same person. Furthermore, their opinions are contextual and may change depending on a host of other factors.

Interaction

All the contextual factors mentioned previously do significantly alter perspectives and opinions. This is not a fault of sexology. It is because sex is not only contextual but also interactive. Classifications of paraphilias need to accurately describe not only the specific interest or act but also with whom the person wants to act. As described in Chapter 10, every paraphilia has an opposite. Most can be defined in terms of persistent interest. But whether the interest is acted on with another person or persons and/or on one's self is an important independent variable. For example, despite the claim in the Fifth edition of the *Diagnostic and Statistical Manual of Mental Disorders* (DSM-5; American Psychiatric Association [APA], 2013, p. 698) that people with multiple victims are pedophilic even if they report no interest, it is now accepted that not all people with pedophilia sexually assault children and vice versa.

Many of the criticisms of the current diagnostic schema (e.g., the DSM or the *International Classification of Diseases* [ICD; World Health Organization, 2004]) result from a failure to adequately account for context (Fedoroff, 2011, Moser, 2011; First, 2014). Some advocate for the elimination of all paraphilias from the DSM and ICD. Is this a good idea? It depends on the context. If the purpose is to protect men with transvestism from losing access to their children, bravo. But isn't this throwing the baby out with the bathwater? Suppose advocates of Einsteinian physics advocated the abolition of conventional wristwatches because we know that time is relative?

What should researchers, clinicians, and people with paraphilias do? The solution is to make context part of the diagnostic criteria. Rather than a diagnosis of "asphyxiophilia," which the DSM-5 defines as "If the individual engages in the practice of achieving sexual arousal related to restriction of breathing" (APA, 2013, p. 694), the diagnosis should specify how important the act is for sexual arousal, who is being asphyxiated, in what context, and for what purpose. In addition to subcategorizing paraphilias on the basis of these criteria, it is possible to subgroup them into three main categories based on apparent motivation.

Taboo

Many people with paraphilias report they are aroused by the knowledge they are "doing something wrong or disgusting." Of course, what one person finds wrong or disgusting depends on multiple other factors. Examples of paraphilias in which taboo plays a prominent part are summarized in Table 11.2. In Tables 11.2–11.4, the "historic" column heading refers to the way that John Money tended to classify the paraphilia.

Table 11.2 Paraphilias Contextually Motivated by Breaching Taboo

Paraphilia	Core Interest/Act	Historic Classification
Heirophilia	Religious objects	Fetish
Homilophilia	Religious speeches/sermons	Sacrificial
Mysophilia	Filth	Fetish
Nosophilia	Terminal illness	Sacrificial
Pecattiaphilia	Sin	Sacrificial

Social and/or Partner Avoidance

Many people are overwhelmed by the societal expectations concerning courtship and sexual intimacy. Strategies to engage in sexual activity while avoiding social contact include more than the so-called courtship disorders. For example, a person who is unable to approach a potential adult partner due to social anxiety or fear of rejection may divert their sexual interests to children. This is not a conscious choice but can be due to a pattern of behaviors in which a person chooses to avoid adult interactions in order to spend time with children who are perceived as less threating and/or less judgmental. Of course, there are many other possible explanations for the onset of pedophilic interests, but consideration not only of the sexual interest in children but also the failure to develop sexual interest and social interaction with adults is also important. Table 11.3 presents paraphilias characterized by impairment in the ability to form consenting sexual interactions with adults.

Autonomic Paraphilias

A third, and perhaps most important, category of paraphilias is shown in Table 11.4—the autonomic paraphilias. As the name implies, these paraphilias are characterized by some act that manipulates the autonomic nervous system to accentuate the sequence of parasympathetic arousal followed by sympathetic arousal that is characteristic of sexual arousal. Parasympathetic arousal can result from distention of organs (e.g., bladder and rectum). A pattern of increasing parasympathic stimulation may be associated with "edging," in which orgasm is intentionally avoided. Becoming aware of functions that are normally under autonomic control (e.g., breathing) can intensify physical sensation. Heightened parasympathetic activity can accentuate sympathetic activity. An example is autoerotic self-asphyxiation, in which sympathetic stimulation is triggered by anoxia, which in turn heightens the sensation of orgasm.

Review of Tables 11.2–11.4 shows that classifications can be overlapping. People may engage in taboo paraphilias precisely because they avoid conventional social contact or because they heighten autonomic activity.

Table 11.3 Social or Conventional Partner Avoidance Paraphilias

Paraphilia	Core Interest/Act	Historic Classification
Pedophilia	Children	Eligibility
Infantophilia	Infants	Eligibility
Gerontophilia	Elderly	Eligibility
Hebephilia	Late adolescent	Eligibility
Ephebophilia	Early adolescent	Eligibility
Necrophilia	Death	Sacrificial
Incest	Relative(s)	Eligibility
Abasiophilia	Disability	Eligibility
Acoustophilia	Sounds	Solicitation/courtship
Acrotomophilia	Amputees	Eligibility/sacrificial
Agalmatophilia	Statues	Fetish
Agnophilia	Fighting (observing)	Predatory
Agrexophilia	Being heard having sex	Solicitation/courtship
Algolagnia	Pain	Sacrificial
Amaurophilia	Blindness	Solicitation/courtship
Anasteemaphilia	Height difference	Eligibility
Andromimetophilia	Women with male features or dressed as men	Eligibility
Anlilagnia	Older women by younger men	Eligibility
Anthropophagy	Eating human flesh	Predatory
Apodysophilia	Undressing	Solicitation/courtship
Apotemnophilia	Becoming an amputee	Sacrificial
Aquaphilia	Water	Fetish
Aretifism	Bare feet	Fetish
Autoandrophilia	Females being males	Eligibility
Autogynephilia	Being female or having female features	Fetish
Autonepiophilia	Wearing diapers	Fetish
Biastophilia	Rape	Courtship/predatory
Candaulism	Spouse with another partner	Multiple
Capnolagnia	Smoking	Fetish
Celebriphilia	Celebrities	Eligibility
Chremastistophilia	Sex for money	Mercantile
Chronophilia	Age discrepancy	Multiple
Devotee	Disability	Eligibility/sacrificial
Dysmorphilia	Discrepant size	Fetish
Ecouteurism	Overhearing sex	Solicitation/courtship
Exhibitionism	Exposing to strangers	Solicitation/courtship
Faunoiphilia	Watching animal mating	Fetish
Feederism	Feeding	Fetish/eligibility
Frotteurism	Rubbing strangers	Solicitation/courtship
Gonophilia	Knees	Fetish
Gynemimetophilia	Male with breasts	Eligibility

Table 11.3 *Continued*

Paraphilia	Core Interest/Act	Historic Classification
Heterophilia	Heterosexuals by a non-heterosexual person	Eligibility
Hodophilia	Foreign venues/vacations	Solicitation/courtship
Iatronudia	Medical doctors	Eligibility
Macrophilia	Giants	Eligibility
Maiesiophilia	Pregnancy	Eligibility
Mask fetishism	Masks or removal of masks	Eligibility
Masochism	Being controlled	Sacrificial
Microphilia	Smallness	Fetish/eligibility
Morphophilia	Discrepant size	Fetish/eligibility
Nanophilia	Short partner	Eligibility
Narratophilia	Erotic talk	Solicitation/courtship
Necrobestialism	Dead animals	Sacrificial
Necrophilia	Corpses	Sacrificial
Pictophilia	Photographs	Solicitation/courtship
Pseudozoophilia	Partner posing as an animal	Furries
Public masturbation	Masturbation in public with no wish to be seen	Solicitation/courtship
Race fetishism	Race	Eligibility
Rhabdophilia	Flagellation	Sacrificial
Sadism	Control	Sacrificial
Saliromania	Degradation of appearance	Mixed
Scoptophilia	Consensual viewing	Solicitation/courtship
Somnophilia	Sleeping sexual partner	Solicitation/courtship
Telephone scatologia	Obscene phone calls	Solicitation/courtship
Timophilia	Wealth or status	Eligibility
Tourcherism	Touching	Solicitation/courtship
Voyeurism	Spying	Solicitation/courtship
Wannabee	To be disabled	Acrotemnophilia (J. Money)
Xenophilia	Strangers/other races	Eligibility
Zoophilia	Animals	Eligibility
Zoosadism	Control of animals/harm	Mixed

Mutability

Tables 11.2–11.4 show that sexual interest is, if nothing else, complex. It is difficult to imagine how anyone could argue that sex is not contextual. Therefore, if sex is both complex and contextual, how can it be immutable? This topic has recently been dealt with in detail in an invited debate (Cantor & Fedoroff, 2018; Fedoroff, 2018). The fact that many well-informed professionals maintain that paraphilias are untreatable, or at least that there is no evidence they are treatable, is testament to the

Table 11.4 Autonomic Paraphilias

Paraphilia	Core Interest/Act	Historic Classification
Acrophilia	Heights	Eligibility
Agnophilia	Fighting (observing)	Predatory
Algolagnia	Pain	Sacrificial
Asphyxiophilia	Asphyxiation	Sacrificial
Autagonistophilia	Being on display	Solicitation/courtship
Autoassassinophilia	Being hunted	Predatory
Autoerotic self-asphyxia	Self-strangulation	Sacrificial
Autohemofetishism	Self-bleeding	Sacrificial
Autophagiophilia	Self-ingestion	Sacrificial
Catherophilia	Catheterization	Fetish
Coprophilia	Feces	Fetish
Dacnolagnomania	Murder	Sacrificial
Dacryphilia	Emotional distress, crying	Sacrificial
Dippoldism	Spanking children of partner	Sacrificial
Emetophilia	Vomiting	Sacrificial
Entomophilia	Insects	Fetish
Eproctophilia	Flatulence	Fetish
Erotophonophilia	Murder	Sacrificial
Harpazophilia	Being robbed	Mercentile
Hybristophilia	Criminals	Eligibility/sacrificial
Hygrophilia	Body fluids	Fetish
Kleptophilia	Stealing	Mercentile
Klismaphilia	Enemas	Fetish
Lactophilia	Lactation	Fetish
Lust murder	Murder	Sacrificial
Melissophilia	Bee stings	Sacrificial
Mucophila	Mucous	Fetish
Odaxelagnia	Biting	Predatory
Olphactophilia	Odors	Fetish
Omorashi	Full bladder	Fetish
Phobophilia	Fear	Sacrificial
Picquerism	Stabbing	Sacrificial
Psychrocism	Being cold or freezing	Fetish
Pyrophilia	Fire	Mixed
Salirophilia	Perspiration	Mixed
Scoptic syndrome	Being castrated (male)	Sacrificial
Stitophilia	Food	Fetish
Symphorophilia	Disasters	Sacrificial
Taphophilia	Buried alive	Sacrificial
Undinsim	Water or urine	Fetish
Urophilia	Urine	Fetish
Vampirism	Blood	Fetish
Vomerophilia	Vomiting	Sacrificial
Vorarephilia	To consume or be consumed	Sacrificial
Zelophilia	Feeling jealous	Eligibility

power of paradigms. In a previous article, the phenomenon of reinterpreting data that do not conform to the current dominant paradigm was described (Fedoroff, Curry, Ranger, & Bradford, 2016). It is important to recall that "paraphilias" are defined by the DSM-5 and elsewhere as persistent sexual interests that are not "normal." To contend that paraphilia interests cannot change, it is also necessary to contend that "normal" cannot change.

"Virtuous" Pedophiles

Much of the debate about the mutability of paraphilias has focused on pedophilia. Paradoxically, some of the strongest opponents to the idea that pedophilic interests can change are members of a self-named group Virtuous Pedophiles (https://www.virped.org). These are people who self-identify as "pedophiles" and who say they are "virtuous" because they have chosen to not have sex with children. Some members of this group have argued that removing the sentence "Pedophilia appears to be a life-long condition" from the DSM-5 would cause harm because it could lead the public to think people with pedophilia have chosen their sexual interest.

In fact, people with pedophilia have the misfortune of being hated by the public because they have a sexual interest that would cause harm to children if it was acted on. When patients with pedophilia in the Sexual Behaviours Clinic (SBC) were informally surveyed about whether they agreed with the Virtuous Pedophilia community, the patients were universally appalled. Most patients in the SBC find that pedophilic interests are changeable and, more importantly, discover that it is possible to acquire sexual interest in consensual adult partners. Many argue that the observation that there is no evidence that pedophilic interests does not match their lived-experience and more importantly does not match their experience of acquiring sexual interest in adults (see Chapter 6, this volume). This is especially important given the lack of any mechanism to explain how sexual interests can be kept from changing.

Self-Identity

The Virtuous Pedophile argument raises two important points. The first is that the notion that paraphilic interests cannot be changed is supported by a subgroup of people with self-diagnosed pedophilia. This is a group that has voluntarily forgone reciprocal sexual activity, or at least whatever their preferred sexual activities were, due to their claim they are now permanently sexually interested in children. They are therefore similar to people who voluntarily choose celibacy. In the case of celibacy, there is often an admission of sexual interest but also a belief that sex (at least for them) is sinful or bad.

"Virtuous pedophiles" self-identify as pedophiles who have chosen to give up sex. In contrast, the men and women who receive treatment in the SBC admit to a wish for sexual activity. They describe a change in sexual interests from children to adults and bring their adult girlfriends and boyfriends to the SBC's Friends and Family group. They report a change in sexual interest from children to adult(s) that is confirmed by their adult sexual partner(s). Many in the Virtuous Pedophile group question the honesty of people who say their sexual interests have changed. But their "proof" rests on their own subjective beliefs that pedophilia is unchangeable. They have committed to this belief to the point that they self-identify as "virtuous" because of it. Given the frequent reports by people with pedophilia that their interests did change (either acquiring a sexual interest in children or experiencing a change to sexual interest in adults), and given the absence of any verifiable mechanism that could explain why sexual interests are the only unchangeable interests that we know of, is it not time to question the claim by some people with pedophilia that they cannot change their sexual interests?

Consent

The second important point raised by Virtuous Pedophiles is their claim that they are virtuous because they have not sexually assaulted children. Although unstated, there is an implication that those who do sexually assault children do so because they are not virtuous. If fact, most people do not sexually assault children not only because they do not have untreated pedophilia but also because non-consensual sex with anyone is abhorrent.

In the SBC, patients are encouraged to change their sexual interests not only toward legal (adult) partners but also to consenting partners (Fedoroff, 2016). The emphasis on consensuality in the SBC begins with the first contact in which prospective patients are asked for their consent to be assessed, to have their information used for ethically approved anonymous research, and before any transmission of information about them occurs. The psychiatric hospital in which the SBC is located belongs to a system in which qualified health care professionals can access any of their patients' electronic medical charts. The SBC fully informs its patients of this fact and after disussiong the risks and benefits routinely assists them to have their names removed from the program if they do not consent. Not only is this ethical but also it demonstrates the SBC's respect for consent, which is crucial in any therapy designed to foster respect for consent, including sexual consent.

Final Words

On the first day of medical school, in the first lecture, Dr. Baker, who was a pediatrician, told us,

> Welcome to med school. I have some bad news for you. Ninety percent of what you learn in the next few years of your life will turn out to be untrue. Unfortunately, I cannot tell you which 90% that will be. My advice is to learn as much as you can, but more importantly, learn to question what you think you know.

It turns out Dr. Baker was more than right. Almost none of the medications prescribed today were even invented when Dr. Baker gave the lecture. When Dr. Baker's professors taught him about paraphilias, the paradigm included a belief that once "set," paraphilias could never change (Krafft-Ebing, 1939/1999). For the reasons reviewed in this book, that paradigm no longer seems viable. Advocacy for a change in paradigms does not mean disrespect for previous (or current) authorities. To the contrary, it is what the best teachers have always insisted should be done. Students should not simply parrot what they were taught. They should question and challenge what they have been taught and consider better paradigms that better explain current data and the data yet to be collected. As Knack, Winder, Murphy, and Fedoroff (2019) note,

> The treatment of paraphilic disorders has become much more sophisticated than it was 30 years ago. But the best is yet to come. No matter how low the recidivism rates of sex offenders become, they will never be low enough because recidivism means relapse. The field is now moving toward treatment of problematic sexual interests *before* they commit any offences.

This book has summarized much of what has been learned about the assessment and treatment of paraphilias and other unconventional sexual interests. Readers and reviewers likely will find some of the statements in this book annoying and some comments that provoke their distain and outrage. Join the club!

Clinicians and researchers should take a breath and together remember that winning academic points in an area as complex as the classification, assessment, and treatment of paraphilic interests is beside the point. People with paraphilias, especially those with paraphilic interests that may lead to illegal or lethal acts, need and want help. Let's combine interests, respect each others' perspectives, and create new paradigms that better explain the data and include legitimate optimism.

References

American Psychiatric Association. (2013). Paraphilic disorders. In *Diagnostic and statistical manual of mental disorders* (5th ed., pp. 685–705). Arlington, VA: American Psychiatric Publishing.

Cantor, J. M., & Fedoroff, J. P. (2018). Can pedophiles change response to opening arguments and conclusions. *Current Sexual Health Reports, 10*(4), 213–220. https://doi.org/10.1007/s11930-018-0167-0

Fedoroff, J. P. (2009). The paraphilias. In M. G. Gelder, N. C. Andereasen, J. J. Lopez-Iber, Jr., & J. R. Beddes (Eds.), *The new Oxford textbook of psychiatry* (2nd ed., pp. 832–842). Oxford, UK: Oxford University Press.

Fedoroff, J. P. (2011a). Forensic and diagnostic concerns arising from the proposed DSM-5 criteria for sexual paraphilic disorder. *Journal of the American Academy of Psychiatry and the Law*, *39*, 238–241.

Fedoroff, J. P. (2011b, September). The pharmacologic treatment of paraphilic sexual disorders. *AAPL Newsletter*, 21–30.

Fedoroff, J. P. (2016). Managing versus successfully treating paraphilic disorders: The paradigm is changing. In S. B. Levine, C. B. Risen, & S. E. Althof (Eds.), *Handbook of clinical sexuality for mental health professionals* (pp. 345–361). New York, NY: Taylor & Francis.

Fedoroff, J. P. (2018). Can people with pedophilia change? Yes they can! *Current Sexual Health Reports, 10*(4), 207–212. https://doi.org/10.1007/s11930-018-0166-1

Fedoroff, P., Curry, S., Ranger, R. C., & Bradford, J. M. W. (2016). Regression to the mean or the Semmelweis reflex? Invited commentary. *Archives of Sexual Behavior, 45*(7), 1869–1870. doi:10.1007/s10508-016-0786-3

First, M. B. (2014). DSM-5 and paraphilic disorders. *Journal of the American Academy of Psychiatry and the Law*, *42*, 191–201.

Knack, N., Winder, B., Murphy, L. & Fedoroff, J. P. (2019). Primary and secondary prevention of child sexual abuse. *International Review of Psychiatry, (2)181-194.* https://doi.org/10.1080/09540261.2018.1541872

Krafft-Ebing, R. von. (1999). *Psychopathia sexualis.* Burbank, California, Bloat Books. ISBN:0-9650324-1-8 (Original work published 1886)

McHugh, P. R., & Slavney, P. R. (Eds.). (1983). *The perspectives of psychiatry* (2nd ed.). Baltimore, MD: Johns Hopkins University Press.

Money, J. (1986). *Lovemaps: Clinical concepts of sexual/erotic health and pathology, paraphilia, and gender transposition in childhood, adolescence, and maturity.* New York, NY: Prometheus.

Money, J., & Lamacz, M. (1989). *Vandalized lovemaps: New concepts in sexuality.* New York, NY: Prometheus.

Moser, C. (2011). Yet another paraphilia definition fails. *Archives of Sexual Behavior, 40*(3), 483–485. doi:10.1007/s10508-010-9717-x

World Health Organization. (2004). ICD-10: international statistical classification of diseases and related health problems: tenth revision, 2nd ed. World Health Organization. https://apps.who.int/iris/handle/10665/42980

Index

For the benefit of digital users, indexed terms that span two pages (e.g., 52–53) may, on occasion, appear on only one of those pages.